Culture, Health and Illness

Second edition

To Vetta and Zoe

Culture, Health and Illness
An Introduction for Health Professionals

Second edition

Cecil G. Helman MB, ChB, Dip. Soc. Anthrop., MRCGP
Lecturer, Department of Primary Health Care, University
College and Middlesex Medical School; Research Fellow,
Department of Anthropology, University College, London

WRIGHT
London   Boston   Singapore   Sydney   Toronto   Wellington

Wright
is an imprint of Butterworth–Heinemann

 PART OF REED INTERNATIONAL P.L.C.

First published by John Wright and Sons Ltd 1984
Paperback edition 1985
   Reprinted 1986
Second edition, 1990
   Reprinted 1990

© **Butterworth–Heinemann Ltd., 1990**

British Library Cataloguing in Publication Data
Helman, Cecil
   Culture, health and illness: an introduction for health
   professionals. 2nd ed.
   1. Man. Health. Social aspects
   I. Title
   362.1042
   ISBN 0-7236-1991-3

Library of Congress Cataloging in Publication Data
Helman, Cecil, 1944–
   Culture, health, and illness: an introduction for health
   professionals / Cecil Helman. -- 2nd ed.
      p.   cm.
   Includes bibliographical references.
   ISBN 0-7236-1991-3
   1. Medical anthropology. 2. Social medicine. I. Title.
   [DNLM: 1. Social Medicine. 2. Sociology, Medical. WA 31 H478c]
   GN296.H45   1990
   306.4'61--dc20
   DNLM/DLC   89-21508

Photoset by Scribe Design, Gillingham, Kent
Printed and bound in Great Britain by Courier International Ltd, Tiptree, Essex

Preface to the second edition

The first edition of this book appeared in 1984, and since then it has been adopted as a course textbook in universities and medical schools in a number of countries. However, the last five years have also seen a significant increase in research into cultural issues in health and illness, and a burgeoning of articles, journals and books on the subject. At the same time there has been a steady growth in interest in medical anthropology, among both social scientists and many health professionals.

In preparing this second edition, I have tried to maintain the essential structure and most of the content of the first edition, but also to add where necessary material that would make the approach of the book more contemporary. In doing this, I have been grateful for the constructive criticisms of many of the reviewers of the earlier edition. Many of them have pointed out, quite rightly, that the book lacked any specific focus on the issues of gender, reproduction and childbirth. I have therefore added a complete chapter (Chapter 6) which deals with anthropological theories of gender; the 'gender cultures' of males and females in different societies; the relation of gender to both health and health care; the relationship between gender and sexuality; and the gradual 'medicalization' of several aspects of the female life-cycle, including menstruation, menopause and childbirth. In the second part of Chapter 6 I have described some of the 'birth cultures' of both modern Western obstetrics and many communities in the developing world; the growth of technological, hospital-based obstetrics, and the dissatisfaction of some women with this development; concepts of fertility and infertility in different communities; attitudes towards abortion, contraception and infanticide; the advantages, and disadvantages, of traditional birth attendants (TBAs) or folk midwives (who deliver two-thirds of the world's babies); and the physical and psychological reactions of many men to the birth of their child.

Another omission, mentioned by some reviewers, was the danger of the concept of 'culture' being misunderstood, or even misused. In the first chapter, therefore, I have described some of these misuses (especially the use of stereotypes, and 'victim blaming'), and elsewhere in the book I have pointed out that cultural factors in health and illness can only be understood in a particular *context* – and this often includes political and economic issues, which may also contribute towards the poor health of an individual or community. In Chapter 3, for example, I have described the role of the political economy of food (including the over-dependence on cash crops) in contributing to malnutrition in some parts of the world. In Chapter 2 I have included new anthropological work on the relation of the individual body to the 'social body' imposed on it by the culture in which it lives, and the relevance of this to health and illness. I have also described the modern metaphor of the mind as a 'computer', and the more traditional notion of the polluting power of menstrual blood. A section has been added on the frequent use of metaphors for illness, especially for acquired immune deficiency syndrome (AIDS), and how these metaphors and prejudices may obstruct the rational diagnosis, treatment and prevention of serious disease. In Chapter 5 I have summarized some of the critiques – from medical sociologists and others – of the Western medical system, and its role in social control and in reproducing some of the inequalities (of gender, class and ethnicity) of the wider society in which it occurs. To illustrate the 'culture-bound' aspect of all health systems I have summarized some of the recent work on cultural differences between the medical systems of Britain, France, Germany, Italy, Spain, the USA and Canada as shown by the different diagnoses given and the types of treatment prescribed in each of these countries. In both Chapter 5 and Chapter 6 I have described the origins and nature of the nursing profession (another omission in the first edition), and its cultural and social role in modern health care. In Chapter 8 I have discussed recent research into smoking behaviour, and the relation of tobacco abuse to wider economic issues, and have also included data on the use of hallucinogenic drugs in a religious context in many parts of the world. In Chapter 10, on cross-cultural psychiatry, more material on psychosomatic and culture-bound disorders has been added, as well as a new section on the growing overlap between family therapy, psychiatry and medical anthropology. Some of the controversial relationships between family dynamics and culture are discussed here in more detail. In Chapter 12 I have added recent work on the relation of cultural factors to the spread of hepatitis B, and to wider ecological issues.

In this second edition, I have continued the orientation towards *applied* medical anthropology. Throughout the text I have tried to illustrate its relevance to health and illness, and to the delivery of health care. New examples have been included, such as the role of cultural factors in people's acceptance of oral rehydration therapy (ORT) for diarrhoeal diseases.

Finally, I would like to thank the reviewers of the first edition for their useful comments, and also to thank Sushrut Jadhav, Jenny Littlewood, Roland Littlewood, Anthony Williams, Ronald Frankenberg, and Sue Deeley of Butterworth Scientific Ltd for their help.

Cecil Helman

Preface to the first edition

The aim of this book is to introduce the reader to some of the basic ideas and research in medical anthropology. Although much has been written on this subject, there is a need, I believe, for a book that outlines its practical relevance to both medical care and preventive medicine. For that reason it has mainly been written for those working in the health professions – doctors, nurses, midwives, health visitors, medical social workers and nutritionists – and for those involved in health education or foreign medical aid. It is also directed towards undergraduate students in these various disciplines, and to those studying anthropology or sociology. I hope that the book will be particularly relevant for those health professionals whose patients come from social or cultural backgrounds different from their own.

Each chapter of the book deals with a particular topic – beginning with a theoretical framework from which the subject can be approached, and including several case histories at various points in the text. These case histories have been selected to illustrate the cultural dimensions of health and illness, and their significance in clinical practice. I have tried to choose examples that shed light on such problems as failures in doctor–patient communication, dissatisfaction with medical care, the patient's experience of ill-health, and the types of healing that people resort to outside the medical profession. References to published material are given throughout the text, and details of this can be found at the end of the book. For those who wish for further background on each topic, I have listed a few key books or journal articles at the end of each chapter. In the Appendix I have included short 'Clinical questionnaires' for each topic. These can be used either to initiate a small research project in medical anthropology, or merely as a way of increasing awareness of the cultural components of health, sickness and medical care.

C.H.

Contents

Chapter 1

Introduction: the scope of medical anthropology

Medical anthropology is about how people in different cultures and social groups explain the causes of ill-health, the types of treatment they believe in, and to whom they turn if they do become ill. It is also the study of how these beliefs and practices relate to biological and psychological changes in the human organism, in both health and disease.

To put this subject in perspective, it is necessary to know something about the discipline of anthropology itself, of which medical anthropology is a comparatively new offshoot. Anthropology – from the Greek, meaning 'the study of Man' – has been called 'the most scientific of the humanities and the most humane of the sciences'.[1] Its aim is nothing less than the holistic study of humankind – its origins, development, social and political organizations, religions, languages, art and artefacts.

Anthropology, as a field of study, has several branches. *Physical anthropology* – also known as 'human biology' – is the study of the evolution of the human species, and is concerned with explaining the causes for the present diversity of human populations. In its investigation of human prehistory it utilizes the techniques of archaeology, palaeontology, genetics and serology, as well as the study of primate behaviour and ecology. *Material culture* deals with art and artefacts of mankind, both in the present and in the past. It includes studies of the arts, musical instruments, weapons, clothes, tools and agricultural implements of different populations, and all other aspects of the technology that human beings use to control, shape, exploit and enhance their social or natural environments. *Social* and *cultural anthropology* deal with the comparative study of present-day human societies and their cultural systems, although there is a difference in emphasis between these two approaches.

In the UK, social anthropology is the dominant approach, and emphasizes the social dimensions of human life. The human being is a social animal, organized into groups that regulate and perpetuate themselves, and it is men and women's experience

1

as members of society that shapes their view of the world. In this perspective, culture is seen as one of the ways that humans organize and legitimize society, and provide the basis for its social, political and economic organization. In the USA, cultural anthropology focuses more on the systems of symbols, ideas and meanings that comprise a culture, and of which social organization is just an expression. In practice, the differences in emphasis of social and cultural anthropology provide valuable and complementary perspectives on two central issues – the ways that human groups organize themselves, and the ways that they view the world they inhabit. In other words, when studying a group of human beings, it is necessary to study the features of both their society and their culture.

Keesing[2] has defined a *society* as: 'A population marked by relative separation from surrounding populations and a distinctive culture'. The boundaries between societies are sometimes vague, but in general each has its own territorial and political identity. In studying any society, anthropologists investigate the ways that members of that society organize themselves into various groups, hierarchies and roles. This organization is revealed in its dominant ideology and religion, in its political and economic systems, in the types of bonds that kinship or close residence creates between people, and in the division of labour between different people from different backgrounds and different genders. The rules that underpin the organization of a society and the ways in which it is symbolized and transmitted are all part of that society's culture.

The concept of 'culture'

What then is *culture*? – a word that will be used on many occasions throughout this book. Anthropologists have provided many definitions of it, perhaps the most famous being E. B. Tylor's[3] definition in 1871: 'That complex whole which includes knowledge, belief, art, morals, law, custom and any other capabilities and habits acquired by man as a member of society'. Keesing,[4] in his definition, stresses the ideational aspect of culture. That is, cultures comprise: 'Systems of shared ideas, systems of concepts and rules and meanings that underlie and are expressed in the ways that humans live'.

From these definitions one can see that culture is a set of guidelines (both explicit and implicit) which individuals inherit as members of a particular society, and which tells them how to *view* the world, how to experience it *emotionally*, and how to *behave* in it in relation to other people, to supernatural forces or gods, and to the natural environment. It also provides them with a way of transmitting these guidelines to the next generation – by the use of symbols, language, art and ritual. To some extent, culture can be seen as an inherited 'lens', through which individuals perceive and understand the world that they inhabit, and learn how to live within it. Growing up within any society is a form of *enculturation*, whereby the individual slowly acquires the cultural 'lens' of that society. Without such a shared perception of the world, both the cohesion and the continuity of any human group would be impossible.

One aspect of this 'cultural lens' is the division of the world, and the people within it, into different *categories*, each with their own name. For example, all cultures divide up their members into different social categories, such as men and women, children or adults, young people or old people, kinsfolk or strangers, upper class or lower class, able or disabled, normal or abnormal, mad or bad, healthy or ill. And all cultures have elaborate ways of moving people from one social category into another (such as from 'ill person' to 'healthy person'), and also of confining people – sometimes against their will – to the categories into which they have been put (such as mad, disabled or elderly[5]).

Anthropologists such as Leach[6] have pointed out that virtually all societies have more than one culture within their borders. For example, most societies have some form of social stratification, into social classes, castes or ranks, and each stratum is marked by its own distinctive cultural attributes, including linguistic usages, manners, styles of dress, dietary and housing patterns, and so on. Rich and poor, powerful and powerless – each will have their own inherited cultural perspective. To some extent, both men and women can have their own distinctive cultures within the same society, and are expected to conform to different norms and different expectations. In addition to such social strata, one can see that most modern complex societies, such as the UK or the USA, include within them religious and ethnic minorities, tourists, foreign students, political refugees, recent immigrants, and migrant workers – each with their own distinctive culture. Many of these groups will undergo some degree of *acculturation*, whereby they incorporate some of the cultural attributes of the larger society. A further subdivision of culture within a complex society is seen in the various professional *subcultures* that exist, such as the medical, nursing, legal or military professions. In each case, they form a group apart, with their own concepts, rules and social organization. Although each subculture is developed from the larger culture, and shares many of its concepts and values, it also has unique, distinctive features of its own. Students in these professions also undergo a form of enculturation, as they slowly acquire the 'culture' of their chosen career. In doing so, they also acquire a different perspective on life from those who are outside the profession. In the case of the medical profession, its subculture also reflects many of the social divisions and prejudices of the wider society (see Chapters 4 and 6), and this might interfere with both health care and doctor–patient communication, as illustrated later in this book.

Cultural background therefore has an important influence on many aspects of people's lives, including their beliefs, behaviours, perceptions, emotions, language, religion, family structure, diet, dress, body image, concepts of space and of time, and attitudes to illness, pain and other forms of misfortune – all of which may have important implications for health and health care. However, the culture into which you are born, or in which you live, is by no means the *only* such influence. It is only one of a number of influences which includes *individual* factors (such as age, gender, size, appearance, personality, intelligence and experience), *educational* factors (both formal and informal, and including education into a religious, ethnic or professional subculture), and *socioeconomic* factors (such as social class, economic status, and the networks of social support from other people).

Furthermore, the concept of culture has sometimes been misunderstood, or even misused, by those who have used it. For example, cultures are never homogeneous, and therefore one should always avoid using generalizations in explaining people's beliefs and behaviours. One cannot make broad generalizations about the members of any human group without taking into account that differences among the group's members may be just as marked as those between the members of different cultural groups. Statements such as 'The members of group X do not do Y' (such as smoking, drinking, or eating meat) may be true of some or even most members of the group, but not necessarily of all. One should therefore differentiate between the rules of a culture which govern how one *should* think and behave, and how people actually behave in real life. Generalizations can also be dangerous, for they often lead to the development of stereotypes, and then usually to cultural misunderstandings, prejudices, and also discrimination. Another reason not to generalize is that cultures are never static; they are usually influenced by other human groups around them, and in most parts of the world they are in a constant process of adaptation and change. What is true of a group one year may not be true of it the next.

An important point in understanding the role of culture is that it must always be seen in its particular *context*. This context is made up of historical, economic, social, political and geographical elements. This means that the culture of any group of people, at any particular point in time, is *always* influenced by many other factors. It may therefore be impossible to isolate 'pure' cultural beliefs and behaviour from the social and economic context in which they occur. For example, people may act in a particular way (such as eating certain foods, living in a crowded house, or not going to a doctor when ill) not because it is their culture to do so, but because they are simply too poor to do otherwise. They may have high levels of anxiety in their daily lives, not because their culture makes them anxious, but because they are suffering discrimination or persecution from other people. Therefore, in understanding health and illness it is important to avoid 'victim blaming' – that is, seeing the poor health of a population as the sole result of its culture – instead of looking also at their economic or social situation. Economic factors in particular are an important cause of ill-health, since poverty and unemployment may result in poor nutrition, overcrowded living conditions, inadequate clothing, psychological stress and alcohol abuse. The unequal distribution of wealth and resources, both between countries and within each country, can lead to this situation. As an example of this, the Black Report[7] of 1982 showed how in the UK health could clearly be correlated with income, and people in the poorer social classes had more illness, and a much higher mortality, than their fellow citizens in the more affluent classes. In the developing world too – whatever the local culture – poor health can usually be correlated with a low income, which in turn influences the sorts of food, water, sanitation and housing that people are able to afford.[8] Thus culture should never be considered in a vacuum, but only as one component of a complex mix of influences on what people believe and how they live their lives.

A final misuse of the concept of culture – especially in medical care – is that its influence may be over-emphasized in interpreting how some people present their symptoms to health professionals. Symptoms or behaviour may be ascribed to the person's culture, when they are really due to an underlying physical or mental disorder.[9]

Research methods in anthropology

In studying societies and cultures in different parts of the world, anthropologists have used two main approaches: the ethnographic and the comparative approach. The *ethnographic* approach involves the study of small-scale societies, or of relatively small groups of people, to understand how they view the world and organize their daily lives. The aim is to discover – in so far as this is possible – the 'actor's perspective'; that is, to see how the world looks from the perspective of a member of that society. To discover this, anthropologists often carry out fieldwork, using the 'participant observation' technique, whereby they live with and observe a group of people, and learn to see the world through their eyes, while at the same time retaining the objective perspective of the social scientist. This often involves quantitative studies, such as counting the population, measuring their diet or income, or listing the inhabitants of various households. Ethnography then leads on to the second stage – the *comparative* approach – which seeks to distil out the key features of each society and culture, and to compare these with other societies and cultures, to draw conclusions about the universal nature of man and his social groupings.

In its earlier years, anthropology was mainly concerned with studies of small-scale tribal societies within, or at the borders of, the colonial empires. Modern anthropology, however, is just as concerned with doing ethnographies in complex, Western societies. The 'tribe' of a modern anthropologist might easily be a sect in New York, a suburb in London, a group of doctors in Los Angeles, or patients attending a clinic in Melbourne. In all these cases, both the ethnographic and the comparative approaches are used – as well as some of the interviewing and measurement techniques of sociology and psychology.

Medical anthropology

Although medical anthropology is a branch of social and cultural anthropology, its roots also lie deep within medicine and other natural sciences, because it is also concerned with a wide range of *biological* phenomena, especially in relation to health and disease. As a subject it therefore lies – sometimes uncomfortably – in the overlap between the social and the natural sciences, and draws its insights from both sets of disciplines. In Foster and Anderson's definition[10] it is: 'A biocultural discipline concerned with both the biological and sociocultural aspects of human behaviour, and particularly with the ways in which the two interact and have interacted throughout human history to influence health and disease'.

Anthropologists studying the sociocultural end of this spectrum have pointed out that in all human societies beliefs and practices relating to ill-health are a central feature of the culture. Often these are linked to beliefs about the origin of a much wider range of misfortune (including accidents, interpersonal conflicts, natural disasters, crop failures, and theft or loss), of which ill-health is only one form. In some of these societies, the whole range of these misfortunes is blamed on supernatural forces, or on divine retribution, or on the malevolence of a 'witch' or 'sorcerer'. The values and customs associated with ill-health are part of the wider culture, and cannot really be studied in isolation from it. One cannot understand how people react to illness, death or other misfortune without an understanding of the type of culture they have grown up in or acquired – that is, of the 'lens' through which they are perceiving and interpreting their world. In addition to the study of culture, it is also necessary to examine the social organization of health and illness in that society (the 'health care system'), which includes the ways that people become recognized as 'ill', the ways that they present this illness to other people, the attributes of those they present their illness to, and the ways that the illness is dealt with. A group of 'healers' is found in different forms in every human society. Anthropologists are particularly interested in the characteristics of this special social group – their selection, training, concepts, values and internal organization. They also study the way that these people fit into the social system as a whole – their rank in the social hierarchy, their economic or political power, and the division of labour between them and other members of the society. In some human groups the healers play roles beyond their healing functions: they may act as 'integrators' of the society, who regularly reassert the society's values (see Chapter 9), or as agents of social control, helping to label and punish socially deviant behaviour (see Chapter 10). Their focus may not be only on the ill individual, but rather on the patient's 'ill' family, community, village or tribe. It is therefore important, when studying how individuals in a particular society perceive and react to ill-health, and the types of health care that they turn to, to know something about both the cultural and the social attributes of the society in which they live. This is one of the main tasks of medical anthropology.

At the biological end of the spectrum, medical anthropology draws on the techniques and findings of medical science, and its various subfields, including microbiology, biochemistry, genetics, parasitology, pathology, nutrition and epidemiology. In many cases it is possible to link biological changes found by these techniques to social and cultural factors in a particular society. For example, a hereditary disease transmitted by a recessive gene may occur at a higher frequency in a particular population because of that group's cultural preference for endogamy – that is, for marrying only within one's family or local kin-group. To unravel this problem one needs a number of perspectives: *clinical medicine* (to identify the clinical manifestation of the disease), *pathology* (to confirm the disease on the cellular or biochemical level), *genetics* (to identify and predict the hereditary basis of the disease and its linkage to a recessive gene), *epidemiology* (to show its high incidence in a particular population in relation to 'pooling' of recessive genes and certain marriage customs), and social or cultural *anthropology* (to explain the marriage patterns of that society, and to identify who may marry whom within it). Medical anthropology tries to solve this type of clinical problem by utilizing not only anthropological findings, but also those of the biological sciences – by being, in other words, a 'biocultural discipline'.

Applied medical anthropology

Within medical anthropology, some researchers have concentrated on its theoretical aspects, while others – especially those involved in clinical practice, health education programmes or foreign medical aid – have focused more on its *applied* aspects in health care and preventive medicine.

Interest in this field of applied medical anthropology has grown steadily in the last few years. Medical anthropologists have become involved in a variety of multidisciplinary projects in many parts of the world, aimed at improving health and health care. They have worked both in the developing world and within the cities and suburbs of Europe and North America.

Some have widened their focus to include the more 'macro' influences on health, such as the political and economic inequality between, and within, many of the societies in today's world.[8] Many of them have worked for international aid agencies, such as the World Health Organisation (WHO), on health problems in various parts of the non-industrialized world.

An example of such a problem is the high incidence of diarrhoeal diseases in the developing world, which according to WHO[11] poses a major health problem world-wide. These diseases are usually associated with poverty, and the resultant malnutrition and infection, and kill about 5–7 million people every year. A long-term solution to this problem does not lie in the hands of medical science, but will involve major structural changes – economic, political and social – both within those countries and in their relation to the rest of the world.[8]

In terms of treatment, oral rehydration therapy (ORT) provides a safe and inexpensive way to prevent and treat the life-threatening dehydration associated with these diseases, in both infants and children. However, in many parts of the world mothers are reluctant to use this relatively simple form of treatment. Anthropological research has found that this is partly due to indigenous beliefs about the causes and dangers of diarrhoeal disease and how they should best be treated.[12]

Case history: Oral rehydration therapy in Pakistan

A recent study by Mull and Mull[13] in rural Pakistan showed widespread ignorance or rejection of ORT by mothers despite the fact that the use of ORT has been promoted on a national level by the Pakistan Ministry of Health since 1983, packets of oral rehydration solution (ORS) are available free of charge through government health outlets, and more than 18 million packets of ORS are produced annually by Pakistan's own pharmaceutical industry. The researchers found that many of the mothers were ignorant of how the ORS should be used, and some of them saw the diarrhoea – which was very common in that area – as a 'natural' and expected part of teething and growing up, and not as an illness. Some believed it was dangerous to try to stop the diarrhoea, lest the trapped 'heat' within it spread to the brain and cause a fever. Others explained infant diarrhoea as due to certain folk illness (see Chapter 5), such as *nazar* (evil eye), *jinns* (malevolent spirits), or *sutt* (a sunken or 'fallen' fontanelle, said to cause difficulty in infant sucking), which should be treated with traditional remedies or by traditional healers without recourse to ORT. Some of these mothers did not connect the fallen fontanelle with severe dehydration, and tried to raise the fontanelle by applying sticky substances to the top of the infant's head, or by pushing up on the hard palate with a finger. Many mothers in the group saw diarrhoea as a 'hot' illness (see Chapter 3), which required a 'cold' form of treatment – such as a change in maternal diet, or giving certain foods and herbs to the infant – to restore the sick infant to a normal temperature. They classified most Western medicines, such as antibiotics and even vitamins, as also 'hot', and therefore inappropriate for a diarrhoeal child. A few mothers even rejected ORS (which contains salt) because they believed that salt 'was bad for diarrhoea'.

As this and other studies illustrate, therefore, health care programmes should always be designed not only to address medical concerns, but also to take into account what the people in the community actually believe about their own ill-health, and how it should be treated[12] – and also the social, economic and political context in which that ill-health occurs.[8]

This book arises from the growing field of applied medical anthropology, which I have briefly described above. Its aim is to demonstrate the clinical significance of cultural and social factors, in illness and in health, and in the delivery of all forms of health care.

Recommended reading

Medical anthropology

Foster, G. M. and Anderson, B. G. (1978) *Medical Anthropology*. New York: Wiley
Kleinman, A. (1980) *Patients and Healers in the Context of Culture*. Berkeley: University of California Press
Landy, D. (ed.) (1977) *Culture, Disease, and Healing*. New York: Macmillan

Social and cultural anthropology

Keesing, R. M. (1981) *Cultural Anthropology*. New York: Holt, Rinehart and Winston
Leach, E. (1982) *Social Anthropology*. Glasgow: Fontana

Research techniques in anthropology

Pelto, P. J. and Pelto, G. H. (1978) *Anthropological Research: the Structure of Inquiry*. Cambridge: Cambridge University Press

Chapter 2

Cultural definitions of anatomy and physiology

To the members of all societies, the human body is more than just a physical organism, fluctuating between health and illness. It is also the focus of a set of beliefs about its social and psychological significance, its structure and function. The term 'body image' has been used to describe all the ways that an individual conceptualizes, and experiences, his or her body, whether consciously or not. In Fisher's definition,[1] this includes 'his collective attitudes, feelings and fantasies about his body', as well as 'the manner in which a person has learnt to organize and integrate his body experiences'. The culture of the group in which we grow up teaches us how to perceive and interpret the many changes that can occur over time in our own bodies – and in the bodies of other people. We learn how to differentiate a 'young' body from an 'aged', one, a 'sick' body from a 'healthy' one; how to define 'a fever' or 'a pain', a feeling of 'clumsiness' or of 'anxiety'; how to perceive some parts of the body as 'public' and others as 'private'; and how to view some bodily functions as socially acceptable and others as morally unclean.

The body image, then, is something acquired by every individual as part of growing up in a particular family or society, though there are, of course, individual variations in body image within a society.

In general, concepts of body image can be divided into three main groups:

1. Beliefs about the optimal shape and size of the body, including the clothing and decoration of its surface.
2. Beliefs about the body's inner structure.
3. Beliefs about how it functions.

All three are influenced by social and cultural background and can have important effects on the health of the individual.

Shape, size, clothing and the surface of the body

In every society, the human body has a *social* as well as a
physical reality. That is, the shape, size and adornments of the
body are a way of communicating information about its owner's
position in society. This includes information about gender,
social status, occupation and membership of certain groups,
both religious and secular. Included in this form of communication are bodily gestures and postures, which frequently differ
between cultures and between different groups within a culture.
The body languages of, for example, doctors, priests, policemen
and salespeople are very different from each other, and convey
different types of messages to other people. Clothing is also of
particular importance in signalling social rank and occupation:
in the Western world mink coats and jewels are worn as
displays of wealth, in contrast to the ill-fitting clothes of the
poor. Similarly, the white coat of the Western doctor or the
starched cap of the nurse have not only a practical aspect –
cleanliness and the prevention of infection – but also a social
function, indicating their membership of a prestigious and
powerful occupational group, with its own specific rights and
privileges (see Chapter 9). A change in social position is often
signalled by a change in clothing: the black dress and shawl
adopted by widows in a Greek village are a public indicator of
their transition from married woman to solitary mourner;
similarly, new graduates at a Western university wear, at least
temporarily, a uniform of academic gown and mortar board.
Thus many aspects of the body's adornments, especially
clothing, have both a social function (signalling information
about the individual's current position in society) and the more
obvious utilitarian function of protecting the body from the
environment.

Artificial changes in the shape, size and surface of the body,
which are widespread throughout the world, can also have a
social function. This applies also to the more extreme forms of
bodily mutilation, which will be mentioned below. Inherent in
most of these are culturally defined notions of beauty, and of the
optimal size and shape of the body. Polhemus[2] has listed some
of the more extreme forms of body alteration practised
historically and, at the present time, among non-industrialized
peoples. These include artificial deformation of the skull during
infancy in parts of Peru; filing and carving of teeth in
pre-Columbian Mexico and Ecuador; scarification of the chest
and limbs in New Guinea and parts of Central Africa; binding of
women's feet in Imperial China; artificial fattening of girls in

parts of West Africa; tattooing of the body in Tahiti and among some American Indians; insertion of large ornaments into the lips and earlobes in Brazil, East Africa and Melanesia; and the wearing of nose rings and earrings among the people of Timbuktu, Mali. The health risks of such bodily mutilations are obvious, but they may also bring benefits to the population. While female circumcision, practised still in parts of Africa, carries with it the dangers of infection, scar tissue formation and difficulty with future childbirth,[3] early male circumcision is believed to be one of the factors protecting women from developing cancer of the cervix.[4] In addition, as has been found among the Mende of Sierra Leone, the use of ritual scarring by a community may make them accept the 'ritual scars' of vaccination more enthusiastically than other groups without these customs (C.P. MacCormack, 1982, personal communication). Both scarification and tattooing (which carry with them the dangers of local infection and serum hepatitis) are now rarely seen in the West, except among sailors and servicemen.

Various forms of self-mutilation or alteration are used in Western industrialized societies, particularly by women, to conform to culturally defined standards of 'beauty'. These include the widespread use of orthodontics to straighten front teeth; plastic surgery to noses, ears and chins; ear piercing; body building regimens; breast prostheses; face-lift surgery; hair implants for baldness; as well as the use of false teeth, eyelashes and fingernails. Also included here are the various forms of dieting used by women to reduce their weight to 'attractive' dimensions. It has been hypothesized that anorexia nervosa is an extreme, pathological form of dissatisfaction with body image, in a society that values and rewards female slimness,[5] and thus it can be understood only within the context of certain cultural values;[6] furthermore, Orbach[7] has suggested that it may even represent a symbolic 'hunger strike' by some women against their oppression in Western society. By contrast, in parts of West Africa, wealthy men frequently sent their daughters to 'fatting-houses' where they were fed on fatty foods, with minimal exercise, to make them plump and pale, a culturally defined shape believed to indicate both wealth and fertility.[8] In the Western world, however, 'obesity' is seen as a major health problem, and also carries with it a significant social stigma. Ritenbaugh[9] points out that medical descriptions of the causes of obesity – over-eating and under-exercising – are often just a modern version of the traditional moral disapproval of gluttony and sloth, as well as of a lack of self-control.

Not only is body shape altered to fit in with culturally

prescribed patterns, but special clothes are worn that make this possible, including women's corsets and other constrictive underwear, and high-heeled or platform shoes, all of which may have a negative effect on health. Cosmetics and deodorants, which may cause skin allergies or contact dermatitis, are also part of the Western mode of communication, where personal odour is considered to be offensive – a belief not shared by some other cultures.

While the body is protected by clothes, and by its covering of skin, some areas of the body surface are sometimes considered to be more vulnerable than others. For example, in my own study[10] of English beliefs about 'chills', 'colds' and 'fevers', the lay body image included certain areas of skin – the top of the head, the back of the neck, and the feet – considered more vulnerable than other parts to penetration by environmental cold, damp or draughts. In this model, one 'caught cold' if one 'went out into the rain without a hat on (or after a haircut)', or 'stepped in a puddle' or on a cold floor. At the same time, fevers were believed to result from the penetration of 'germs', 'bugs' or 'viruses' through other breaks in the body's surface – the orifices, such as the anus, urethra, throat, nostrils or ears.

Thus, as the section above illustrates, each human being has, in a sense, *two* bodies: an *individual* body-self (both physical and psychological) which is acquired at birth, and also the *social* body that it needs in order to live within a particular society.

The social body is an important part of body image, as it provides each person with a framework for perceiving and interpreting his or her own physical and psychological experiences.[11] It is also the means whereby the physiology of the individual is influenced and controlled by the rules of the society in which it lives. This larger society – or 'body politic' – exerts a powerful control over all aspects of the individual body: its shape, size, clothing, diet and postures; its behaviour in sickness and in health; and its reproductive, work and leisure activities.[12]

The inner structure of the body

To most people the inner structure of the body is a matter of speculation. Without the benefit of anatomical dissections, charts of the skeletal and organ structures, or radiographs, beliefs about how the body is constructed are based on inherited folklore, books and magazines, personal experience and theorizing. The importance of this 'inside-the-body' image is that it influences people's perception and presentation of bodily complaints. It also influences their responses to medical treatment. For example, a 20-year-old London woman was told, on the basis of her history, that she was suffering from 'heartburn', and an antacid mixture was prescribed. A week later, with the same symptom, she admitted to me that she had not taken any antacid. Asked why she hadn't followed the first doctor's advice she replied, 'Of course I didn't take his mixture. How could he know I had heartburn if he didn't even listen to my heart?'

Several studies have been carried out on lay conceptions of what lies inside the body. Boyle[13] studied 234 patients, with the aid of multiple-choice questionnaires, to discover their knowledge of bodily structure and function, and then compared these with a sample of 35 doctors. He found a wide discrepancy between the two sets of answers, especially on the location of internal organs. For example, 14.9% of the patients placed the heart as occupying most of the thoracic cavity; 58.8% located the stomach as occupying the entire abdomen, from waist to groin; 48.7% located the kidneys low down in the groin; and 45.5% saw the liver as lying in the lower abdomen, just above the pelvis. In another study of 81 men and women in hospital awaiting major abdominal surgery, Pearson and Dudley[14] found that out of a total of 729 responses dealing with organ location only 28% were correct, 14% were only vague answers, and 58% were incorrect. Fifteen per cent equated the stomach with the abdominal cavity, 14% marked in two livers on opposite sides of the body, and 18% said the gallbladder was concerned with urine, or located it in the lower pelvic area, or both. Such bodily perceptions obviously influence how patients interpret, and present, certain bodily symptoms. For example, a vague discomfort anywhere in the chest may be interpreted as 'heart trouble', whether the doctor confirms this or not. A patient complaining of 'a pain in the stomach' may be referring to virtually anywhere in the abdominal cavity.

Conceptions of what lies inside the body are not static, however. They can vary with certain physical and psychological states, and seem to vary with age. A study by Tait and Ascher[15] examined these conceptions in 107 hospitalized psychiatric patients, 105 candidates for admission to a Naval Academy, 55 military men hospitalized in medical or surgical wards, and 22 sixth-grade pupils in New York. Many of the drawings of the psychotics 'exhibited disorderly arrangement, confusion, vagueness and pronounced and bizarre distortions of shape, relative size and position of (bodily) parts'. In the children's drawings the sexual organs were omitted, and the skeletomuscular system was prominently emphasized. In medical and surgical patients there was a tendency to emphasize the organ or system involved in the illness for which they were hospitalized, such as the lung, the kidneys, or the skeletomuscular system. One patient, with 'neurodermatitis', drew the skin surface of the body with only the faintest indication of ribs as the inside of the body.

Illness may also involve reifying a diseased organ or bodily part – thinking of it as though it were an 'it', something partly alien to the body and only partially under its control. In this way unpleasant or worrying bodily experiences can be denied, or separated from the type of body image now idealized in the modern world – a body which is healthy, happy, independent, and in full control of all its faculties.[16] In one study of psychosomatic disorders,[17] for example, patients put the blame for their embarrassing symptoms – such as unexpected vomiting or diarrhoea – on a part of their body that was 'weak', unreliable, and only partly under their control, such as an 'irritable colon', a 'nervous stomach', or a 'weak chest'.

The effect of body image in clinical diagnosis is also seen in the presentation of non-organic – that is, psychogenic – signs and symptoms. Waddell et al.[18] studied the distribution of physical signs for which no organic cause could be found in 350 British and American patients with low back pain. The distribution of these signs (such as numbness, weakness or tremor) did not match accepted neuroanatomical distribution, but corresponded rather to lay divisions of the body into regions such as knee, groin or waist. In another study by Walters,[19] 'hysterical pain' or 'psychogenic regional pain' was found to occur in distributions that matched patients' body images, especially their beliefs about parts of the body supplied by a particular 'nerve', rather than their actual anatomical innervation. Examples of this are the 'glove' or 'stocking' distribution of hysterical pain, numbness or paralysis.

Case history: Body image

Kleinman et al.[20] describe a case that illustrates the clinical significance of patients' beliefs about their bodies, and how these beliefs can affect their behaviour, and the reaction of clinicians to them. A 60-year-old white woman was admitted to a medical ward in Massachusetts General Hospital suffering from pulmonary oedema secondary to atherosclerotic cardiovascular disease and chronic congestive heart failure. As she began to recover, her behaviour became increasingly bizarre: she forced herself to vomit and urinated frequently in her bed. A psychiatrist was called in to give an opinion on her. On close questioning he discovered that, from her point of view at least, her behaviour made sense. She had been told by the doctors that she had 'water in the lungs'. She was the wife and daughter of plumbers, and according to her concept of the structure of the body the chest was connected by 'pipes' to the mouth and the urethra. She was therefore trying to remove as much of the water in the lungs as possible by vomiting and urinating frequently. She compared the latter to the effect of the 'water pills' that she had been prescribed, and which she had been told would get rid of the water in her chest by making her urinate. Once it had been explained to her with the aid of diagrams, how the 'plumbing' of the human body actually worked, her bizarre behaviour immediately ended.

The functioning of the body

Although beliefs about the body's structure can have clinical importance, those about how it functions are probably more significant in their effect on people's behaviour. Beliefs about function usually deal with one or more interrelated aspects of the body:

1. Its inner workings.
2. The effect on these of outside influences, such as diet or environment.
3. The nature (and disposal) of the by-products of the body's functioning, such as faeces, urine and menstrual blood.

Out of the wide range of lay theories of physiology that have been studied, I have selected a few for closer examination.

Balance and imbalance

In all these theories, the healthy working of the body is thought to depend on the harmonious *balance* between two or more elements or forces within the body. To a lesser or greater extent, this balance is dependent on external forces, such as diet, environment or supernatural agents, as well as on internal influences such as inherited weakness, or state of mind. The most widespread of these theories is the *humoral* theory, which has its roots in ancient China and India, but which was elaborated into a system of medicine by Hippocrates, who was born in 460 BC. In the Hippocratic theory, the body contained four liquids or humours: blood, phlegm, yellow bile and black bile. Health resulted from these four humours being in optimal proportion to one another, ill-health from an excess or deficiency of one of them. Diet and environment could affect this balance, as could the season of the year. Treatment for imbalance/disease consisted of restoring the optimal proportion of the humours by removing excess (by bleeding, purging, vomiting, starvation), or by replacing the deficiency (by special diets, medicines, etc.). It also included a theory of personality types, based on the predominance of one of the humours, the four types being sanguine (excess blood), phlegmatic (excess phlegm), choleric (excess yellow bile) and melancholic (excess black bile). Hippocratic medicine was restored and further elaborated by Galen (AD 130–200), a Greek physician living in Rome. In the centuries that followed, Galen's work gradually diffused throughout the Roman world and into the Islamic world. In the ninth century, under the Abbasid Dynasty of Baghdad, large portions of his work were translated into Arabic. During the Moorish occupation of the Iberian Peninsula, much of this humoral medicine was taken over by Spanish and Portuguese physicians, and later carried by their descendants to South and Central America and to the Philippines (though some anthropologists have found traces of indigenous humoral beliefs in Latin America that preceded the European conquest).[21] Today, humoral medicine remains the basis of lay beliefs about health and illness in much of Latin America, is prominent in the Islamic world, and is a component of the Ayurvedic medical tradition in India.

In Latin American folk medicine, the humoral theory – often called the 'hot–cold theory of disease' – postulates that health can be maintained (or lost) only by the effect of heat or cold on the body.[22] As Logan[23] points out, 'hot' and 'cold' here do not pertain to actual temperature, but to a symbolic power contained in most substances, including food, herbs and medicines. In addition, *all* mental states, illnesses, natural and supernatural forces are grouped in a binary fashion into hot or cold categories. To maintain health, the body's internal

'temperature' balance must be maintained between the oppos-
ing powers of hot and cold, especially by avoiding prolonged
exposure to either quality. In illness, health is restored by
re-establishing the internal temperature balance by exposing
oneself to, or ingesting, items of an opposite quality to that
believed to be responsible for the illness. Certain illnesses are
hot illnesses, believed to result from over-exposure to sun or fire
or from ingesting hot foods or beverages. Both pregnancy and
menstruation are considered to be hot states, and like other hot
conditions are treated by the ingestion of cold foods and
medicines, or by cold treatments such as spongeing with cool
water. Such beliefs can have dangerous effects on women's
health. For example, postpartum or menstruating women from
parts of Latin America may avoid certain fruits and vegetables,
which they classify as cold and liable to clot their hot menstrual
blood. The avoidance of such foods, in women who already
have a diet deficient in vitamins, may eliminate even more of
these vitamins from their diet. In one American study,[24] some
postpartum Puerto Rican women believed that if the lochia was
'clotted' by cold foods it would be reabsorbed to cause
nervousness, or even insanity. As a preventive measure, they
drank tonics containing hot foods, such as chocolate, garlic and
cinnamon.

Humoral medicine is still one component of the pluralistic
medical system in Morocco, as described by Greenwood,[25] but
most of the emphasis is now placed on two of the humours:
blood and phlegm. As in Latin America, this lay theory of health
and illness relates the inner workings of the body to outside
influences such as diet and environment. There are hot and cold
foods and environmental factors, the imbalance of which in the
body can cause hot or cold illnesses that are treated by foods of
the opposite quality. Food is commonly used as treatment as
most foods are considered hot and most illnesses cold. Excess
blood is seen as a feature of hot illnesses, and excess phlegm in
the body as a feature of cold ones. Most hot illnesses are caused
by over-exposure to sun, heat, hot winds, or eating excess foods
in summer. The 'heat' then enters the blood, which 'rises to the
head' causing flushing, fever and other symptoms. Treatment,
in this Moroccan humoral model, is by removing the 'excess' hot
blood by cooling the body's surface, eating cold foods, and also
using cupping and leeching at the neck to draw off some of the
blood.

In the ancient Indian Ayurvedic system, there are similar
highly complex concepts of the physiology of the body that

equate health with balance. As described by Obeyesekere,[26] there are five *bhūtas* or basic elements in the universe: ether, wind, water, earth and fire. These are the basic constituents of all life, and also make up the three *dōsas* or humours (wind, bile and phlegm) and the seven *dhātus* or components of the body. Food which contains the five elements is 'cooked' by fires in the body and converted into bodily refuse, and into a refined portion which is successively transformed into the seven basic components of the body: food juice, blood, flesh, fat, bone, marrow and semen. The five elements also go to make up the three humours in the body: the wind element becomes wind, or flatulence, fire appears as bile, and water as phlegm. The harmonious working of the body results from an optimal balance of these three humours, and illness results from relative excess or deficiency of one or more of the humours. As in Latin America there are 'cooling' and 'heat-producing' foods, which are used to reduce the excess of a humour; hot foods can cause excess bile, and thus illness must be treated by a diet of cold food and other medication. Ayurveda also includes a theory of temperament and its relationship to ill-health. For example, a patient whose temperament results from an excess of bile is believed to be especially vulnerable to illness caused by an excess of this humour, and thus should avoid heat-producing food which may increase even further the amount of bile in the body.

Like Ayurveda, traditional Chinese medicine also saw health as a harmonious balance, in this case between two contrasting cosmic principles: *yin*, described as dark, moist, watery and female, and *yang* which is hot, dry, fiery and male. The organs of the body were either predominately *yin* (such as the heart, lungs, spleen, kidneys and liver), or *yang* (such as the intestines, stomach and gallbladder). Illness was believed to result from an imbalance, usually an excess of one principle within an organ, which might then have to be removed by acupuncture or moxibustion.[27]

The humoral concept has largely disappeared from the UK and other European societies, but concepts of restoring health by counteracting one element in the body by another still persist. In English lay beliefs about colds and chills, which are conceptualized as being due to the penetration of environmental cold or damp into the body, a common lay treatment was to counteract cold by heat. Heat was administered in the form of warm drinks, warm foods (which help generate the body's own heat) and rest in a warm bed. The aphorism 'feed a cold, starve a fever' sums up this approach. To prevent colds and chills a variety of patent 'tonics' were used, such as Cod Liver Oil and Malt Extract, to generate heat inside the body. As one elderly patient put it, if you went outdoors after having taken a tonic 'you felt warm inside', for the tonic was an internal protection against excess cold.[10]

Humoral medicine has, of course, also disappeared from modern scientific medicine. Nevertheless, modern physiology does include numerous examples of diseases that are caused by a deficiency, or excess, of certain substances in the body, such as hormones, enzymes, electrolytes, vitamins, trace elements and blood cells, which can be corrected by replacing the deficient substance, or counteracting the excess. The concept of the negative feedback loop in endocrinology, whereby the rise of one hormone in the bloodstream results in a decline in another, might also be seen as a balance/imbalance view of ill-health, though it also includes notions simultaneously of deficiency/ excess.

The 'plumbing' model of the body

Many contemporary concepts of the body's structure and function, at least in the Western world, seem to be borrowed partly from the worlds of science and technology. Familiarity with drainage systems in the home, electricity, machines and the internal combustion engine all provide the models in terms of which people conceptualize and explain the structure and workings of the body. A common version of this might be termed the 'plumbing' model. The body is conceived of as a series of hollow cavities or chambers, connected with one another, and with the body's orifices, by a series of pipes or tubes. The major cavities are usually 'the chest' and 'the stomach', which almost completely fill the thoracic and abdominal spaces respectively.

This type of subdivision of the body into large volumes with a single name was demonstrated in Boyle's study,[13] mentioned above, where 58.8% of the sample saw the stomach as occupying all of the abdominal cavity. Lay vocabulary of ill-health also reflects this conception, e.g. 'I've got a cold on my chest' or 'My chest's full of phlegm'. The cavities are connected to each other, and to the orifices, by pipes such as 'the intestines', 'the bowel', 'the windpipe', 'the blood vessels'. Central to this model is the belief that health is maintained by the uninterrupted *flow* of various substances – including blood, air, food, faeces, urine and menstrual blood – between cavities, or between a cavity and the exterior of the body via one of the orifices. Disease, therefore, is the result of 'blockage' of an internal tube or pipe.

The clinical implications of this model were well demonstrated in the case history quoted above from Kleinman et al.[20] A further example, in the UK, is the widespread lay concept of the dangers of constipation; that is, of a 'blockage in the bowels'. The retained faeces are thought to diffuse into the bloodstream and contaminate it with 'impurities' and 'toxins', which then affect the general health as well as the skin's complexion. Self-prescribed laxatives are still widely used[28] to achieve a 'good clear out', and so preserve good health and a good complexion. The notion of a good clear out is also applied to menstrual and postpartum blood, and will be described more fully below.

The plumbing model does not necessarily cover all aspects of the body's physiology and anatomy, but mostly deals with the respiratory, cardiovascular, gastrointestinal, and genitourinary functions of the body. It is not a coherent or internally consistent system, but rather a series of metaphors used to explain the body's functioning. Often different physiological systems are lumped together if they occur in the same area (e.g. 'the chest'); a patient with nasal catarrh and cough, for example, described his self-treatment as: 'I gargled with salt water to get the catarrh out – and I always swallow a bit of it to loosen the cough'.[10]

The model can also be used to express emotional states, especially lay notions of 'stress' or 'pressure', in images borrowed from the Age of Steam – 'I blew my top', 'I need to let off steam', 'I almost burst a boiler'.

The body as machine

The lay conceptualization of the body as an internal combustion engine, or as a battery-driven machine, has become more common in Western society. These machine and engine metaphors are increasingly encountered by nurses and doctors, who may in turn reinforce them, especially by the use of such explanatory phrases as: 'Your heart isn't pumping so well', 'You've had a nervous breakdown', 'The current isn't flowing so well along your nerves', or 'You need a rest – your batteries need recharging'. Central to the body-as-machine concept is the idea of a renewable fuel or battery power needed to provide energy for the smooth working of the body. 'Fuels' here include various foodstuffs or beverages, such as tea or coffee, and the large number of self-prescribed tonics, vitamins, and other patent remedies. Some people may conceive of alcohol, tobacco or psychotropic drugs as forms of essential fuel, without which they could not function in everyday life.

The machine model includes the idea that the individual parts of the body, like the parts of a motor car, may fail or stop working, and may sometimes need to be replaced. Modern 'spare part surgery', with its widespread usage of organ transplants (heart, lungs, liver, kidney, nerves, skin, bone, larynx and cornea) and various prostheses (artificial joints, bones, arteries, heart valves and teeth), as well as the use of electronic aids such as heart pacemakers and transistor hearing-aids all help to reinforce the image of the body as a machine, with treatment consisting of 'new parts for old'.[29] Certain diagnostic procedures, such as electrocardiographs or electroencephalograms, which measure the body's 'electric currents' or waves, as well as the use of fetal monitors in obstetrics (see Chapter 6), may all reinforce this metaphor in the minds of both patients and health professionals.

Allied with this image of the body-as-machine is that of the mind as a *computer*. The increasing use of computers has influenced the ways many people in the Western world think about themselves. We now live in a new psychological culture, in what Turkle[30] calls a 'computational culture', with new metaphors for the mind as mainly a processor and storehouse of information. In this model, thoughts, ideas, creativity, memory and personality are all seen as forms of 'software' or 'programs', hidden inside the 'hardware' of the brain and the skull. Thus mental illness or deviant behaviour can be now conceived of as only faulty 'wiring' or 'programming' of the individual brain, to be cured by merely 'reprogramming' or 'rewiring' that brain – and this new and simplified image of human thought and behaviour has important social implications.

The body during pregnancy

All cultures share beliefs about the vulnerability of the mother and fetus during pregnancy; to a variable extent, this extends after birth, usually throughout the early postpartum or lactation period. Cultural concepts of the physiology of pregnancy are often evoked after the child is born, in order to explain *post hoc* any unwanted outcomes of pregnancy such as a deformed, ailing or retarded child. In most cultures it is believed that the mother's *behaviour* – her diet, physical activity, state of mind, moral behaviour, use of drink, drugs or tobacco – can directly affect the physiology of reproduction and cause damage to the unborn child. Anthropologists have argued that not all the taboos and restrictions surrounding pregnant women can be explained as protecting the mother and fetus from physical damage: the pregnant woman is also in a state of *social* vulnerability and ambiguity. She is in a state of transition between two social roles – that of wife and that of mother.[31] In this marginal state, as in other states of social transition (see Chapter 9), the person involved is seen as somehow in an ambiguous and 'abnormal' state, dangerous both to herself and to others. The rituals and taboos surrounding pregnancy therefore serve both to mark this transition and to protect mother and fetus during this dangerous period.

Several studies have been carried out into lay beliefs about the physiology and dangers of pregnancy by Snow *et al*. at Michigan State University. In many cases these beliefs were markedly different from those of clinicians involved in antenatal care. In one study of 31 pregnant women attending a public antenatal clinic in Michigan,[32] 77% of them believed that the fetus could be 'marked' – that is, permanently disfigured or even killed – by strong emotional states on the part of the mother, divine punishment for behavioural lapses, the 'power of nature', or the evil intentions of others. The Mexican American women in the sample believed that too much sleep or rest during pregnancy would harm the baby by causing it to 'stick to the uterus' and make delivery difficult or impossible. They also feared the effect on the child if they saw a lunar eclipse, believing that if a pregnant woman goes out unprotected at this time her child may be born dead, or with a cleft palate, or with part of the body missing. Wearing a key suspended around the waist was thought to be adequate protection at this time. Many in the study also believed that excessive emotion in the mother – fear, hate, jealousy, anger, sorrow, pity – could all be dangerous to the unborn child. If the pregnant woman saw something that frightened her – like a cat, or a fish – the child might be born resembling that object; one woman who had been frightened by a fish during pregnancy gave birth to a child that 'has two holes in the roof of her mouth and can swim like a fish'. Behavioural lapses on the part of the mother could also result in fetal damage – making fun of a cripple or retarded person during pregnancy could result in God afflicting the infant with a similar disability. Finally, the malevolence of another person could cause fetal damage, and even death. Similar lay beliefs are found throughout the world, with local variations.

Beliefs about the effects on the fetus of maternal diet were also studied at the public clinic in Michigan.[24] In a sample of 40 women, 90% thought that pregnant women should change their diets in some way, while 38% believed that food cravings could 'mark' the child permanently if these cravings were not satisfied. One woman thought that if a pregnant woman craved chicken, but did not get it, the baby could be born 'looking like a chicken'. Other beliefs related to the effect of particular types of food on the fetus: for example, a baby might be born with 'red spots' if the mother ate too many cherries or strawberries during pregnancy, or have a 'chocolate mark' if she ate (or even sat upon) any chocolate. Snow points out that some of these dietary beliefs may be dangerous in pregnancy as they may provide the rationale for undesirable eating habits by the women. Another factor, among some Latin American women, is the use of 'hot' or 'cold' foods in pregnancy, irrespective of their nutritional properties, in order to maintain their internal 'balance'. Similar beliefs are found among women from the Indian subcontinent. Homans[31] quotes a British-born Asian woman as saying, 'my mother said not to have "hot" things, not to sit in front of the heater and not to have Coca Cola. . . The body acquires too much heat and this can lead to miscarriage'.

Beliefs about the state of the uterus during pregnancy can also affect a pregnant woman's health. In the Michigan study,[33] a widely held belief was that the uterus was a hollow organ that was 'tightly closed' during pregnancy to prevent the loss of the fetus. One woman believed that pregnant women could not contract venereal disease (and therefore did not need to take precautions against it), as during pregnancy 'the uterus is closed and germs cannot enter'.

Beliefs about the physiology and dangers of pregnancy have both social and physical aspects. They set pregnant women apart, as a special category of person, surrounded by what their culture tells them are protective taboos and customs; and they help to explain retrospectively any physical damage or deformity in newborn children. Both aspects, as illustrated above, may have damaging effects on both the pregnant woman and her unborn child.

Beliefs about blood

To illustrate further some of the clinical implications of cultural conceptions of physiology, a number of beliefs about the nature and function of human blood are described below. The human experience of blood – as a vital liquid circulating within the body, and which appears at the surface at times of injury, illness, menstruation or childbirth – provides the basis for lay theories about a variety of illnesses. In general, these illnesses are ascribed to changes in its *volume* ('high blood', due to too much blood), *consistency* ('thin blood', causing anaemia), *temperature* ('hot illnesses' caused by 'heat in the blood' in Morocco), *quality* ('impurities' in the blood, from constipation), or *polluting power* (menstrual blood causing 'weakness' in men). It should also be remembered that lay concepts of blood deal with much more than its perceived physiological actions; blood is a potent image for a number of things, social, physical and psychological. It is what Victor Turner[34] calls 'a multivocal symbol', that is signifying a number of elements at the same time. Among the cluster of meanings associated with blood cross-culturally are: as an *index* of emotional state (blushing or pallor), personality type ('hot blooded', 'cold blooded'), illness (flushed or feverish), kinship ('blood is thicker than water'), social relationships ('bad blood between us'), physical injury (bleeding, bruises), gender (menstruation), danger (menstrual and postpartum blood), and diet ('thin blood' from a bad diet). The clinician should thus be aware of the possible hidden symbolism in any lay conceptualizations of blood.

Case history: Beliefs about menstruation in South Wales, UK

Skultans[35] studied the beliefs about menstruation among women in a mining village in South Wales. She found two types of belief about menstrual blood. First, a belief that menstrual blood is 'bad blood', and menstruation the process by which the system is purged of 'badness' or 'excess'. The emphasis was on losing as much blood as possible, as this was the method whereby 'the system rights itself'. The women said they felt huge, bloated, slow and sluggish 'if they do not have a period or if they do not lose much'. One woman felt 'really great' after a heavy period, and most insisted on the value of having a monthly 'good clearance'. Skultans found that this group had relatively undisturbed and stable married lives, and regarded the menstrual process as 'essential to producing and maintaining a healthy equilibrium' by regular purging of the badness. These women also saw menstruation as a state of increased vulnerability, and particularly feared anything that might stop the flow; this would obviously give them a pessimistic attitude towards the menopause, while at the same time they might not worry about menorrhagia or an exceptionally heavy bleed, regarding it instead as a 'good clearance'. The second group of women believed that menstruation was damaging to their overall health, and were fearful of 'losing their life's blood'. They wished to cease menstruating as early as possible, and unlike the first group were much more positive about the menopause and its attendant symptoms. Skultans found that this group, who viewed periods as 'a nuisance', seemed to be associated with irregular or disturbed conjugal relationships.

Case history: Beliefs about menstruation among the Zulu of South Africa

Ngubane[36] describes beliefs about menstrual blood among the Zulu people of Southern Africa. Menstruating women are believed to have a contagious pollution, which is dangerous both to other humans and to the natural world. Men's virility may be weakened by this blood, especially if they have intercourse with a menstruating woman. She should also avoid sick people or their medicines during her period, and crops may be ruined or cattle fall ill if she walks among them. In other African societies, women may be confined each month to an isolated 'menstrual hut' to protect the community from their dangerous pollution. Similiar beliefs about the 'uncleanness' and polluting powers of menstrual blood are found, especially among men, in cultures and religious groups in many parts of the world.[37]

Case history: Beliefs about menstruation in Michigan, USA

Snow and Johnson[24,33] examined the views of low-income women in a public clinic in Michigan. Many of the women saw menstruation as a method of ridding the body of 'impurities' that might otherwise cause illness or poison the system. They saw the uterus as a hollow organ that is tightly closed between periods while it slowly fills with 'tainted blood', and then opens up to allow the blood to escape during the period. As a result they reasoned that one could become pregnant only just before, during or just after the period, while the uterus is still open. While the uterus was open, the women believed themselves to be particularly vulnerable to illness, caused by the entry of external forces such as cold air or water, 'germs' or witchcraft. One woman in the group speculated that one should not attend a funeral during menstruation, lest the germs that caused the deceased's death enter the open uterus and cause disease. A recurrent fear among the women studied was of stopped or impeded menstrual flow, or of the flow of blood in the postpartum or postabortion period. Latin American women, in particular, feared that certain 'cold' foods (or cold water or air) might clot the 'hot' blood, and interrupt the flow. The stopped flow might then 'back up' in the body and cause a stroke, cancer, sterility, or 'quick TB'. Cold foodstuffs included fresh fruits, especially citrus fruits, tomatoes and green vegetables. As one Mexican American woman put it *Le da mucha friadad a la matriz* ('Such things make the womb very cold').[24] The researchers point out that avoidance of such foods during the vaginal bleeding associated with menstruation, postabortion or postpartum states can eliminate much-needed vitamins from a diet which, for many low-income women, is already deficient in vitamins. The fear of impeded menstruation may also lead some women to avoid some methods of contraception (oral contraceptives, intrauterine contraceptive devices) that may cause changes in menstruation.

Case history: 'High blood' in the Southern United States

Snow[38] has described a common lay belief among low-income patients in the Southern United States, both black and white, called 'high blood'. The central belief is that the blood goes up or down in *volume*, depending on what one eats or drinks, and this can cause either high blood or low blood. 'Low blood' is believed to result from eating too many 'acid' or astringent foods, such as lemon juice, vinegar, pickles, olives, sauerkraut and Epsom salts. Low blood causes lassitude, fatigue and weakness: it is thought to occur particularly in pregnant women, and should be treated by ingesting certain red food or drink – beets, grape juice, red wine, liver and red meat. 'High blood', by contrast, results from eating too much rich food, especially red meat. Home remedies include taking lemon juice, vinegar, sour oranges, Epsom salt, and the brine from pickles or olives. The clinical implications of this belief are not only the effects on health of this type of diet (for example, one with a very high salt content), but also the effect on compliance with a doctor's instructions by one who confuses 'high blood' with 'high blood pressure'. A patient who interprets a diagnosis of high blood pressure as high blood may increase the amount of salt in their diet and reduce the intake of red meat from a diet which may already be deficient in protein.

Case history: 'Sleeping blood' in the Cape Verde Islands

Like and Ellison[39] described the case of a 48-year-old woman from the Cape Verde Islands who was admitted to a neurology ward in a hospital in the USA. She was suffering from paralysis, numbness, pain and tremor of her right arm. It was discovered that two years previously she had suffered bilateral Colles' fractures of her wrists, and after that her neurological symptoms gradually appeared. No physical cause for her illness could be found, until it was realized that she believed herself to be suffering from a Cape Verdean folk illness, 'sleeping blood' (*sangue dormido*). In this lay model, traumatic injuries (in this case, her wrist fractures) may cause a person's normal 'living blood' (*sangue vivo*) to leak out into the skin, turn black (i.e. form a haematoma), and become sleeping blood. It is feared that deeper deposits of blood develop between the muscles and bones, and if not removed its volume may expand over time and obstruct the circulation distal to the traumatized area. In addition, the internal living blood may dam up, and cause various disorders such as pain, tremor, paralysis, convulsions, stroke, blindness, heart attack, infection, miscarriage and mental illness. The patient explained her neurological disabilities as due to the 'blockage' resulting from the sleeping blood. She was eventually treated by withdrawing 12 ml of blood from her right wrist (the *sangue dormido*) on two occasions, and by the application of cold packs, after which her tremor, paralysis and pain completely disappeared.

Case history: Blood as a non-regenerative liquid

Foster and Anderson[40] point out that the belief that blood is a *non*-regenerative liquid which, when lost through injury or disease, cannot be replaced and leaves the victim permanently weakened is common in many parts of the world. In Latin America 'people are most reluctant to part with their precious blood', and this may be one of the reasons why blood banks are less successful in getting donations of blood than in the USA.

Recommended reading

Boyle, C. M. (1970) Differences between patients' and doctors' interpretation of some common medical terms. *Br. Med. J.* ii, 286–289

Fisher, S. (1968) Body image. In: Sills, D. (ed.) *International Encyclopaedia of the Social Sciences*. New York: Free Press, pp. 113–116

Polhemus, T. (ed.) (1978) *Social Aspects of the Human Body*. Harmondsworth: Penguin. A collection of basic readings on the subject.

Scheper-Hughes, N. and Lock, M.M. (1987) The mindful body: a prolegomenon to future work in medical anthropology. *Med. Anthropol. Q.* (New Series) **1**, 6–41. A comprehensive review of the modern literature on body image.

Chapter 3
Diet and nutrition

Food is more than just a source of nutrition. In all human societies it plays many roles, and is deeply embedded in the social, religious and economic aspects of everyday life. For people in these societies it also carries with it a range of symbolic meanings, both expressing and creating the relationships between man and man, man and his deities, and man and the natural environment. Food, therefore, is an essential part of the way that any society organizes itself – and of the way that it views the world it inhabits.

The anthropologist Claude Lévi-Strauss[1] has argued that just as there is no human society which does not have a spoken language, so also there is no human group which does not in some way process some of its food supply through cooking. In fact, the constant transformation of raw into cooked food is one of the defining features of all human societies, a key criterion of 'culture' as opposed to 'nature'.

Anthropologists have further pointed out how cultural groups differ markedly from one another in many of their beliefs and practices related to food. For example, there are wide variations throughout the world in what substances are regarded as food and what are not. Foodstuffs that are eaten in one society or group are rigorously forbidden in another. There are also variations between cultures as to how food is cultivated, harvested, prepared, served and eaten. Each culture usually has a set of implicit rules which determine who prepares and serves the food and to whom; which individuals or groups eat together; where, and on what occasions, the consumption of food takes place; the order of dishes within a meal; and the actual manner of eating the food. All of these stages in food consumption are closely patterned by culture, and are part of the accepted way of life of that community.

In most parts of the world the actual preparation of food is usually the task of women,[2] but in many societies they are also closely involved in the production of food – milking animals, caring for poultry and livestock, and planting, tending and harvesting a wide variety of crops. In many rural parts of the

Third World women also play a leading role in the marketing of food – such as the famous 'market women' of West Africa, the Caribbean and parts of Latin America.

Food classification

Because of the central role of food in daily life, especially in social relationships, dietary beliefs and practices are notoriously difficult to change, even if they interfere with adequate nutrition. Many well-meaning nutritionists, nurses and doctors have discovered this fact in dealing with cultures other than their own. Before these beliefs and practices can be modified or improved, it is important to understand the way that each culture views its food, and the way that it *classifies* it into different categories. In general, five types of food classification system can be identified, though in practice several of them usually coexist within the same society. They are:

1. Food *versus* non-food.
2. Sacred *versus* profane foods.
3. Parallel food classifications.
4. Food used as medicine, and medicine as food.
5. Social foods (which signal relationships, status, occupation, gender or group identity).

Their clinical significance is that they may severely restrict the types of foodstuffs available to people – and that diet may be based on cultural, rather than nutritional criteria.

Food *versus* non-food

Each culture defines which substances are edible and which are not, although this definition often leaves out substances that *do* have a nutritional value. In the UK, for example, snakes, squirrels, otters, dogs, cats and mice are all edible, but are rarely classified as food. In France, snails and frogs' legs are food, but they are usually not so classified in the UK. In some cases, the definition of substances as non-food may be due to their historical associations; for example, Jelliffe[3] suggests that the spleen is rarely eaten in the UK because, in the ancient Galenic humoral system, it was the prime seat of the 'melancholic' humour. Definitions of what is considered edible and what is not tend to be flexible, however, especially under conditions of famine, economic deprivation and foreign travel. In addition, there is a spectrum among the substances defined as food between those which are regarded as nutritious, and are eaten during meals, and those eaten between meals as snacks. In some cases the manufacturers of certain of these snacks, such as sweets, chocolates and cakes, have sought to promote their products as a nutritious food, something that 'fills the energy gap' between proper mealtimes.

Whatever the origins of these definitions, classifying a substance as non-food on cultural grounds may leave out useful nutriments from the diet, and this seems to be a universal phenomenon. As Foster and Anderson[4] put it, 'No group, even under conditions of extreme starvation, utilizes all available nutritional substances as food.'

Sacred *versus* profane foods

I .1ave used the term 'sacred foods' to refer to those foodstuffs the use of which is validated by *religious* beliefs, while foodstuffs expressly forbidden by the religion can be termed 'profane'. This latter group is usually the subject of strict taboos that not only prohibit ingestion of the food but also forbid physical contact with it. In most cases, this profane food is also seen as 'unclean' and dangerous to health. The sacred/profane dichotomy applies to much more than food, since it is usually part of a wider moral framework. Dress, behaviour, speech and certain ritual actions can also be divided into the sacred and the profane. Religious groups that have strong food taboos tend also to have strict observances and rituals which separate the sacred from the profane aspects of daily life, such as regular prayers, or ritual bathing and other rites of purification. The priestly castes and officiators within these groups are more likely to be subject to these strict rules – which maintain their purity and holiness – than the average worshipper. On certain occasions or fasts, all – or certain – foodstuffs are considered profane, and must be avoided. Examples of this are the Jewish *Yom Kippur* (a 25-hour fast) and the Muslim fast of *Ramadan* where, for the ninth month of the lunar year, food and drink are avoided between dawn and sunset by all Muslims above the 'age of responsibility' (15 years for boys, 12 for girls). Regular food abstentions are also a feature of Hinduism, and according to Hunt[5] many observant Hindus spend two or three days a week 'fasting'; that is, eating only 'pure' foods such as milk, fruit, nuts, and starchy root vegetables like cassava and potatoes.

Strict taboos against certain types of food are characteristic of a number of religious faiths:

1. *Hinduism*. Orthodox Hindus are forbidden to kill or eat any animal, particularly the cow. Milk and its products may be eaten, since they do not involve taking the animal's life. Both fish and eggs are infrequently eaten.
2. *Islam*. Neither pork nor any pig products may be eaten. The only meat permitted is that from cloven hooved animals that chew the cud, and it must be *halal* or ritually slaughtered. Only fish that have fins and scales may be eaten, and shellfish and eels are therefore forbidden.
3. *Judaism*. As with Islam, all pig products are forbidden, and also fish without fins or scales, birds of prey, and carrion. Only animals that chew the cud, have cloven hooves, and have been ritually slaughtered are *kosher* and may be eaten. Meat and milk dishes are never mixed within the same meal.
4. *Sikhism*. Beef is strictly forbidden, but pork is allowed – though it is rarely eaten. The meat must also be slaughtered in a special, ritual way.
5. *Rastafarianism*. Many Rastafarians are vegetarian, although some follow dietary restrictions similar to those of Judaism.[6] As with many other religious groups, alcohol is strictly prohibited.

A more secular example of food taboos is found in the contemporary whole food movement in the UK and the USA. Here the sacred/profane dichotomy is between the 'natural' and the 'artificial', between *whole foods* on the one hand and 'junk foods' on the other. Junk foods are associated with ideas of uncleanness and danger, especially from their additives, dyes, preservatives and other pollutants. Similarly, the modern movement of *vegetarianism* – which Twigg[7] sees as offering 'a this-worldly form of salvation in terms of the body' – sees meat and its various products as dangerous and 'profane'. They associate a vegetarian diet with purity, lightness, wholeness, and spirituality while, by contrast, meat and blood are associated with aggressiveness, base sexual instincts, an 'animal nature', and a disharmonious world.

In all these cases of food taboos, classifying a foodstuff as profane, and therefore forbidden, may exclude much-needed nutriments from the diet, as will be illustrated below.

Parallel food classifications

The division of all foodstuffs into two main groups, usually called 'hot' and 'cold', is a feature of many cultural groups in the

Islamic world, the Indian subcontinent, Latin America and China. In all these cultures, this binary system of classification includes much more than food: medicines, illnesses, mental and physical states, natural and supernatural forces, are all grouped into either 'hot' or 'cold' categories. The theory of physiology on which this is based, and which equates health with *balance* between these two categories, has been fully described in the previous chapter.

In many cases this view of health and illness represents a survival of the humoral theory of physiology, especially in Latin America and North Africa. In China and India, while hot/cold dichotomies are also found, they have a different genealogy – from the Yin–Yang and Ayurvedic systems respectively. The notions of hot and cold do not refer to actual temperature, but rather to certain symbolic values associated with each category of foodstuffs. Because 'health' is defined as a balance between these categories, ill-health is treated by adding hot or cold foods or medicines to the diet to restore the balance. For example, among some Latin American groups living in the USA, a cold disease like arthritis may be treated by hot foods or medications, while in Morocco hot illnesses like sunstroke are treated by cold substances. In most cases, these parallel food classifications are not based on a logically consistent principle, nor are foodstuffs that are classified as hot in one culture necessarily seen as hot in another.

Local historical and cultural factors, as well as personal idiosyncrasies, may play a part in assigning foods to these two categories. For example, in his study in Morocco, Greenwood[8] found significant differences among his informants as to what foods were hot and what were cold, although they all agreed on the tastes, physiological effects and therapeutic value expected of the two categories. In some cases the choice of category was based mainly on personal experience; one man, for example, noted that goat meat tasted sour and caused indigestion and joint stiffness (cold conditions), and that goats could not tolerate being outside in the winter, while cattle could, and therefore goat meat was cold while beef was hot.

Parallel food classifications sometimes include intermediate categories, such as 'cool' or 'neutral', so that there is a spectrum between hot and cold, rather than a clear division. An example of this form of classification was described by Harwood[9], among a group of Puerto Ricans in New York City. Although diseases were grouped by them into hot or cold categories, foodstuffs and medications were divided into hot (*caliente*), cool (*fresco*) or cold (*frio*). Arthritis, colds, menstrual periods and joint pains

Table 3.1 Hot–cold classification of foods among New York Puerto Ricans

Hot (caliente)	Cool (fresco)	Cold (frio)
Alcoholic beverages	Barley water	Avocado
Chilli peppers	Bottled milk	Bananas
Chocolate	Chicken	Coconut
Coffee	Fruits	Lima beans
Corn meal	Honey	Sugar cane
Evaporated milk	Raisins	White beans
Garlic	Salt-cod	
Kidney beans	Watercress	
Onions		
Peas		
Tobacco		

Reproduced from Harwood[9] by permission

were all cold diseases, while constipation, diarrhoea, rashes, tenesmus and ulcers were all hot. The hot medicines included aspirin, castor oil, penicillin, cod liver oil, iron and vitamins, while cold medicines were bicarbonate of soda, mannitol, nightshade and milk of magnesia.

The three categories of foods are shown in Table 3.1, although this division is not necessarily typical of all Puerto Ricans, both in New York and elsewhere. Harwood notes how the classification he described is not based on relative temperatures – iced beer, for example, is still considered hot as it is an alcoholic beverage. Cold illnesses are sometimes blamed on eating too many cold foods, which cause a stomach chill or *frialdad del estomago*; similarly, a person with a cold may refuse to drink the fruit juices recommended by his physician as these are also classified as cold.

During pregnancy a woman in this group would avoid hot foods or medications (including iron and vitamin supplements) lest her child be born with a hot illness, such as a rash. After delivery – and during menstruation – cold foods are avoided, lest they clot the blood and impede the flow, causing it to go backwards into the body and cause nervousness or insanity.

Hunt[5] has described the hot–cold classification system among some Asian immigrants (from India, Pakistan and Bangladesh) living in the UK, including both Hindus and Muslims. The Indian classification of foodstuffs into hot and cold is shown in Table 3.2. As with the Puerto Rican example, illnesses were treated by restoring the balance of hot and cold forces within the body; a febrile illness, for instance, is treated by cold foods such as rice, green gram and buttermilk.

Table 3.2 Hot–cold classification of foods among Indians in the UK

Hot	Cold
Wheat	Rice
Potato	Plantains
Buffalo milk	Cows' milk
Fish	Buttermilk
Chicken	Green gram
Horse gram	Peas
Groundnut	Beans
Drumstick	Onions
Bitter gourd	Green tomatoes
Carrot	Pumpkin
Radish	Spinach
Fenugreek	Ripe mango
Garlic	Bananas
Green mango	Guava
Pawpaw	Lemons
Dates	

Reproduced from Hunt[5] by permission

In another study, by Tann and Wheeler,[10] a group of London Chinese mothers believed that their diet should be modified according to the general health of the infant receiving their breast milk. If the baby had a cold illness, they avoided cold foods which might turn the breast milk cold and thus aggravate the illness. In some cases, this led to a considerable restriction in the sources of nutrition available to the mother. In this case, as in others, parallel food classifications are usually used by patients as a form of self-medication which in some circumstances may prove damaging to their health.

Food as medicine, medicine as food

This category system usually overlaps with parallel food classifications, when the two coexist in the same society, as in the cases of Morocco, India and Puerto Rico quoted above. However, in other societies, special diets may also be seen as a form of medicine for certain illnesses or physiological states. Some examples of this have been quoted in the previous chapter, such as 'feed a cold, starve a fever' in the case of common viral or bacterial infections, or the use of certain foods or vitamins (a form of concentrated 'food') to prevent colds and chills. In the case of special physiological states, such as pregnancy, lactation and menstruation, certain foods are sometimes avoided, or else prescribed to aid in the physiological process. The effect of hot and cold foods on these states have already been described in the case of women from Latin America. In a study[11] of 40 women attending a public clinic in Michigan, 11 believed the fetus could be 'marked' if the mother's food cravings were not satisfied, 12 thought that the diet should be altered in the postpartum period, and four believed it should be changed during lactation. Twelve women in the sample admitted to having eaten starch, clay or dirt during pregnancy – as one pregnant woman put it, it was a good idea to eat earth since it acts as 'a scrub brush through the organs'. One woman believed that during lactation the supply of breast milk could be increased by drinking red raspberry tea and avoiding acid foods and cabbage. In many of these cases, cultural prescriptions about the appropriate food or drink to treat or advance a physiological process may have negative effects on the patient's health.

The American folk illness 'high blood' (and its opposite 'low blood'), described in Chapter 2, is a further example of the use of food as medicine. High blood is treated by taking lemon juice, vinegar, sour oranges, pickles, olives or sauerkraut while the treatment of low blood involves an increased consumption of beets, grape juice, red wine, liver and red meat. Where patients confuse the diagnosis of 'high blood pressure' with 'high blood', they may cut out much-needed sources of protein from their diet, and replace them with foods with a high salt content – which may be dangerous in a case of hypertension.

Etkin and Ross[12] studied the use of plants, both as medicine and as food, among the Hausa people of Northern Nigeria. They found that many of the plants were used as folk medicines *and* as food. For example, cashew nuts were chewed for treatment of intestinal worms, diarrhoea and dyspepsia, but were also added to soups and used as a condiment in vegetable foods. By analysing both the nutritional and the pharmacological properties of many of these substances, they conclude that many plants taken as medicine may in fact also have nutritional value, while some of the plants used mainly as food also have a medicinal effect; only by examining all the many uses of plants can an estimation of their overall nutritional value be made. They also suggest that agricultural development programmes that attempt to reduce crop diversity to maximize calorie and protein availability may reduce the range of nutrients available to food-producing populations, as well as the plants available both as medicines and as dietary constituents.

Medicines, whether medically or self-prescribed, may also come to be regarded as a form of food or nutriment, without which the patient might weaken or die. Examples of this are certain cardiac or hypotensive drugs, insulin therapy, and thyroid and other hormone replacement therapy. When these drugs are regularly taken at mealtimes, they may become incorporated into the meal as a symbolic form of food. Other substances such as vitamins and 'tonics', alcohol, tobacco and psychotropic drugs, if taken regularly, might also come to play this role (see Chapter 8).

Social foods

Social foods are those consumed in the presence of other people, and which have a *symbolic* as well as a nutritional value for all those concerned. A snack eaten in private is not a social food, but the contents of a family meal or religious feast usually are. In every human society food is a way of creating, and expressing, the *relationships* between people. These relationships may be between individuals, between the members of social, religious or ethnic groups, or between any of these and the supernatural world. Food used in this way has many of the properties of the ritual symbols described later in this book (Chapter 9). In particular, when food is consumed in the formalized atmosphere of a communal meal, it carries with it many associations, telling the participants much about their relationships with one another and with the outside world. Most meals have a ritual aspect, in addition to their purely practical role in providing nutrition for a number of people at the same time. Like all ritual occasions, they are tightly controlled by the norms of a particular culture or group. These norms, or rules, determine who prepares and serves the food, who eats together, and who clears up afterwards. They also determine the times and setting of meals, the order of dishes within the meal, the cutlery or crockery used, and the precise way in which the food may be consumed – or 'table manners'. The food itself is subject to cultural patterning, which determines its appropriate size, shape, consistency, colour, smell and taste. Both the formal occasion of a meal and the types of food served within it can therefore be viewed as a complicated *language*, which can be decoded to reveal much about the relationships and values of those sharing in the food. Each meal is a restatement, and re-creation, of these values and relationships.

Different types of meal convey different messages to those taking part in them. Farb and Armelagos[13] point out that in North America cocktails without a meal are for acquaintances or people of lower social status; meals preceded by alcoholic drinks are for close friends and honoured guests; a cold lunch is 'at the threshold of intimacy', but not quite there; social intimacy is symbolized by invitation to a complete meal, with a sequence of courses contrasted by hot and cold; the buffet, the 'cookout' and the barbecue extend friendship to a greater extent than an invitation to morning coffee, but less so than an invitation to a complete sit-down meal.

Meals can also be used to symbolize social *status*, often by serving rare and expensive dishes – what Jelliffe[3] calls 'prestige foods'. According to him they are usually protein (and often animal), are difficult to obtain or prepare (as they are rare, expensive or imported), and are often linked historically with a dominant social group (such as venison, which was the preserve of the upper classes in Europe during the Middle Ages). Among the prestige foods that can be identified are venison and game birds in Northern Europe, the T-bone steak in America, the camel hump among Bedouin Arabs, and the pig in New Guinea. Status can also be acquired by giving enormous feasts, where large amounts of food are conspicuously eaten or wasted. A well known example of this, from the anthropological literature, is the *potlach* feast, used by the Indians of the North-Western United States and Canada. Different families competed with one another to throw huge, lavish feasts, each one greater than the next, and at which large amounts of food were wasted. The aim was to humiliate rival families by throwing a feast that could not be matched by them.

In other societies, the display and sharing of food is also used to obtain prestige, but without the wastage characteristic of the *potlach*. In the Trobriand Islands off Papua-New Guinea, for example, a farmer who has produced much food during a season is regarded as having shown great skill and prowess in farming, and to have been especially favoured by the supernatural powers. He is now able to demonstrate his success, and increase in status, by displaying large piles of food he has grown at any of the tribal group ceremonies (such as harvest or mourning rituals), and to distribute this food to relatives and friends whom he wishes to honour. Belshaw[14] points out that this does not result in a gluttonous feast, since the food, when distributed, is cooked and eaten in the home of the recipient.

In other social systems, such as the Hindu caste system in India, social rank is usually marked by the types of food prepared and eaten by each caste. The highest prestige is given to raw foods, which are considered suitable for the priestly Brahmins and other upper castes. Cooked food is less valued unless it contains *ghee,* a form of butter from which the water has been removed. Inferior cooked foods include pickles, cheap curries and barley cakes, each of which lacks ghee. Food may not be accepted from, or prepared by, the members of lower castes, though food can travel downwards in the caste system as payment for goods or services. In this society, food functions both as a form of currency and as an indicator of social position.

In many parts of the world light-coloured foods, such as white bread or white rice, have a higher status than dark-coloured foods. In Europe, it was the peasants who ate rough, brown bread, while the aristocracy ate white bread or cakes, and the same pattern existed elsewhere. In the Third World, as Trowell and Burkitt[15] note, Westernization has led to the increased status of white bread and rice. Cereals are increasingly refined to produce low-fibre white wheat flour and polished white rice, resulting in a decreased intake of dietary fibre, especially cereal fibre. Some of the Western diseases that possibly result from this change will be mentioned below.

As well as signalling status, food can be used as a badge of *group identity* – whether the group is based on regional, familial, ethnic or religious criteria. Each country has its national dish, and often regions within those countries are known by their local cuisine. Food produced and eaten locally is closely identified with the sense of continuity and cohesion of the community, and its dietary practices are often carried to other countries when members of the community emigrate. In their new countries, the immigrants may continue to eat their traditional diet – with its familiar taste, smells and mode of preparation – or merely revert to it on special occasions. For example, Jerome[16] studied the changes in diet and the pattern of meals in black Americans who had migrated from rural areas in the South to large cities in the North. The traditional Southern pattern consisted of two meals: breakfast, which comprised fried meats of various kinds, rice, grits, biscuits, gravy, fried sweet Irish potatoes, coffee and milk; and the 'heavy boiled dinner', which took place in the mid-afternoon, and comprised boiled vegetables or dry legumes, seasoned with a variety of meat items. This main dish was accompanied by cornbread, potatoes, a sweet beverage or milk, and an occasional dessert or fruit. In the Northern urban environment, under the influence of occupational schedules, the pattern changed, with the heavy boiled dinner now served at 4–6 p.m. and renamed 'supper'. The heavy breakfast usually persisted for about 18 months after migration, with 'lunch' consisting of leftovers from it. Eventually, a new pattern was established with three meals: breakfast, comprising eggs, or bacon or sausage with eggs, hot biscuits, 'light' bread and coffee; a lunch of sandwiches, soup, crackers, raw fruits and a fruit drink; and dinner, of either 'heavy boiled' or fried food. The traditional heavy breakfasts were reserved for weekends, 'off-days' and holidays.

As Jerome's study illustrates, the internal structure and content of meals can be remarkably uniform within a social or cultural group. A similar study, on working-class British meals, was carried out by Douglas and Nicod.[17] They found that meals, unlike 'snacks', were highly structured events, with certain combinations of foods served in the appropriate sequence. Breakfast, where the dishes were served in any order, was usually not regarded as a 'meal'. At meals, careful combinations were made between salty and sweet, moist and dry, and hot and cold foods. When food was very hot, it had to be accompanied by a cold drink, while a dessert taken with a hot beverage had to be cold, dry and solid (cake or biscuits). Douglas and Nicod were able to decipher the underlying, recurrent 'grammar' of these meals, and point out that improvement in their nutritional qualities had to take this structure into account, instead of imposing on it the opinions of the middle-class dietitian.

Because of their central role in defining and recreating group identity and cohesion, communal meals or feasts mark many of the important occasions in the life of the group. Examples of this are feasts associated with weddings, christenings, wakes, *barmitzvahs* and religious festivals and services. Foods consumed during religious occasions are more likely to have a symbolic, rather than a nutritional significance – for example the Communion wafer or Host, or the Passover *matzoh*. Consuming these foods confirms and re-establishes the relationship between man and his deity, as well as between man and man. More secular group festivals, where the group's history and experiences are celebrated, also utilize special foods, such as the turkey eaten at the American Thanksgiving. Farb and Armelagos[18] note how the pumpkin, originally a commonly used vegetable, has gradually assumed more symbolic, and less nutritional, significance as a decoration at Halloween or

Thanksgiving. They estimate that every autumn nearly three million pumpkins are sold in Massachusetts, and that 90% of them will never be eaten, being carved instead into jack-o-lanterns or used to decorate front porches, window sills and dining tables.

A further example of a social food with ritual significance is the British wedding cake. Charsley[19] suggests that the wedding cake – comprising three tiers, each one covered with smooth white icing and surrounded by elaborate ornaments and decorations (silver or gold horseshoes, slippers or flowers) – is symbolic of the bride herself, in her long white dress and veil. Furthermore, the joint cutting of the 'virginal white' cake by the new bride and groom has a sexual significance – symbolic of the couple now 'becoming one flesh'.

These many examples of social foods illustrate the multiple roles that food plays in human society: creating and sustaining social relationships; signalling social status, occupation and gender roles; marking important life changes, anniversaries and festivals; and reasserting religious, ethnic or regional identities. Because of their many social roles, dietary beliefs and practices are sometimes difficult to discard, even when they are dangerous to health.

Culture and malnutrition

The five systems of food classification described above illustrate how food may be eaten for cultural as well as nutritional reasons. From a clinical perspective, these cultural influences may affect nutrition in two ways:

1. They may exclude much-needed nutriments from the diet (by defining them as non-food, profane, alien or lower-class food, or food on the wrong side of a hot/cold dichotomy).
2. They may encourage the consumption of certain foods or drinks (by defining them as food, sacred, medicine, or as a sign of social, religious or ethnic identity) which are actually injurious to health.

When both of these influences coexist there is likely to be an increased risk of *malnutrition*, manifesting either as *under*nutrition (a deficiency of vitamins, proteins, energy sources or elements) or as *over*nutrition (especially obesity and its consequences). Other cultural factors can also have an indirect effect on nutrition – such as beliefs about the structure and functioning of the body, its optimal size and shape, and the role of diet in health and disease.

However, it should always be remembered that cultural influences alone do *not* account for most cases of malnutrition world-wide, though they may be one of the factors contributing towards them. To be fully understood, malnutrition should also be placed in its wider social, political, economic and environmental context. For example, various forms of *deprivation* – that is, the lack of available food, or of the means to obtain what food there is – accounts for most cases of *under*nutrition, especially in the developing world. Such deprivation may result from a number of factors, including: *poverty*, due to the unequal distribution of resources within a society, or between societies; *natural disasters*, such as floods, tidal waves, tornadoes and drought; *wars*, especially civil wars, and other forms of violent social upheaval; and *crop failures* due to locusts and other insects or parasites. Another factor, fully described by Keesing,[20] is the international *political economy* of food production and consumption. He notes how in many parts of the Third World, both under colonialism and afterwards, people were encouraged (and sometimes forced) to grow commodities for export – such as tobacco or cotton – rather than staple foods for internal consumption. In large areas of the developing world, more and more land was devoted to producing these 'cash crops' for export. In the 1970s, for example, cash crops occupied an estimated 55% of the cropland in the Philippines, 80% in Mauritius, and 50% of all cultivated land in Senegal. Many developing countries are therefore at the mercy of fluctuations in the world market for their cash crops, and are also increasingly reliant on imported food for subsistence. Furthermore, advertising from firms in the industrialized countries has promoted the use of less nutritious, and more expensive, artificial foods such as soft drinks, canned foods and infant formula feeds (see below).

In each case of malnutrition, therefore, cultural factors – as well as personal factors, such as ignorance or idiosyncrasy – are only one part of the mix of influences on the individual, which determine whether his or her diet is nutritionally adequate or not.

To illustrate the contributory role of culture in malnutrition, three topics are discussed below, with examples.

Immigrants and ethnic minorities in the UK: some nutritional problems

Most immigrant groups bring with them their own 'dietary culture' – their traditional beliefs and practices relating to food. Not only does this ensure a sense of cultural continuity with their countries of origin, but it also plays many symbolic, religious and social roles in their daily lives. Food habits are one of the important indicators of acculturation. Together with dress, behaviour and family structure they are often among the last cultural traits to go, if immigrants seek to discard their original cultures. In addition to dietary habits, other factors – beyond the control of the immigrants themselves – may affect their health and nutrition. These include: discrimination or rejection by the host community; unemployment; physical violence or racial harassment;[21] substandard or overcrowded living conditions; low incomes; little leisure time and long working hours; social isolation; and the stressful effects of culture-change itself (see Chapter 11).

Stroud[22] has reviewed the commonest nutritional problems of Asian (from India, Pakistan and Bangladesh) and West Indian immigrants in the UK. These include osteomalacia and rickets among Asians; various forms of anaemia among both Asians and West Indians; and overnutrition (obesity) in some West Indian infants. Another study, by Ward et al.,[23] also identified rickets among some of the children of West Indian Rastafarians.

Considerable research has been done on Asian rickets in the UK, which has a much higher incidence than among the white population. It is especially common among those aged 9 months to 3 years and 8–14 years and among pregnant and lactating Asian women. Several factors have been blamed for this high incidence, including: a deficiency of vitamin D in the Asian vegetarian diet; the phytase content of Asian diets (in chapattis), which binds with calcium and prevents its absorption; skin pigmentation (due to absorption of ultraviolet light by skin pigments, with consequent reduction in vitamin D production); genetic factors; and a lack of exposure to ultraviolet light (due to poor housing, confinement of women indoors, and types of female dress that cover large areas of skin surface).[24,25] While the lack of dietary vitamin D is not the sole cause of rickets (one should include, for example, the fear of racial attacks which may keep some Asian women indoors[21]), it is still an important cause of the condition. Hunt[5] points out that the Asian diet supplies about 1.5 μg of vitamin D daily, compared with 2.9 μg daily in the rest of the British population. The British population derive most of their vitamin D from margarine and fish, both of which are hardly used by the Asians. Hindus reject fish for religious reasons, while some Muslims believe that margarine contains pork fat. The lack of dietary vitamin D is especially important in girls during their growth spurt at puberty and in pregnant women – in both cases, social seclusion and dress also play a part. Rickets in infancy has also been blamed on the Asian practice of weaning babies directly onto cows' milk without using vitamin drops or vitamin D enriched baby foods. Stroud[22] points out that cows' milk and human milk contain 20–40 iu/l of vitamin D, while the recommended allowance for infants is 400 iu/day, so that a baby fed entirely on human or non-proprietary cows' milk will have much less than the recommended daily allowance. Vitamin D supplements have been suggested both for infants and for pregnant Asian women. According to the *Lancet*[24] doctors should 'regard all pregnant Asian women as potentially osteomalacic and ensure that they receive adequate supplementary vitamin D (400 iu daily) throughout pregnancy and lactation'. More recently, Mares *et al.*[26] have argued against this over-emphasis on the role of Asian diet in causing rickets. They suggest that only about a quarter of British Asians are, to a lesser or greater extent, vegetarian; that many Asians do in fact eat large amounts of dairy products; and that the positive role of vegetarian diets in protecting against heart disease should also be emphasized.

Nutritional rickets has also been described among West Indian infants whose parents belong to the Rastafarian religion. Ward *et al.*[23] have described four cases of children aged between 11 and 20 months who were found to have clinical rickets. Their parents were strict Rastafarians and ate a vegetarian diet, which also excluded fish. They were breast fed until the second half of the first year of life, when they were weaned on an essentially vegetarian diet known as I-tal. None had received vitamin supplements during infancy or had completed a full course of immunizations. Like many Asians, they had low incomes, and lived in depressed inner city areas where opportunities for outdoor play are few, and exposure to sunlight is likely to be limited.

Stroud[22] also reports higher rates of iron-deficiency anaemia among both Asian and West Indian infants and children. Part of this may be caused by prolonged breast feeding or weaning directly onto cows' milk since both types of milk are deficient in iron, containing 0.3 and 1.0 mg/l respectively. According to

Hunt,[5] the diet of adult Asians is devoid of easily assimilated iron from animal sources. Although iron is added to chapatti flour, only about 3% of it is absorbed when eaten as part of an Asian diet. In some cases, the anaemia may result from hookworm (*Ancylostoma*) infestations, because of the demands such infestation may make on body proteins, though according to Stroud this is rare in the UK in all communities. Hunt also points out that megaloblastic anaemias – due to folic acid or vitamin B_{12} deficiency – are more common among Asians in the UK, especially Hindus. Asian cooking habits may destroy much of the folic acid, for example by boiling pulses for about an hour, or by the prolonged gentle heating of finely cut up foods. In addition, the habit of boiling the milk, tea leaves and water together for five minutes when making tea is thought to destroy much of the vitamin B_{12}, which is especially important in Hindus, whose vegetarian diet lacks other sources of vitamin B_{12}.

A final problem among immigrants in the UK is that of overnutrition, a condition which is by no means confined to immigrant or ethnic minority communities. In Stroud's opinion, West Indian children in the UK are in more danger from obesity than from undernutrition. Since many of their families come from communities where malnutrition was common, 'many of the West Indian mothers seem to have a very deep-seated desire to see their children as big, fat babies, and are not satisfied with their average growth along the fiftieth centile'.

Infant feeding practices in the UK: a comparison of different communities

The care and feeding of infants is a central concern in every cultural group. There are widespread differences, however, in the techniques of infant feeding, whether breast, bottle or artificial feed is used, and in the age and technique of weaning. Despite medical advice that for a variety of physiological and emotional reasons 'breast is best', breast feeding has declined in most countries in the world this century. This is particularly the case in urban, industrialized societies or in non-Western societies undergoing modernization. As Farb and Armelagos[27] put it, 'mothers in many parts of the world often consider breast feeding to be a vulgar peasant custom, to be abandoned as soon as the bottle can be afforded'. This decline in human lactation has been described as the greatest nutritional crisis in today's world.[20] Several reasons have been advanced for this shift from breast to bottle, including urbanization and the increased employment of women outside the home. A further factor in some developing countries, especially in Africa, are the huge advertising campaigns in favour of bottle feeding, promoted by Western manufacturers of artificial infant foods. These campaigns have been heavily criticized for depriving babies of the nutritional and immunological advantages of breast milk, and for increasing the dangers of malnutrition and the risk of diarrhoeal diseases. In many areas, mothers may not have the facilities to prepare the infant feeds with properly boiled water and sterilized bottles, thus increasing their babies' risk of infection.[28]

A reverse trend is appearing in many industrialized countries, as the last few years have seen a gradual return to breast feeding among many mothers in the upper socioeconomic classes.

In the UK, several studies have been done on infant feeding practices among different communities in different parts of the country, and four of these are described below.

Case history: Infant feeding practices in Glasgow, UK

Goel et al.[29] studied the infant feeding practices of 172 families from various communities in Glasgow. These included 206 Asian, 99 African, 99 Chinese and 102 Scots children. It was found that, after arrival in the UK, most immigrant mothers did not want to breast feed their babies. Those immigrant children born outside the UK were more likely to have been breast fed than those born within Britain: 83.7% of Asian, 79% of African and 81% of Chinese children born abroad had been breast fed, while of those born in the UK only 20.9% of the Asian, 48% of the African, and 2% of the Chinese children had been breast fed. Of the Scots children, 99% had been exclusively bottle fed. The commonest reasons given by the immigrant mothers for not breast feeding were embarrassment, inconvenience and insufficient breast milk. Two-thirds of the breast-fed Asian children were fed for at least 6 months, only 5% of the African babies were breast fed for more than 1 year, but Chinese mothers often fed for 1–3 years, and many of their children were not given solid foods until they were 1 year or over. Asian children born in the UK usually had solids by 6 months (but were given these at 1 year if they had been born abroad). Both African and Scots children were given solids at 6 months. The authors suggest that all Asian children be given vitamin D supplements, since 12.5% of the Asian children in the sample were found to have rickets.

Case history: Breast feeding *versus* bottle feeding in London, UK

Jones and Belsey[30] surveyed 265 mothers of 12-week-old infants in the London borough of Lambeth. Of these mothers, 62% had attempted to breast feed (compared with 16% in Dublin, 39% in Newcastle and 52% in Gloucestershire). The different communities showed different rates of breast feeding: British 58%, African 86%, West Indian 84%, Asian 77%, European 59%, and Irish 64%. The ethnic background of the mothers was an important influence here, as in many communities breast feeding was the accepted norm. Several reasons were given for not breast feeding, especially that they 'disliked the thought of breast feeding': 54% of the bottle feeders said this, while 44% thought bottle feeding more convenient, as it required less privacy than breast feeding. Only 13% of the bottle feeders thought the method they had chosen was healthiest for the baby, compared with 85% of the breast feeders. Social as well as ethnic factors were important in the choice of feeding technique, though the two were related: mothers were more likely to continue breast feeding after 6 weeks if they had friends who had breast fed. African and West Indian mothers more often had friends who had breast fed successfully than mothers in other ethnic groups, as did women in the upper socioeconomic classes. Little evidence was found that either antenatal or postnatal medical advice affected the type of feeding chosen by mothers.

Case history: Feeding patterns in London Chinese children

Tann and Wheeler[10] assessed feeding patterns and growth rates of 20 London Chinese children, aged between 1 and 24 months, over a period of 6 months. All the families had originated from the New Territories, a rural area of Hong Kong. With one exception, all the children were bottle fed, and soft canned food and rusks of the British type were introduced at between 1 and 6 months. Subsequent to this, at 6–10 months, most mothers introduced *congee*, a traditional Chinese weaning food prepared by boiling rice in large quantities of watery meat broth. Soft boiled rice was introduced at about 10 months, and then gradually the full range of Chinese foods was introduced. The mothers had chosen not to breast feed mainly because of the 'inconvenience', although in Hong Kong nearly 60% of mothers wholly or partially breast feed their children. Most of the sample believed that milk quality was affected by the quality of food eaten by the mother after delivery: in Hong Kong, Chinese mothers were usually confined at home for 30 days after delivery, during which 'nutritious' (i.e. meaty) food was served to them by female relatives. In London, they could not afford such a 'luxurious' period after confinement, as they had to get on with work or household chores. As a result, they believed they were not sufficiently well nourished to produce good milk for the babies. Meat served in hospital after delivery was not considered nourishing enough, since it should be cooked in a traditional way with special spices, herbs and wines. The authors found that, despite this, all the Chinese children in the sample were well nourished. The role of 'hot–cold' foods in the mother's diet has been mentioned earlier.

Case history: Feeding patterns in infants in Sheffield, UK

Taitz[31] studied 261 normal full-term infants born in Sheffield, at birth and at 6 weeks old. Only 21 of the babies were breast fed. It was found that the majority of the artificially fed infants were substantially overweight at 6 weeks, in relation to their expected weight at that age. For example, 40.4% of the boys and 37.3% of the girls were above the 90th percentile for their age on Tanner centile charts. Taitz ascribes this overnutrition to encouragement by doctors, welfare clinics, health visitors and grandmothers, and to 'the popular notion of the "bonny" baby with bloated cheeks and limbs, protuberant belly, and the various signs of the "Michelin Tyre Man" syndrome'. In addition, 'the apparently low resistance of present-day mothers to the crying infant and the tendency to provide instant gratification in a caloric form may also play its part'. Taitz points out the danger of overnutrition in infancy, which may result in obesity in later childhood and adulthood.

These four studies indicate the range of infant feeding practices among different communities in England and Scotland, and the effects this may have on the babies' health. However, as noted above, the effects of cultural factors on maternal diet, and therefore on the infant's health, are also relevant. For example, both fetal and neonatal rickets among

Asian babies have been reported in the UK as a result of maternal vitamin D deficiency.[24] The reasons for choosing one type, or amount, of infant feeding over another are many; some of these reasons have been described above, but they include cultural conceptions of what a healthy, 'bonny' baby should look like, the types of lifestyle the mother should follow after delivery, and whether public breast feeding is socially acceptable or not. It should also be remembered that in some parts of the world lactation is seen as an effective contraceptive, and this may influence the choice of type of infant feeding. In some of these societies, this is backed up by taboos which prohibit sexual intercourse until the infant is weaned. Where breast feeding is optional and other forms of contraceptive are available, cultural beliefs and fashions, as well as economic factors, will determine whether most mothers choose this form of infant feeding or not.

Dietary changes and diseases of Western civilization

Burkitt[32] has examined many of the diseases which have become common in the Western world, particularly in Europe and the USA, in the past century. These same diseases are rare or unknown in traditional, non-Western societies, but they increase in frequency under the influence of culture change – that is, where Western customs and lifestyles are adopted. These 'new' diseases include appendicitis, diverticular disease, benign colonic tumours, cancer of the large bowel, ulcerative colitis, varicose veins, deep vein thrombosis, pulmonary embolism, haemorrhoids, coronary heart disease, gallstones, hiatus hernia, obesity and diabetes.

Burkitt sees obesity as 'the commonest form of malnutrition in the West', and it is also associated with some of the other 'Western diseases'. He estimates that over 40% of people in the UK are overweight, and the problem is just as serious in the USA. He relates the dramatic increase in frequency of the various diseases to dietary changes in the past century. During the years 1860–1960, fat consumption increased by less than 50%, while sugar consumption doubled. Over the past 100 years the quantity of fibre consumed in the diet has markedly dropped. In 1860 the fibre content of white flour was 0.2–0.5% and the amount of fibre supplied daily in bread was between 1.1 and 2.8 g. With bread consumption halved, and the fibre content of white flour reduced to 0.1–0.01%, the daily fibre intake in bread is about 10% of the pre–1860 level. In addition, porridge oats, which have a high fibre content, have gone out of fashion, and have been replaced by low-fibre packaged cereals. In non-Western societies that become 'Westernized', traditional diets are usually changed by the addition of sugar, substituting white bread for high-fibre cereals, and often an increase in meat consumption. Burkitt points out that in none of the Western diseases is fibre deficiency a *sole* causative factor, but that it might be one important aetiological factor.

Burkitt's study indicates how changes in technology and dietary culture may be related to the increased incidence of certain diseases. Food fads and the high prestige given in some cultures to white bread and rice all contribute to this effect.

Diet and cancer

The study of a culture's dietary patterns and preferences are not only important in the search for malnutrition, or for any of the Western diseases listed by Burkitt. A number of studies suggest that, in some cases, diet and nutrition may be linked to certain forms of cancer. Lowenfels and Anderson,[33] in reviewing the evidence for this hypothesis, found that differences in food intake patterns can be positively correlated with differences in the incidence of various cancers in world populations. This is especially the case in colonic and gastric cancer. In addition to the food consumed, such variables as total caloric intake, nutritional excess or deficit, exposure to carcinogens, and consumption of alcohol also increase the risk of cancer. Many of these dietary factors, as noted earlier, may be affected by cultural beliefs and practices. In another review of the subject, Newberne[34] also cites the evidence linking dietary patterns to a number of cancers, including cancers of the stomach, colon, oesophagus and breast (which has been linked to an increased intake of fat in the diet). He points out that, in the USA, food habits have gradually changed in the past 40 years, a period in which cancer has increased in some populations. A further study, by Kolonel et *al.*,[35] examined the incidence rate of stomach cancer in four populations: Japanese in Japan, Japanese in Hawaii, Caucasians in Hawaii, and all American whites. The highest rates were in the Japan Japanese, followed by the Hawaii Japanese, with the white groups at a much lower level. There was a positive association of high rates of stomach cancer with consumption, early in life, of the traditional Japanese foods: rice, pickled vegetables, and dried or salted fish. It was postulated that stomach cancer might be caused by endogenous nitrosamines formed from dietary precursors – the nitrates, nitrites and secondary amines that are at high levels in the Japanese diet.

As the examples in this chapter indicate, a large number of diseases can be linked to dietary beliefs and practices, although these cultural factors are mainly relevant where enough food is available for nutrition in the first place. Attempts to modify or improve diets should therefore take into account the important cultural roles that food plays in all societies and cultural groups.

Recommended reading

Farb, P. and Armelagos, G. (1980) *Consuming Passions: The Anthropology of Eating.* Boston: Houghton Mifflin. An excellent guide to nutritional anthropology.

Keesing, R.M. (1981) *Cultural Anthropology.* New York: Holt, Rinehart and Winston. See pages 459–466 for a discussion of the political economy of food production.

Lennon, D. and Fieldhouse, P. (1979) *Community Dietetics.* London: Forbes. See Chapter 9 on the nutritional problems of immigrants to the UK.

Snow, L. F. and Johnson, S. M. (1978) Folklore, food, female reproductive cycle. *Ecol. Food Nutr.* 7, 41–49

Chapter 4

Caring and curing: the sectors of health care

In most societies people suffering from physical discomfort or emotional distress have a number of ways of helping themselves or of seeking help from other people. They may, for example, decide to rest or to take a home remedy; or ask advice from a friend, relative or neighbour; or consult a local priest, folk healer or 'wise person'; or consult a doctor, provided that one is available. They may follow all of these steps, or perhaps only one or two of them, and may follow them in any order. The larger and more complex the society in which the person is living, the more of these therapeutic options are likely to be available, provided the individual can afford to pay for them. Modern urbanized societies, whether Western or non-Western, are more likely, therefore, to exhibit *medical pluralism.* Within these societies there are many groups or individuals, each offering the patient their own particular way of explaining, diagnosing and treating ill-health. Although these therapeutic modes coexist, they are often based on entirely different premises, and may even originate in other cultures, such as Western medicine in China, or Chinese acupuncture in the modern Western world. To the ill person, however, the origin of these treatments is less important than their efficacy in relieving suffering.

Social and cultural aspects of medical pluralism

Anthropologists have pointed out that any society's medical system cannot be studied in isolation from other aspects of that society, especially its social, religious, political and economic organization. It is interwoven with these, and is based on the same assumptions, values and view of the world. Landy[1] points out that a medical system has two interrelated aspects: a *cultural* aspect, which includes certain basic concepts, theories, normative practices and shared modes of perception; and a *social*

54

aspect, including its organization into certain specified roles (such as 'patient' and 'doctor') and rules governing relationships between these roles in specialized settings (such as a hospital or a doctor's office). In most societies, one form of health care, such as scientific medicine in the West, is elevated above the other forms, and both its cultural and social aspects are upheld by law. Besides this 'official' medical system – which includes the medical and nursing professions – there are usually smaller, alternative systems, such as homeopathy, herbalism and spiritual healing in the UK, which might be termed *medical subcultures*. Each has its own way of explaining and treating ill-health, and the healers in each group are organized into professional associations, with rules of entry, codes of conduct and ways of relating to patients. Medical subcultures may be indigenous to the society, or they may be imported from elsewhere; in many cases, immigrants to a society often bring their folk healers along with them to deal with their ill-health in a culturally familiar way. In the UK, examples of this are the Muslim *hakims* or Hindu *vaids* sometimes consulted by immigrants from the Indian subcontinent. In looking at medical pluralism, wherever it occurs, it is important to examine both the cultural and the social aspects of the types of health care available to the individual patient.

In this chapter I will examine the pluralistic health care systems of complex societies to illustrate:

1. The *range* of therapeutic options available in these societies.
2. How and why *choices* are made between the various options.

I will also discuss medical pluralism in the UK, and the implications of this for the delivery of health care.

The three sectors of health care

Kleinman[2] has suggested that, in looking at any complex society, one can identify three overlapping sectors of health care: the *popular* sector, the *folk* sector, and the *professional* sector. Each sector has its own ways of explaining and treating ill-health, defining who is the healer and who is the patient, and specifying how healer and patient should interact in their therapeutic encounter.

The popular sector

This is the lay, non-professional, non-specialist domain of society, where ill-health is first recognized and defined, and health care activities are initiated. It includes all the therapeutic options that people utilize without any payment and without consulting either folk healers or medical practitioners. Among these options are: self-treatment or self-medication; advice or treatment given by a relative, friend, neighbour or workmate; healing and mutual care activities in a church, cult or self-help group; or consultation with another lay person who has special experience of a particular disorder, or of treatment of a physical state. In this sector, the main arena of health care is the family; here most ill-health is recognized and then treated. It is the real site of primary health care in any society. In the family, as Chrisman[3] points out, the main providers of health care are women, usually mothers or grandmothers, who diagnose most common illnesses and treat them with the materials at hand. It has been estimated[4] that about 70–90% of health care takes place within this sector, in both Western and non-Western societies.

People who become 'ill' typically follow a 'hierarchy of resort', ranging from self-medication to consultation with others. Self-treatment is based on lay beliefs about the structure and function of the body, and the origin and nature of ill-health. It includes a variety of substances and treatment, such as patent medicines, traditional folk remedies or 'old wives' tales, as well as changes in diet or behaviour. Food can be used as a form of 'medicine' (see Chapter 3), for example, in folk illnesses such as 'high blood' in the southern USA, where certain foods are used to reduce the excess volume of blood which is believed to cause the condition, or in Latin America, where certain foods are used to counteract 'hot' or 'cold' illnesses and to restore the body to equilibrium. In both the UK and the USA, self-prescribed vitamins are commonly used to restore health when one is 'feeling low'. The changes in behaviour that accompany ill-health range from special prayers, rituals, confession or fasting to resting in a warm bed for a chill or a cold.

The popular sector usually includes a set of beliefs about *health maintenance*. These are usually a series of guidelines, specific to each cultural group, about the 'correct' behaviour for preventing ill-health in oneself and in others. They include beliefs about the 'healthy' way to eat, drink, sleep, dress, work, pray and generally conduct one's life. In some societies, health is also maintained by the use of charms, amulets and religious medallions to ward off 'bad luck', including unexpected illness, and to attract 'good luck' and good health.

Most health care in this sector takes place between people

already linked to one another by ties of kinship, friendship, co-residence or membership of work or religious organizations. This means that both patient and healer share similar assumptions about health and illness, and misunderstandings between the two are comparatively rare.[3] The sector is made up of a series of *informal* and unpaid healing relationships, of variable duration, which occur within the sufferer's own social network, particularly the family. These therapeutic encounters occur without fixed rules governing behaviour or setting; at a later date the roles may be reversed, with today's patient becoming tomorrow's healer. There are certain individuals, though, who tend to act as a source of health advice more often than others. These include:

1. Those with long experience of a particular illness, or type of treatment.
2. Those with extensive experience of certain life events, such as women who have raised several children.
3. Paramedical professionals (such as nurses, pharmacists, physiotherapists or doctors' receptionists) who are consulted informally about health problems.
4. Doctors' wives or husbands, who share some of their spouses' experience, if not training.
5. Individuals such as hairdressers, salespeople or even bank managers, who interact frequently with the public and sometimes act as lay confessors or psychotherapists.
6. Organizers of self-help groups.
7. Members or officiants of certain healing cults or churches.

All of these people may be considered resources of advice and assistance on health matters by their friends or families. Their credentials are mainly their own experience rather than education, social status or special occult powers. A woman who has had several pregnancies, for example, can give informal advice to a newly pregnant younger woman, telling her what symptoms to expect and how to deal with them. Similarly, a person with long experience of a particular medication may 'lend' some to a friend with similar symptoms.

Individuals' experiences of ill-health are sometimes shared within a self-help group, which may act as a repository of knowledge about a particular ailment or experience, to be used both for the benefit of other members, and for the rest of society. Self-help groups can bring many other benefits to members, such as sharing advice on lifestyle or coping strategies, or acting as a refuge for isolated individuals – especially those suffering from stigmatized conditions, such as obesity, alcoholism or homosexuality.

Experiences of ill-health and suffering may also be shared within a healing cult or church. For example, McGuire[5] has described some of the healing groups that are now found in middle-class, suburban America. These include movements such as Christian Science and the Unity School of Christianity, various other Christian groups (such as charismatic Catholic and Protestant pentacostal groups), human potential groups (such as Scientology, EST, Progoff Process and Cornucopia), Eastern meditation and yoga groups (based on Zen or Tibetan Buddhism, Jainism or Hinduism), and the many types of spiritualist church and 'healing circle' that practise occult or psychic healing for their members. In non-Western societies, too, self-help groups often have a religious basis. 'Spirit possession' cults, for example, are common in parts of Africa, especially among women. In these cults, women who have been 'possessed' and made ill by a particular spirit form what Turner[6] calls 'a community of suffering', the members of which ritually diagnose and treat those in the rest of society suffering from possession by the same malign spirit. Lewis[7] sees some of these spirit possession cults, like the Hausa *bori* cult in Northern Nigeria, as essentially women's protest movements against their social disadvantages. Membership of the cult brings prestige, healing power and special attention from their menfolk, who lavish gifts on them to appease the possessing spirits.

All aspects of the popular sector (and of the other two sectors) may sometimes have negative effects on people's mental and physical health. The family, for example, may either facilitate or impede health care. In Taiwan, according to Kleinman,[8] the family's usual response to a sick member is to attempt to contain him, his sickness, and the social problems that it generates, within the circle of the family, instead of sharing it with an outsider, such as a medical practitioner.

In general, ill people move freely between the popular and the other two sectors, and back again, especially when treatment in that sector fails to relieve physical discomfort or emotional distress.

The folk sector

In this sector, which is especially large in non-Western societies, certain individuals specialize in forms of healing which are either *sacred* or *secular*, or a mixture of the two. These healers are not part of the 'official' medical system, and occupy an intermediate position between the popular and professional sectors. There is a wide variation in the types of folk healer found in any society, from purely secular and technical experts like bone-setters, midwives, tooth extractors or herbalists, to spiritual healers, clairvoyants and shamans. Folk healers form a heterogeneous group, with much individual variation in style and outlook, but sometimes they are organized into associations of healers, with rules of entry, codes of conduct, and the sharing of information.

Most communities include a mixture of sacred and secular folk healers. For example, in her study of black folk healers in urban America, Snow[9] has described: 'herb doctors', 'root doctors', spiritualists, 'conjure' men or women, Voodoo *houngans* or *mambos*, healing ministers and faith healers, neighbourhood 'prophets', 'granny women' and vendors of magical herbs, roots and patent medicines. Spiritual healers, who operate out of temples, churches or 'candle shops', are particularly common, and deal with illnesses believed to be due to sorcery (hexing) or to divine punishment. More secular illnesses are dealt with by self-medication or by neighbourhood granny women or herb doctors. In practice, though, there is some overlap between their approaches and techniques. In another community, the Zulu of Southern Africa, there is also an overlap between sacred and secular healers. While sacred divination is carried out by female *isangomas*, treatment by African herbal medicines is by male *inyangas*; both, though, will gather information about the social background of the victim, as well as details of the illness, before making a diagnosis.[10]

An example of a purely secular healer is the *sahi*, or health worker, as described by Underwood and Underwood[11] in Raymah, Yemen Arab Republic. These healers have only appeared in Yemen in recent years, and their practice consists mainly of giving injections of various Western drugs. They have little training (usually a brief association with a health professional, in one case a month's work as a hospital cleaner), limited diagnostic skills, and they utilize little counselling or psychological skills. To the inhabitants of Raymah, however, the *sahi* practices what is considered to be the quintessence of Western medicine – the treatment of illness by injections. Other examples of this trend in the Third World have been described by Kimani[12] in Kenya. There untrained 'bush doctors' adminis-ter medicines and injections, and 'street and bus-depot doctor boys' hustle antibiotic capsules, acquired through the black market.

Most folk healers share the basic cultural values, and world view, of the communities in which they live, including beliefs about the origin, significance and treatment of ill-health. In societies where ill-health and other forms of misfortune are blamed on social causes (witchcraft, sorcery or Evil Eye) or on supernatural causes (gods, spirits or ancestral ghosts), sacred folk healers are particularly common. Their approach is usually a holistic one, dealing with *all* aspects of the patient's life, including relationships with other people, with the natural environment, and with supernatural forces, as well as any physical or emotional symptoms. In many non-Western societies, all these aspects of life are part of the definition of 'health', which is seen as a *balance* between man and his social, natural and supernatural environments. A disturbance of any of these (such as immoral behaviour, conflicts within the family, or failure to observe religious practices) may result in physical symptoms or emotional distress and require the services of a sacred folk healer. Healers of this type, when faced with ill-health, often enquire about the patient's behaviour before the illness, and about any conflicts with other people. In a small-scale society, the healer may also have first-hand knowledge of a family's difficulties through local gossip, and this may be useful in reaching a diagnosis. As well as gathering information about the patient's recent history and social background, the healer may employ a ritual of *divination*. There are many forms of this world-wide, including the use of cards, bones and special stones (the random arrangement of which is interpreted by the healer), the examination of the entrails of certain animals or birds, and direct consultation with spirits or supernatural beings by going into a trance. In each case, the divination aims to uncover the supernatural cause of the illness (such as witchcraft or divine retribution) by the use of supernatural techniques.

Trance divination is common in non-industrialized societies (but is also found in the West among 'mediums' and 'channellers'). The Zulu *isangoma*, for example, is consulted by the relatives of a sick person, who remains at home. Her diagnosis is made by going into a trance and 'communicating with spirits' who tell her the cause and treatment of the illness.[10] Another form of this is the *shaman*, who is found in many cultures. In Lewis's definition,[12] a shaman is 'a person of either sex who has mastered spirits and can at will introduce them into his own body'. Divination takes place in a seance, in which the healer allows the spirits to enter him, and through him diagnose the illness and prescribe treatment. In some cases, he may only enter his trance with the aid of powerful hallucinogenic drugs (see Chapter 8). This, and other forms of divination, sometimes take place in the presence of the patient's family, friends and other social contacts. In this public setting, the diviner aims to bring conflicts within a community – which may have led to witchcraft or sorcery between people – to the surface, and to resolve these conflicts in a ritual way. Sacred healers also provide explanations and treatment for subjective feelings of guilt, shame or anger, by prescribing, for example, prayer, repentance or the resolution of interpersonal problems. They may also prescribe physical treatments or remedies at the same time.

For those who utilize it, folk healing offers several advantages over modern scientific medicine. One of these is the frequent involvement of the family in diagnosis and treatment. For example, as Martin[14] has pointed out, in Native American healing the patient's sickness places a responsibility on both patient *and* family to participate in healing rites. The focus of attention is not only the patient (as in Western medicine), but also the reaction of the family and others to the illness. The healer is usually surrounded by 'helpers', who take part in the ceremony, give explanations to the patient and the patient's family, and answer any of their queries. From a modern perspective, this type of Native American healer with his or her helpers, together with the patient's family, provides an effective primary health care team, especially in dealing with psycho-social problems. Fabrega and Silver[15] have examined the advantages to the patient of another type of folk healer, the *h'ilol* in Zinacantan, Mexico, over Western doctors. In particular, there is a shared world view, closeness, warmth, informality and the use of everyday language in consultations; the family and other community members are involved in treatment; the *h'ilol* is a crucial figure in the community, and is believed to act for the benefit of the patient and the community, as well as the gods; he can influence society at large, particularly the patient's social relationships; he can influence the patient's future behaviour, by pointing out the influence of past actions on his present illness; and his healing takes place in a familiar setting, such as the home or a religious shrine. Because folk healers such as the *h'ilol* articulate and reinforce the cultural values of the communities in which they live, they have advantages over Western doctors, who are often separated from their patients by social class, economic position, gender, specialized education, and sometimes cultural background. In particular, these healers are better able to define and treat 'illness' – that is, the social, psychological and moral dimensions associated with ill-health, as with other forms of misfortune (see Chapter 5). They also provide culturally familiar ways of explaining the *causes* and timing of ill-health and its relation to the social and supernatural worlds.

In general, folk healers have little formal training equivalent to the Western medical school. Skills are usually acquired by apprenticeship to an older healer, experience of certain techniques or conditions, or by the possession of inborn or acquired 'healing power'. People can become folk healers in a number of ways, such as:

1. Inheritance – being born into a 'healing family'.
2. Position within a family, like the 'seventh son of a seventh son' in Ireland.
3. Signs and portents at birth, like a birthmark or 'crying in the womb', or being born with the amniotic membrane across the face (the 'caul' in Scotland).
4. Revelation – discovering one 'has the gift', which may occur as an intense emotional experience during an illness, dream or trance. In extreme cases, as Lewis[13] points out, the vocation may be announced by 'an initially uncontrolled state of possession: a traumatic experience associated with hysteroid, ecstatic behaviour'.
5. Apprenticeship to another healer – a common pattern in all parts of the world, although the apprenticeship may last for many years.
6. Acquiring a particular skill on one's own, like the Yemeni *sahi* or the Kenyan 'bush doctors'.

In practice, these pathways into folk healing tend to overlap: for example, someone born of a healing family and with certain signs and portents at birth may still need to refine their 'gift' by a lengthy apprenticeship to an older healer.

While most folk healers work individually, informal networks or associations of healers do exist, and these provide for the exchange of techniques and information, and monitoring of each other's behaviour. Such a network among Zulu diviners or *isangomas* is described by Ngubane;[10] meetings take place regularly between diviners to share ideas, experiences and techniques. Each diviner has the opportunity to meet the ex-students, teacher and neophyte of each of her neighbouring diviners, as well as more distant ones. It is estimated that, over a period of 3–5 years, a diviner might make contact with over 400 fellow diviners, all over Southern Africa. In other settings, such as some low-income black neighbourhoods in the USA, several healers might be ministers of a spiritualist church, which also acts as an association of healers. In the suburban healing circles described by McGuire,[5] almost all the participants have the chance to be both healer and patient at various times; therefore these groups overlap the boundary between folk and popular healing, and also provide a venue for the exchange of information and experiences among a group of healers.

The relationships between folk and professional healers tend to be marked by mutual distrust and suspicion. In the Western world, modern medicine views most folk healers as quacks, charlatans or 'medicine men', who pose a danger to their patients' health. While folk healing does have obvious shortcomings and dangers, it does have advantages to the patient, especially in dealing with psychosocial problems. Other advantages of traditional folk medicine for the under-doctored Third World have been recognized by the World Health Organisation.[16] In 1978 they recommended that traditional healing be integrated, where possible, with modern medicine and stressed the necessity 'to ensure respect, recognition and collaboration among the practitioners of the various systems concerned'. The manpower resources that WHO hope to enlist in the folk sector include: traditional birth attendants (TBAs); Ayurvedic, Unāni or Yoga practitioners; Chinese traditional healers, such as acupuncturists; and various others.

The professional sector

This comprises the organized, legally sanctioned healing professions, such as modern Western scientific medicine, or *allopathy*. It includes not only physicians of various types and specialities, but also the recognized *para*-medical professions such as nurses, midwives or physiotherapists. In most countries, scientific medicine is the basis of the professional sector but, as Kleinman notes, traditional medical systems may also become 'professionalized' to some extent; examples of this are the 91 Ayurvedic and ten Unāni medical colleges in India, which receive governmental support. It is important to realize that Western scientific medicine provides only a small proportion of health care in most countries of the world. Medical manpower is often a scarce resource, with most health care taking place in the popular and folk sectors. The World Health

Table 4.1 Relation of physicians and hospital beds to population in selected countries

Country	Population per physician	Hospital beds per 10 000 population
Ethiopia	73 043	3.0
Malawi	47 638	17.4
Bangladesh	12 378	2.3
India	3 652	7.8
Jamaica	3 505	38.9
Mexico	1 251	11.6
Japan	845	106.0
England and Wales	659	86.3*
France	613	63.0
USA	595	63.0
USSR	289	121.3

* Average of figures for England and Wales.
(Source: WHO[17].)

Organisation statistics in 1980[17] illustrate the huge variations in the availability of doctors and hospital beds throughout the world (Table 4.1).

These figures probably overestimate the numbers of doctors involved in direct patient care, as many are involved in research or administration. In addition, the distribution of doctors is not uniform; in many non-industrialized societies they tend to cluster in cities, where facilities are better and practice more lucrative, leaving many in the countryside to rely on the popular and folk sectors of care.

In most countries the practitioners of scientific medicine form the only group of healers whose positions are upheld by law. They enjoy higher social status, greater income, and more clearly defined rights and obligations than other types of healers. They have the power to question or examine their patients, prescribe powerful and sometimes dangerous treatments or medication, and deprive certain people of their freedom – and confine them to hospitals – if they are diagnosed as psychotic or infectious. In hospital, they can tightly control their patients' diet, behaviour, sleeping patterns and medication, and can initiate a variety of tests, such as biopsies, radiographs or venesection. They can also label their patients (sometimes permanently) as ill, incurable, malingering, hypochondriacal, or fully recovered – a label which may conflict with the patient's perspective. These labels can have important effects, both social (confirming the patient in the sick role) and economic (influencing health insurance or pension payments).

The medical system

As mentioned earlier, the dominant system of health care of any society cannot be studied in isolation from other aspects of that society, because the *medical system* – or professional sector of health care – does not exist in a social or cultural vacuum. Rather, it is an expression of – and to some extent a miniature model of – the values and social structure of the society from which it arises. Different types of society therefore, depending on their dominant ideology – whether this is capitalist, welfare state, socialist or communist – produce different types of medical system, and different attitudes to health and illness. One society may see free (or relatively inexpensive) health care as a basic right of citizenship, or the basic right only of the very poor or the very old, while another may see medical care as a commodity to be bought only by those who can afford it. In the latter case, the pursuit of profits in health care will exclude many of the poorer members of society who do not have the resources to pay for it. Whatever the type of society, the medical system not only reflects these basic values and ideologies, but in turn helps also to shape and maintain them.[18]

As an example of this, critics of the medical systems in the USA and the UK have pointed out how the internal organization of the professional sector reflects some of the basic inequalities in those societies, especially in relation to gender, social class and ethnic background. Within the medical system most doctors are men (and usually white) and, as in the wider society, occupy many more of the prestigious, powerful and well paid jobs than do women doctors and nurses.[19] Also, the personnel within this sector are arranged in hierarchies similar to the social strata of the wider society. In its dealings with the population, the medical system may reproduce many of the underlying prejudices of society, as well as cultural assumptions as to what constitutes 'good' and 'bad' behaviour. For example, Littlewood and Lipsedge[20] suggest that racial prejudice plays an important role in how some Afro-Caribbean patients in the UK are classified by psychiatrists as 'mad', even when there is evidence to the contrary (see Chapter 10), and Wing[21] suggests that a similar process operates in the USSR, in state psychiatry's attitude to political dissent.

Other critiques of the Western medical system include those by Illich,[22] who has claimed that high-technology modern medicine has become increasingly dangerous to the population's health by reducing their autonomy, making them dependent on the medical profession, and damaging their health by the side-effects of drugs and surgical interventions. In addition, the medical system is in a symbiotic relationship with the manufacturers of pharmaceuticals and medical equipment, and this relationship is not necessarily in the patient's interest.

Like Illich, other critics of the medical system have maintained that modern medicine, as well as controlling micro-organisms, also seeks to control the behaviour of the population, especially by 'medicalizing' deviant behaviour, as well as many of the normal stages of the human life-cycle. Stacey[23] and others have suggested that this phenomenon is particularly evident in the case of women, especially during pregnancy and childbirth (see Chapter 6). Furthermore, much of the ill-health in Western society which may be caused by other factors – such as poverty, unemployment, economic crises, pollution or persecution – is often ignored by the medical system because its main focus is increasingly on the *individual* patient and the 'risk factors' in his or her own lifestyle.[24]

Thus, in understanding any medical system, one must always see it in the context of the basic values, ideology, political organization and economic system of the society from which it arises. In that sense, the professional sector of health care – like the other two sectors – is always to some extent 'culture-bound'.

Comparison of medical systems
One can illustrate this culture-bound aspect in the case of Western medicine by comparing the medical systems of different Western countries with similar levels of economic development. Obviously these countries vary in whether health care lies mainly in the private or the public sectors, in the distribution of medical resources, in their arrangements for health insurance, and so on, but their professional sectors are all rooted in the same tradition of Western scientific medicine, and there is considerable exchange of medical data and techniques between them.

Various studies have illustrated significant differences in the types of diagnosis given, and the treatment prescribed, between different Western medical systems. For example, in 1984 a comparison of the patterns of prescribing in five different European countries (the UK, Germany, Italy, France and

Spain)[25] found marked variations between them which could *not* be explained solely by disparities in the health of their populations. The study examined the 20 leading diagnostic categories and 20 leading types of drug prescribed in each of these countries. In the UK, for example, the major group of drugs prescribed was the tranquillizers, hypnotics and sedatives (8.6% of the total number of prescriptions), compared with 6.8% in France, 6.0% in Germany, 3.1% in Italy and 2.0% in Spain. In the UK, 'neuroses' were among the commonest of diagnoses (5.1% of the total number of diagnoses given), compared with 4.1% in France, 3.2% in Italy, and 1.7% in Spain. These differences may represent not only differences in morbidity between the five countries, but also major differences in nomenclature, in the criteria of diagnosis, and in *cultural* attitudes towards certain types of behaviour and how they should be dealt with. Other studies, some of which are described later in this book, have shown differences between UK and US psychiatrists in the criteria they use to diagnose schizophrenia and affective disorders (see Chapter 10); differences between UK, Canadian and US rates of various surgical operations, including Caesarian sections (see Chapter 12); and differences in the medical use of spas and hydrotherapy (*la thermalisme*) in France and in Germany (the *kur*)[26] but not in countries like the UK or the USA.

A closer look at these national differences in the perception, diagnosis, naming and treatment of disease may suggest some of the cultural values that underly those differences. For example, Payer[27] has examined the medical systems of the USA, France, Germany and the UK. She has described some of the diagnostic categories that have no clear equivalents in other countries, such as the *crise de foie* and *spasmophilia* in France, *Herzinsuffizienz* and *Kreislaufkollaps* in Germany, or *chillblains* or 'bowel problems' in the UK. Furthermore, in understanding these variations, she has related certain medical beliefs and practices to core cultural values in each of those societies. In the USA, for example, she sees a relation between the high rate of coronary bypass operations and other types of surgery, and the American view of the body as a repairable 'machine' – and one that needs to be 'repaired' and 'overhauled' at regular intervals. She describes the dominant attitude of US doctors to sickness as an 'aggressive' and 'can-do' approach, part of the legacy of the frontier spirit: 'Americans not only want to *do* something, they want to do it *fast*, and if they cannot they often become frustrated'. As a result, US doctors do more diagnostic tests on their patients, and perform surgery more often, than do doctors from the other three countries. According to Payer, they often eschew drug treatment in favour of more aggressive surgery, and if they do use drugs tend to use higher doses than their European colleagues. In psychiatry, for example, the doses of some drugs used in the USA are up to ten times higher than those used elsewhere. The reasons for these approaches to medical care are various, including the types of payment US doctors receive for their services, and the threat of malpractice suits against them. However, like doctors from the three European countries, it is the underlying *cultural* values of their society that play a part in determining how ill-health is both diagnosed and then treated.

The medical profession

Within the medical system, those who practice medicine form a group apart, with their own values, concepts, theories of disease and rules of behaviour, as well as organization into a hierarchy of healing roles. This group therefore has both cultural and social aspects. They can be regarded – like lawyers, architects and engineers – as *professionals*. Foster and Anderson[28] define a profession as being 'based on, or organized around, a body of specialized knowledge (the content) not easily acquired and that, in the hands of qualified practitioners, meets the needs of, or serves, *clients'*. It also has a *collegial organization* of conceptual equals, which exists to maintain *control* over their field of expertise, promote their common interests, maintain their monopoly of knowledge, set qualifications for admission (such as the licensing of new physicians), protect themselves from incursions or competition by outsiders, and monitor the competence and ethics of their members. Although conceptually equal, the profession is arranged in hierarchies of knowledge and power, such as professors, consultants, registrars and house officers. Below them are the paramedical professionals: nurses, midwives, physiotherapists, occupational therapists and medical social workers. Each paramedical group has its own body of knowledge, clients, collegial organization and control over an area of competence, but overall has less autonomy and power than the physicians. The doctors themselves are divided into specialized subprofessions, which duplicate on a smaller scale the structure of the medical profession as a whole. Examples of this are surgeons, paediatricians, gynaecologists and psychiatrists. Each have their own unique perspective on ill-health, their own area of knowledge, and their own hierarchy from experts down to novices.

Pfifferling[29] has examined some of the assumptions and premises underlying the medical profession in the USA. In his view, it is:

1. Physician centred – the doctor, and not the patient, defines the nature and boundary of the patient's problem; diagnostic and intellectual skills are valued above communication skills; settings for health care, such as doctors' offices, are often located for the benefit of doctors, far from their patients' homes.
2. Specialist orientated – specialists, rather than generalists, receive the highest prestige and rewards.
3. Credentials orientated – those with higher credentials can rise in the medical hierarchy and are considered to possess greater clinical skills and knowledge.
4. Memory based – feats of memory (of medical facts, cases, drugs, discoveries, etc.) are rewarded by promotion and the respect of one's peers.
5. Single-case centred – decisions are made on a single case of a disease, based on cumulative descriptions of previous clinical cases.
6. Process orientated – evaluations of doctors' clinical skill are made by measuring their impact on quantifiable biological processes in the patient, over time (such as a fall in blood pressure).

One could add to this list the increasing emphasis on diagnostic technology, rather than clinical evaluations, and the growing influence of the corporate takeover of many hospitals throughout the country, and its implications for health care. Many of these points are now beginning to apply equally to physicians in other Western countries, such as the UK.

In most countries, the main institutional structure of scientific medicine is the *hospital*. Unlike in the popular and folk sectors, the ill person is removed from family, friends and community at a time of personal crisis. In hospital they undergo a standardized ritual of 'depersonalization' (see Chapter 9), becoming converted into a numbered 'case' in a ward full of strangers. The emphasis is on their physical disease, with little reference to their home environment, religion, social relationships, moral status, or the meaning they give to their ill-health. Hospital specialization ensures that they are classified, and allocated to different wards, on the basis of *age* (adults, paediatrics, geriatrics), *gender* (male, female), *condition* (medical, surgical or other), *organ or system* involved (ENT, ophthalmology, dermatology), or *severity* (intensive care units, accident and emergency departments). Patients of the same sex, similar age range and similar illnesses often share a ward. All of these have been stripped of the props of social identity and individuality, and clothed in a uniform of pyjamas, nightdress or bathrobe. There is a loss of control over one's body, and over personal space, privacy, behaviour, diet and use of time. Patients are removed from the continuous emotional support of family and community, and cared for by healers whom they may never have seen before. In hospitals, the relationship of health professionals – doctors, nurses, technicians – with their patients is largely characterized by distance, formality, brief conversations and often the use of professional jargon. Hospitals have been seen by anthropologists such as Goffman[30] as 'small societies', with their own implicit and explicit rules of behaviour. Patients in a ward form a 'temporary' community of suffering', linked together by commiseration, ward gossip, and discussion of one another's condition. However, this community does not resemble, or replace, the communities in which they live; and, unlike the members of self-help groups, their afflictions do not entitle them to heal others, at least not within the hospital setting.

In most countries the professional sector is also composed of local general practitioners or family physicians, who are often deeply rooted within a community. There is some resemblance between these doctors (and nurses) and healers in the folk sector, particularly in their familiarity with the social, familial and psychological aspects of ill-health, even though their healing is based on entirely different premises.

Therapeutic networks

People who become ill, and who are not helped by self-treatment, make choices about whom to consult in the popular, folk or professional sectors for further help. These choices are influenced by the context in which they are made, which includes the types of helper actually available, whether payment for their services has to be made, whether the patient can afford to pay for these services, and the explanatory model that the patient uses in explaining his ill-health. This model, which is described in Chapter 5, provides explanations for the aetiology, symptoms, physiological changes, natural history and treatment of the illness. On this basis, patients choose what seems to be the appropriate source of advice and treatment for the condition. Illnesses such as colds are treated by relatives; supernatural illnesses (such as 'spirit possession') by sacred folk healers and 'natural' illnesses by physicians – especially if they are very severe. If, for example, the ill-health is ascribed to divine punishment for a moral transgression then, as Snow[9] points out, 'Prayer and repentance, not penicillin, cure sin' – although both may be used simultaneously: a doctor is used for physical symptoms, a priest or faith healer for the cause.

In this way, ill people frequently utilize several different types of healer at the same time, or in sequence. This may be done on the pragmatic basis that 'two (or more) heads are better than one'. For example, Scott[31] describes the case of a black woman from South Carolina, living in Miami, Florida. Believing that she had been 'fixed' (bewitched), she treated herself with olive oil and drops of turpentine on sugar cubes. When this failed to relieve her symptoms (abdominal pain), she consulted: two 'root doctors', who gave her magical powders, and candles to burn, and prayed over her; a 'sanctified woman', who massaged her and prayed for her; and two local hospitals, for radiography and gastrointestinal tests to 'find out what is down there'. At one stage she was following the advice of all three folk healers simultaneously. As Scott points out, her contacts with doctors were not for curative purposes, but rather 'to check the effectiveness of the folk therapy' at each stage. Each of these healers may redefine the patient's problem in their own idiom, such as 'peptic ulcer' or 'witchcraft'.

Ill people are at the centres of *therapeutic networks*, which are connected to all three sectors of the health care system. Advice and treatment pass along the links in this network, beginning with advice from family, friends, neighbours, friends of friends, and then moving on to sacred or secular folk healers, or physicians. Even after advice is given, it may be discussed and evaluated by other parts of the patient's network, in the light of their own knowledge and experience. As Stimson[32] has noted, a doctor's treatment is often evaluated 'in the light of his past performance, with what other people have experienced, and compared with what the person expected the doctor to do'. In this way, ill people make choices, not only between different types of healer (popular, professional or folk), but also between diagnoses and advice that *make sense* to them and those that do not. In the latter case the result may be 'non-compliance', or a shift to another part of the therapeutic network.

Medical pluralism in the UK

In the UK, as in other complex societies, there is a wide range of therapeutic options available for the alleviation of physical discomfort or emotional distress, and popular, folk and professional sectors of health care can be identified. This section will concentrate mainly on the popular and folk sectors. The professional sector has already been examined in detail by medical sociologists, such as Stacey[33] and Levitt.[34] An overview of the three sectors of health care in the UK illustrates the full range of options available for the management of misfortune, including ill-health.

The popular sector

Two studies by Elliott-Binns,[35,36] which are quoted below, are among the few dealing with lay therapeutic networks in the UK. Other studies have concentrated on the phenomenon of self-medication. For example, in Dunnell and Cartwright's large study[37] in 1972 the use of self-prescribed medication was twice as common as the use of prescribed medicines. Self-medication was most commonly taken for temperature, headache, indigestion and sore throats. These and other symptoms were common in the sample, but while 91% of adults reported one or more 'abnormal' symptoms during the previous 2 weeks, only 16% of them had consulted a doctor for this. Self-medication was often used as an alternative to consulting the doctor, who was expected to deal with more serious conditions. The idea of using a particular self-prescribed patent medicine came from a number of sources, including: spouses (7%), parents and grandparents (18%), other relatives (5%), friends (13%) and the doctor (10%). Fifty-seven per cent of the sample thought the local pharmacist a good source of health advice for many conditions. This is confirmed in Sharpe's study[38] of a London pharmacy where, in a 10-day period, 72 requests for advice were received, especially for skin complaints, respiratory tract infections, dental problems, vomiting and diarrhoea. In another study, by Jefferys et al.,[39] in a working-class housing estate, two-thirds of people interviewed were taking some self-prescribed medication, often in addition to a prescribed drug. Laxatives and aspirins were most commonly self-prescribed. The aspirins, and other analgesics, were used for many symptoms, including 'arthritis and anaemia, bronchitis and backache, menstrual disorders and menopausal symptoms, nerves and neuritis, influenza and insomnia, colds and catarrh, and of course for headaches and rheumatism'.

Hoarding and exchanging of medication, both patent and prescribed, are common in the UK. People who have been ill sometimes act as what Hindmarch[40] terms 'over-the-fence physicians', sharing their prescribed drugs with a friend, relative or neighbour with similar symptoms. Warburton,[41] in Reading, found that 68% of young adults in his study admitted having received psychotropic drugs from friends or relatives. In his Leeds study, Hindmarch[40] also found that an average of 25.9 prescribed tablets or capsules *per person* were hoarded by people living in a selected street. Decisions whether to take prescribed drugs are also part of popular health culture, and lay evaluation of the drug as 'making sense' or not may, as Stimson[32] suggests, influence *non-compliance*. The incidence of this phenomenon has been estimated by him at 30% or more.

Few studies have been done on the efficacy of British popular health care. Blaxter and Paterson,[42] in their study of working-class mothers in Aberdeen, found that common children's illnesses, such as a discharging ear, were often ignored if they did not interfere with everyday functioning. However, in another study by Pattison et al.,[43] the findings were very different, and it was found that mothers were able to recognize their babies' illnesses and seek medical help, even with their first children.

An important component of the popular sector is the wide range of *self-help* groups, which have blossomed in the UK since World War II. Like other parts of the popular sector, members' *experience*, not education, is important, especially experience of a specific misfortune. The total number of members of these groups is not known, though they number many thousands. In 1982 the medical magazine *Pulse*[44] listed 335 groups loosely labelled 'self-help' in the UK or Ireland, and there are several other directories of groups available. These groups can be classified on the basis of why people join them; that is:

1. *Physical problems* (British Migraine Association, Laryngectomy Clubs, Back Pain Association).
2. *Emotional problems* (Depressives Associated, Phobics Society, National Schizophrenia Fellowship).

3. *Relatives* of those with physical or emotional problems (Association of Parents of Vaccine Damaged Children, Adult Children of Alcoholics).
4. *Family problems* (Family Welfare Association, Parents Anonymous, Organisation for Parents under Stress).
5. *Addiction problems* (Alcoholics Anonymous, Tranx, Accept, Action on Smoking and Health).
6. *Social problems* including:
   (a) *sexual non-conformity* (Lesbian Line, Gay Switchboards),
   (b) *one-parent families* (Gingerbread, National Council for the Single Woman and her Dependants),
   (c) *life changes* (Pre-retirement Association, National Association of Widows),
   (d) *social isolation* (Friends by Post, Solo Clubs, Meet-a-Mum Association).
7. *Women's groups* (Women's Health Concern, Rape Crisis Centres, Mothers' Union).
8. *Ethnic minority groups* (Caribbean House Group, Cypriot Advisory Service, Asian Women Community Workers Group).

In practice, though, many of these categories tend to overlap.

Most self-help groups have, as Levy[45] notes, one or more of the following activities:

1. Information and referral.
2. Counselling and advice.
3. Public and professional education.
4. Political and social activity.
5. Fund-raising for research or services.
6. Providing therapeutic services under professional guidance.
7. Mutual supportive activities in small groups.

Many groups are 'communities of suffering', where experience of a type of misfortune is the credential for membership. For example, Depressives Associated describe themselves as 'a self-help organization run for the depressed by those who have been depressed and know better than most what it's like to have one's mind temporarily out of order'.[46] In Levy's[45] study of 71 groups, 41 had membership reserved for people suffering a particular affliction, while in eight membership was mainly composed of relatives of those afflicted. Some groups overlap with the professional sector, like the Psoriasis society; its 4000 members include sufferers and their relatives, doctors, nurses and cosmetic and pharmaceutical companies.[46] Others are hostile to orthodox medicine and have an anti-bureaucratic and anti-professional stance.

Robinson and Henry[47] give a number of reasons for the growth of these groups in the popular sector, including: the perceived failure of the existing medical and social services to meet people's needs; the recognition by members of the value of mutual help; and the role of the media in publicizing the extent of shared problems in the community. Other reasons might be: the nostalgia for 'community' – especially the caring community of the extended family – in an impersonal, industrialized world; as a coping mechanism for those with stigmatized conditions, or marginal social status; and as a way of explaining and dealing with misfortune in a more personalized way.

The folk sector

In the UK, as in other Western societies, this sector is small and ill-defined. While local faith healers, gipsy fortune tellers, clairvoyants, herbalists, and 'wise women' still exist in many rural areas, the forms of diagnosis and healing characteristic of the folk sector are more likely to be found in urban areas, especially in 'alternative' or 'complementary' medicine. In 1987, a study[48] estimated that 13% of the British population seek help from a complementary practitioner every year. As in non-Western societies, many of them aim at a holistic view of the patient, which includes psychological, social, moral and physical dimensions, as well as an emphasis on health as balance. For example, a pamphlet from the National Institute of Medical Herbalists[49] states: 'The herbal practitioner regards disease as being a disturbance of the physiological and mental/emotional equilibrium which is the state of good health and, being aware of the forces of healing within the body, directs the treatment towards restoring that balance'. And similarly, from the Community Health Foundation:[50] 'Health is more than just the absence of pain or discomfort. Good health is a dynamic relationship between the individual, friends, family and the environment within which we live and work.'

Herbalism, faith healing and midwifery probably have the deepest roots in the UK. The first description of herbal remedies dates from AD 1260, and numerous other 'herbals' have been published in the last 400 years.[51] In 1636, for example, a herbal compiled by John Parkinson contained details of the medicinal use of 3800 plants. Midwifery, another traditional form of health care, has been absorbed into the professional sector, especially since compulsory registration was required under the 1902 Midwives' Act. Other forms of healing have been imported from abroad, such as acupuncture, homeopathy and osteopathy.

The folk sector includes both sacred and secular healers. An example of the former are the National Federation of Spiritual Healers (NFSH), who define spiritual healing as 'all forms of healing of the sick in body, mind and spirit by means of the laying-on of hands or by either prayer or meditation whether or not in the actual presence of the patient'.[52] Since 1965, under an agreement with more than 1500 National Health Service Hospitals, NFSH 'Healer Members' may attend those patients in hospital who request their services.[52] In addition, there are a number of Spiritualist Churches and healing circles in the UK that practise spiritual healing through prayer or the laying-on of hands; these include Christian Science Churches and some Caribbean Pentecostalist Churches. Christian healing is encouraged by the Christian Fellowship of Healing, the Churches Council of Health and Healing, and the Guild of St. Raphael.[53] An unknown number of 'Wicca' or 'white magic' groups or covens practise 'magical healing'; writing in Doctor magazine, de Jonge[54] has claimed that there are 7000 'covens' in the UK, with a total membership of 91 000.

As a form of alternative healing, homeopathy has a special position in the UK. The principles of homeopathy were first enunciated in Germany by Samuel Hahnemann in 1796, and the first homeopathic hospital in the UK was founded in London in 1849. There has been a long association between the British Royal Family and homeopathy; in 1937 Sir John Weir was appointed homeopathic physician to King George VI, and this link with Royalty remains. In 1948 the homeopathic hospitals were incorporated into the National Health Service. There are now NHS homeopathic hospitals in London, Liverpool, Bristol and Tunbridge Wells, and there are two in Glasgow. It was estimated that in 1971 there were about 383 available beds in homeopathic hospitals, and 51 037 attendances at homeopathic medical out-patients clinics.[55] These hospitals are staffed by doctors qualified in orthodox medicine, who undertake post-graduate training in homeopathy. Although it is based on different premises from allopathy, homeopathy in the UK enjoys greater legitimacy than other forms of alternative healing. From an anthropological perspective, it spans both folk and professional sectors of health care.

There is a two-way influence between these two sectors. Many orthodox doctors, for example, practise one or more forms of alternative healing. They are organized into collegial organizations such as the British Homeopathic Association, the British Society of Medical and Dental Hypnosis, the Chiropractic Medical Association, the Osteopathic Medical Association, the Psionic Medical Society, and the British Association for the Medical Application of Transcendental Meditation. Similarly, alternative healers have been influenced, to a variable degree, by the training, organization, techniques, credentials and self-presentation of orthodox doctors, and are increasingly forming professional organizations with an educational structure and registers of accredited members. Some are organized on a *collegial* basis, like other British professions: for example, the British Acupuncture Association, the National Institute of Medical Herbalists, the Society of Homeopaths, and the General Council and Register of Osteopaths. In 1979, the British Acupuncture Association offered a 2-year training for a Licentiate, and a further year's study for a Bachelor's degree in acupuncture. It had 100 students in the UK, with 33 medically qualified and 420 non-medically qualified members on its register (Secretary, British Acupuncture Association and Register Ltd, 1979, personal communication).

At the other end of the spectrum are the more individual forms of folk healing, including clairvoyants, astrologers, psychic healers, clairaudients, palmists, Celtic mediums, Tarot readers, Gipsy fortune tellers and Irish seers, whose advertisements appear in the popular press, magazines, handouts, and such publications as *Old Moore's Almanack*. Many of these act as lay counsellors or psychotherapists: 'Do you have a health worry that you cannot get help on? Have you a personal or family worry you need advice on? Then maybe I can help you with both. I was born the Seventh Son of a Seventh Son.'[56] Most of this group utilize some form of *divination*, using coins, dice or Tarot cards to decipher the supernatural and cosmic influences on the individual, and reveal the causes of unhappiness, ill health, or other misfortune. From the patient's perspective, this approach may have the advantage of placing responsibility for misfortune beyond the individual's control; 'fate', 'bad luck' or birth sign, not the patient's behaviour, are the causes of misfortune.

In recent years, there has been a growing criticism of conventional medicine in some quarters, a parallel increase in interest in all forms of complementary and alternative medicine, and a burgeoning of organizations connected with it. For example, the Council for Complementary Medicine was founded 'to promote and maintain the highest standards of training, qualification and treatment in complementary and alternative medicine and to facilitate the dissemination of information relating to it.'[57] The Research Council for Complementary Medicine, as well as fostering research in this area, aims to raise standards of training, and to develop 'a policy for eventual integration of such methods with existing medical services.'[58] The Institute for Complementary Medicine now has 80 professional organizations affiliated to it, and is developing a register of trained practitioners.[59] The British Holistic Medical Association, one of the oldest of these organizations, has 1159 members, both medical and lay, about two-thirds of whom are practising health professionals (such as doctors, nurses, social workers and complementary practitioners). The BHMA sees the emergence of holistic medicine as representing 'an attempt to heal medical science itself by re-integrating psychological and spiritual dimensions into healthcare'.[60]

No precise statistics exist about the total numbers of non-orthodox healers in the UK. One major study, privately commissioned by the Threshold Foundation,[61] was carried out in the early 1980s. They estimated that in 1980–81 there were 7800 full-time and part-time professional alternative practitioners in the UK, and about 20 000 men and women who practise spiritual or religious healing. There were also 2075 doctors who practised one or more alternative therapy, though with the exception of homeopathy their training was 'minimal'. The alternative healers (both medical and lay) included 758 acupuncturists, 540 chiropracters, 303 herbalists, 360 homeopaths, 630 hypnotherapists and 800 osteopaths. They also estimated that alternative practitioners spend, on average, eight times longer with their patients than do orthodox doctors. Many of these practitioners practice more than one form of therapy; in a study in 1984 of 411 practitioners, 51% also practised a second therapy, and 25% a third.[59]

In 1989, the Institute for Complementary Medicine (Institute for Complementary Medicine, 1989, personal communication) estimated that there are about 15 000 alternative practitioners in the UK, who are in professional practice. They defined a 'practitioner' as an individual who was 'in full time practice, who is a member of a professional organization with a code of ethics and practice and a disciplinary committee to enforce them, and who is covered by personal indemnity and a third party liability.' On this basis, their figures included 7000 spiritual healers, 1500 osteopaths, 1500 acupuncturists, 1000 massage practitioners, 500 hypnotherapists, 350 nutritionists, 350 chiropracters, 300 reflexologists, and 250 aromatherapists.

Overall, it has been estimated by Wadsworth *et al.*[62] that in the UK about 75% of abnormal symptoms are treated outside the professional health care sector. Doctors, therefore, see only the 'tip of the iceberg of illness'. Most of the remaining ill-health is dealt with in the popular and folk sectors of health care.

The professional sector

This includes the wide range of medical and paramedical professionals, each with their own perceptions of ill-health, forms of treatment, defined area of competence, internal hierarchy, technical jargon and professional organizations. The Office of Health Economics[63] estimated the numbers of all health professionals within the NHS in 1980 as: 23 674 general practitioners, 31 421 hospital medical staff, 301 081 hospital nursing staff, 17 375 hospital midwives, 32 990 community health nurses, and 2949 community health midwives. In 1981 the community nurses included 9244 health visitors (Department of Health and Social Security, 1982, personal communication). In addition there are a large number of chiropodists, physiotherapists, occupational therapists, pharmacists and hospital technicians. Each of these categories offers some form of defined professional care, but they may also be called upon for informal advice about illness as part of the popular sector.

In the UK there are two complementary forms of professional medical care – the National Health Service and private medical care – although there is an overlap of personnel between the two.

The National Health Service

Since 1948 the NHS has offered free and unrestricted access to health care in the UK, at both the general practitioner and hospital levels. These two forms of medical care have different genealogies, and different perspectives on ill-health. The precursors of the general practitioners (GPs) were specialized tradesmen called apothecaries. From 1617 they were licensed only to sell drugs prescribed by physicians. By 1703 they were entitled to see patients and prescribe for them. They became the GPs of the poor and middle classes. Physicians had a higher status initially than surgeons or apothecaries, and for centuries were the only 'real' doctors. Both physicians and surgeons enhanced their position during the growth of the hospital sector which began about 1700. To some extent, the split and difference in status between GP and hospital medicine persists, and is reflected in the allocation of resources. In England and Wales in 1972, for example, more than half the NHS budget was spent on the hospital sector, even though only 2.3% of patients were annually cared for as hospital in-patients.[64] The NHS remains one of the largest employers in the country, with about 1 million employees; of these, 3% are general practitioners, 4% hospital doctors, and 43% nurses and midwives.[65]

The hospital sector
Many of the organizational and cultural aspects of hospitals have already been described, especially that of specialization. In 1974, according to Levitt[66] there were 42 recognized clinical specialties within the NHS hospital service. There are also numerous specialty hospitals, such as eye, ENT (ear, nose and throat), heart or maternity hospitals. The hospital is the place where 99% of people in the UK are born,[65] and most will die. Between those two points, many people associate it with more severe forms of ill-health, which cannot be dealt with by GPs or by the popular or folk sectors. As in other Western societies, the emphasis is on the individual patient, as a 'case' or 'problem' to be solved in as short a time as possible, and with maximum efficiency. To a large extent, the social, familial, religious and economic aspects of the patient's life are invisible to the hospital staff, though attempts are made to gather this information via social workers. The emphasis is mainly on the identification and treatment of physical disease, though this is less true of psychiatric hospitals. Looked at in perspective, the hospital service deals mostly with acute, severe or sometimes life-threatening episodes of ill-health, as well as birth and death. It is less orientated towards dealing with the subjective *meanings* associated with illness, which are usually dealt with in the popular or folk sectors or by ministers of religion.

The general practitioner service
Unlike in the USA, this area of health care is largely separated from hospital medicine. For example, out of the 482 782 hospital beds allocated in England, Scotland and Wales in 1976, only 13 665 (2.8%) were 'general practitioner beds'; 5406 of these were obstetric beds.[67] In 1978, in England and Wales, there were only 350 GP-run cottage hospitals, with an average of 20–40 beds each.[68] While GPs can visit the wards and discuss management

of their patients with the hospital medical staff, most of the responsibility for medical care rests with the hospital.

Each GP has, according to Levitt,[34] an average of 2347 patients on his or her 'list'; general practice medicine is home- and community-based, and social, psychological and familial factors are considered relevant in making a diagnosis. As Harris[69] puts it, 'all diagnoses have a social component, whether or not there are social problems', and 'in general practice it is easy to appreciate how a patient's illness and social circumstances are related, because the social circumstances are visible'. Similarly, Hunt[70] believes that GPs should 'put care of the patient's mind before that of his body', and 'the family doctor's awareness of what patients think and feel is vitally important for the whole of his or her work'. Unlike most hospital doctors, the British GP is often a familiar figure in the community. Most live locally, take part in local community activities, dress in civilian clothes, and use everyday language in their consultations. As well as caring for ill people, they are associated with many of the natural milestones of life: they carry out antenatal and postnatal examinations, do check-ups on infants, give immunizations and contraceptive advice, deal with marital and school problems, and counsel bereaved families. Unlike hospital doctors (and most folk healers) they make home visits, and also deal with more than one generation of a family. And, in distinction to the hospital sector, the illnesses they deal with tend to be relatively minor; in one study of the morbidity of 2500 patients in an NHS family practice in 1 year, 1365 had 'minor illnesses', 588 'chronic illness', and only 288 'major illness'.[71] According to Levitt, the GP is the first point of contact for about 90% of those who do seek professional medical help under the NHS, though consultations last only about 5–6 minutes on average.[72]

The NHS GP, in association with the rest of the 'primary health care team', shares some of the attributes of the folk sector, particularly the emphasis on 'illness' (see Chapter 5); that is, the social, psychological and moral dimensions of ill-health.

The nursing service

Nurses and midwives form the largest professional group within the NHS; in 1981 they numbered 476 300, or 43% of its total personnel.[65] The majority of the nursing service is staffed by women, while the majority of doctors are men. Most of the nurses work in the hospital sector, the remainder in the community. Within the hospitals, nurses spend many more hours in direct patient care than do any of the medical hierarchy, and yet they have a lower income and lower prestige than the doctors. Like the medical staff, the nurses are organized into their own professional hierarchies. In English hospitals, this hierarchy ranges from Chief Nurse Adviser down to the various grades of Senior Nurse Manager, Ward Sister, Staff Nurse, ordinary Registered General Nurse (RGN), State Enrolled Nurse (SEN) and Nursing Auxiliary. Many hospital nurses specialize in different branches of medicine, or techniques of patient care, such as stoma or incontinence care nursing, or paediatric, surgical and dental nursing. Nurses working in intensive care units, and in several other hospital departments, usually have a 2-year extra qualification, in addition to their basic training. Within the community, some nurses work as District Nurses, others as Community Midwives, Health Visitors, School Nurses, Practice Nurses (working within a GP practice), or as hospital-based Community Psychiatric Nurses. Some of the features of the nursing profession are described in Chapter 6.

Private medical care

This form of health care preceded the National Health Service, and now coexists with it. It is rapidly growing, partly due to cutbacks in the NHS which have reduced the number of hospital beds and increased waiting lists for operations and out-patient appointments, but it still provides the minority of health care. In 1983 it was estimated that only 7% of the population were insured for private medical care, only 6% of all hospital beds were in private hospitals, and only 2% of hospital beds for acute cases were in private hospitals.[65] There is a considerable overlap in personnel between the two, though some doctors practise private medicine only. There are several private hospitals and clinics, and a number of large health funds. Also, with the exception of homeopathy, all forms of alternative or folk healing are in the private sector. From some patients' perspective, private medicine offers more control over *time* and *choice* of treatment when they are ill. That is, consultation times are longer in the private sector, and this provides more time for explanations of the diagnosis, aetiology, prognosis and treatment of their condition. There are also shorter waiting lists for consultations with specialists, or for surgical operations. The patient also has a choice of specialist and of hospital. Control over time and choice when ill is largely confined to those with

Table 4.2 Professional, folk and popular healers in the UK

Hospital doctors (NHS)	Healing churches and cults
General practitioners (NHS)	Christian healing guilds
Private doctors (hospital or GP)	Church counselling services
Nurses (hospital, school and	Hospital and other chaplains
community)	Probation officers
Midwives	Citizens' Advice Bureaux
Health visitors	Alternative healers (lay and medical)
Social workers	Acupuncture
Physiotherapists	Homeopathy
Occupational therapists	Osteopathy
Pharmacists	Chiropractic
Dietitians	Radionics
Opticians	Herbalism
Dentists	Spiritual healing
Hospital technicians	Hypnotherapy
Nursing auxiliaries	Naturopathy
Medical receptionists	Massage
Local authority health clinics	etc.
Clinical psychologists and	Diviners
psychoanalysts	Astrologers
Counsellors (marriage, child-	Tarot readers
guidance, pregnancy,	Clairvoyants
contraception)	Clairaudientes
Alternative psychotherapists	Mediums
(gestalt, primal therapy, etc.)	Psychic consultants
Group therapists	Palmists
Samaritans and other phone-in	Fortune tellers
counsellors	etc.
Self-help groups	Lay health advisers (family, friends,
Yoga and meditation groups	neighbours, acquaintances,
Health food shops' salespeople	voluntary or charitable workers,
Media healers (advice columnists in	salespeople, hairdressers, etc.)
newspapers and magazines, TV	
and radio doctors)	
Ethnic minority healers	
Muslim *hakims*	
Hindu *vaids*	
Chinese acupuncturists and	
herbalists	
West Indian healing churches	

sufficient income to afford private health insurance, or those who work for large organizations who provide their employees with such insurance.

The NHS and private sectors are not watertight; as with other areas of the health care system, there is a considerable flow of ill people between them, and many doctors work within both systems.

The range of healers

To view the British health care system in perspective, I have listed most of the available sources of health care or advice in Table 4.2. 'Healer' here refers to all those who, either formally or informally, offer advice and care for those suffering from physical discomfort and/or psychological distress. This list spans, therefore, all three sectors of health care in the UK – popular, folk and professional.

Case history: Sources of lay health advice in Northampton, UK

Elliott-Binns[35] studied 1000 patients attending a general practice in Northampton, England. The patients were asked whether they had previously received any advice or treatment for their symptoms. The source, type and soundness of the advice was noted, as well as whether the patient had accepted it. It was found that 96% of patients had received some advice or treatment before consulting their GP. Each patient had had an average of 2.3 sources of advice, or 1.8 excluding self-treatment; that is, 2285 sources, of which 1764 were outside sources, and 521 self-advice. Thirty-five patients received advice from five or more sources; one boy with acne received it from 11 sources. The outside sources of advice for the sample were: friend (499), spouse (466), relative (387), magazines or books (162), pharmacists (108), nurses giving informal advice (102), nurses giving professional advice (52). Wives' advice was evaluated as being among the best, that from mothers and mothers-in-law among the worst. Male relatives usually said, 'Go to the doctor', without offering practical advice, and rarely gave advice to other men. Advice from impersonal sources, such as women's magazines, home doctor books, newspapers and television, were evaluated as the least sound. Pharmacists, consulted by 11% of the sample, gave the soundest advice. Home remedies accounted for 15% of all advice, especially from friends, relatives and parents.

Overall, the best advice was given for respiratory complaints, the worst for psychiatric illness. One example of the patient sample was a married village shopkeeper with a persistent cough. She received advice from her husband, an ex-hospital matron, a doctor's receptionist, and five customers, three of whom recommended a patent remedy 'Golden Syrup', one a boiled onion gruel, and one the application of a hot brick to the chest. One middle-aged widower had come to see the doctor complaining of backache. He had consulted no-one because he 'had no friends and anyway if I got some ointment there's no-one to rub it in'.

Elliott-Binns[36] repeated this study 15 years later on 500 patients in the same practice in Northampton. Surprisingly, the pattern of self-care and lay health advice had remained largely unchanged. Now 55.4% of patients treated themselves before going to the doctor, compared with 52.0% in 1970. The only significant changes were an increase in impersonal sources of advice on health – such as home doctor books and television – and a decline in the use of traditional home remedies (though they still accounted for 11.2% of health advice). In addition, the use of advice from pharmacists increased from 10.8% in 1970 to 16.4% in 1985. Overall, the study suggests that in the UK self-care still remains the chief source of health care for the average patient.

Recommended reading

Sectors of health care

Kleinman, A. (1980) *Patients and Healers in the Context of Culture.* Berkeley: University of California Press. See Chapters 2 and 3 for a discussion of the three sectors of health care, and the cross-cultural comparison of health care systems.

Folk and popular sectors

Dunnell, K. and Cartwright, A. (1972) *Medicine Takers, Prescribers and Hoarders.* London: Routledge and Kegan Paul. A study of self-medication in the UK.
Fulder, S. (1988) *Handbook of Complementary Medicine.* London: Oxford University Press. A survey of alternative and complementary healing in modern Britain.
Janzen, J.M. (1978) *The Quest for Therapy: Medical Pluralism in Lower Zaire.* Berkeley: University of California Press. An African example of medical pluralism.
MacGuire, M.B. (1988) *Ritual Healing in Suburban America.* New Brunswick: Rutgers University Press
Robinson, D. and Henry, S. (1977) *Self-help and Health: Mutual Aid for Modern Problems.* London: Martin Robertson. Self-help groups in the UK.
Snow, L. F. (1978) Sorcerers, saints and charlatans: black healers in urban America. *Cult. Med. Psychiatry* **2**, 69–106

Chapter 5

Doctor–patient interactions

Doctors and their patients, even if they come from the same cultural background, view ill-health in very different ways. Their perspectives are based on different premises, employ a different system of proof, and assess the efficacy of treatment in a different way. Each has its strengths, as well as its weaknesses. The problem is how to ensure some *communication* between them in the clinical encounter between doctor and patient. To illustrate this problem, the differences between medical and lay views of ill-health – between, that is, 'disease' and 'illness' – will be described in some detail.

'Disease' – the doctor's perspective

As described in the previous chapter, those who practice modern scientific medicine form a group apart, with their own values, theories of disease, rules of behaviour, and organization into a hierarchy of specialized roles. The medical profession can be seen as a healing subculture, with its own particular world view. In the process of medical education, students undergo a form of 'enculturation' whereby gradually they acquire a perspective on ill-health that will last throughout their professional lives. They also acquire a high social status, high earning power, and the socially legitimated role of healer, which carries with it certain rights and obligations. The basic premises of this medical perspective can be described as:

1. Scientific rationality.
2. Emphasis on objective, numerical measurement.
3. Emphasis on physicochemical data.
4. Mind–body dualism.
5. The view of 'diseases' as entities.
6. Emphasis on the individual patient, rather than on the family or community.[1]

Medicine, like Western science generally, is based on scientific *rationality*; that is all, assumptions and hypotheses must be capable of being tested, and verified, under objective, empirical and controlled conditions. Phenomena relating to health and sickness only become 'real' when they can be *objectively* observed and measured under these conditions. Once they have been observed, and often quantified, they become clinical 'facts', the cause and effect of which must then be discovered. All facts have a cause, and the task of a clinician is to discover the logical chain of causal influences that led to a particular fact. For example, iron-deficiency anaemia may result from loss of blood, which may be the result of a bleeding stomach tumour, which may have been caused by certain carcinogens in the diet. Where a specific causal influence cannot be isolated, the clinical fact is labelled 'idiopathic' – that is, it has a cause, but that cause has yet to be discovered. Where a phenomenon cannot be objectively observed or measured – for example, a person's beliefs about what caused them to be ill – it is somehow less 'real' than, say, the level of blood pressure, or white cell count. Because blood pressure and white cell count can be measured, and agreed upon by several observers, they form the sorts of clinical facts upon which diagnosis and treatment will be based.

These facts, therefore, arise from a *consensus* among the observers, whose measurements are carried out in accordance with certain agreed guidelines. The assumptions underlying these guidelines – which determine what phenomena are to be looked for, and how they are to be verified and measured – is termed a conceptual *model*. As Eisenberg[2] points out, models 'are ways of constructing reality, of imposing meaning on the chaos of the phenomenal world', and 'once in place, models act to generate their own verification by excluding phenomena outside the frame of reference the user employs'. The 'model' of modern medicine is mainly directed towards discovering and quantifying physicochemical information about the patient, rather than less measurable social and emotional factors. As Kleinman et al.[3] put it, the modern Western doctor's view of clinical reality 'assumes that biologic concerns are more basic, "real", clinically significant, and interesting than psychological and sociocultural issues'.

This emphasis on physiological facts means that a doctor confronted with a patient's symptoms tries first of all to relate these to some underlying *physical* process. For example, if a patient complains of a certain type of chest pain, the doctor's approach is likely to involve a number of examinations or tests to try to identify the physical cause of the pain – such as coronary heart disease. If no physical cause can be found after exhaustive investigation, the symptom might be labelled 'psychogenic' or 'psychosomatic', but this diagnosis is usually made only by excluding a physical cause. Subjective symptoms, therefore, become more 'real' when they can be explained by objective, physical changes. As Good and Good[4] put it, 'Symptoms achieve their *meaning* in relationship to physiological states, which are interpreted as the referents of the symptoms. . . Somatic lesions or dysfunctions produce discomfort and behavioural changes, communicated in a patient's complaints. The critical task of the physician is to "decode" a patient's discourse by relating symptoms to their biological referents in order to diagnose a disease entity.' These somatic or biological referents are discovered by the doctor's examination, and sometimes by the use of specialized tests.

In Feinstein's view[5] there has been a shift in recent years in how doctors collect information about underlying disease processes. The traditional method was by listening to the patient's symptoms and how they developed (the History), and then searching for objective physical signs (the Examination). Increasingly, though, modern medicine has come to rely on diagnostic technology to collect and measure clinical facts. This implies a shift from the subjective (the patient's subjective symptoms, the physician's subjective interpretation of the physical signs) towards the notionally objective forms of diagnosis. The underlying pathological processes are now firmly identified by blood tests, radiographs, scans and other investigations, usually carried out in specialized laboratories or clinics. One result of this is the increasing use of *numerical* definitions of health and disease. Health or normality is defined by reference to certain physical and biochemical parameters, such as weight, height, circumference, blood count, haemoglobin level, levels of electrolytes or hormones, blood pressure, heart rate, respiratory rate, heart size or visual acuity. For each measurement there is a numerical range – the 'normal value' – within which the individual is normal and 'healthy'. Above or below this range is 'abnormal', and indicates the presence of 'disease'. Disease, then, is seen as a deviation from these normal values, accompanied by abnormalities in the structure or function of body organs or systems. For example, below the normal value of thyroid hormone in the blood is *hypo*thyroidism, above it is *hyper*thyroidism, and between the two the thyroid is 'functioning normally'.

The medical definition of ill-health, therefore, is largely based on objectively demonstrable physical changes in the body's structure or function, which can be quantified by reference to 'normal' physiological measurements. These abnormal changes, or *diseases*, are seen as 'entities', with their own specific 'personality' of symptoms and signs. Each disease's personality is made up of a characteristic cause, clinical picture (symptoms and signs), results of hospital investigations, natural history, prognosis and appropriate treatment. For example, tuberculosis is known to be caused by a particular bacillus, to reveal itself by certain characteristic symptoms, to display certain physical signs on examination, to show up in a particular way on chest radiographs and sputum tests, and to have a likely natural history, depending on whether it is treated or not. As Fabrega and Silver[6] point out, the medical perspective assumes that diseases are 'universal in form, progress, and content', and that they have a 'recurring identity'; that is, it is assumed that tuberculosis will be the same disease, in whatever culture or society it appears. It will always have the same cause, clinical picture, treatment, and so on. However, this perspective does not include the social and psychological dimensions of ill-health, and the context in which it appears, which determine the *meaning* of the disease for individual patients, and for those around them. Because modern medicine focuses more on the physical dimensions of illness, factors such as the personality, religious belief, and socioeconomic status of the patient are often considered irrelevant in making the diagnosis or prescribing treatment. Engel[7] sees this approach as further evidence of 'mind–body dualism', a medical way of thinking which focuses on identifying physical abnormalities, while often ignoring 'the patient and his attributes as a person, a human being'; reducing him, that is, to a set of abnormal physiological parameters. This conceptual dualism can be traced back at least to Descartes in the seventeenth century, who divided man into 'body' (to be studied only by science), and 'mind' or 'soul' (to be studied by philosophy and religion). In more recent times, the mind has been handed over to psychiatrists and behavioural scientists to study (rather than priests), while the body – seen increasingly as an animated machine – has been handed over to medical science and its diagnostic technology, so that in modern medicine the basic dualism still remains.

The medical model, however, should not be seen as homogeneous and consistent. There is really no such thing as a uniform 'Western' or 'scientific' medicine, because as illustrated in the previous chapter there is enormous variation in how medicine is practiced both in different Western countries and in other parts of the world. To a large extent the medical model is always 'culture-bound', and varies greatly depending on the context in which it appears. Furthermore, when a doctor trained in modern scientific medicine makes a diagnosis, he or she usually employs a number of different models or perspectives, each of which looks at the problem in a particular way. As Good and Good[4] note, 'any physician or medical discipline has a repertoire of interpretive models – biochemical, immunological, viral, genetic, environmental, psychodynamic, family interactionist and so on' – each with its own unique perspective on the disease. In some cases these perspectives, or models, might be very different from one another. For example, Eisenberg[2] points out that in psychiatry 'multiple and manifestly contradictory models' are used by different psychiatrists in explaining the psychoses. These include:

1. The *organic* model, which emphasizes physical and biochemical changes in the brain.
2. The *psychodynamic* model, which concentrates on developmental and experiential factors.
3. The *behavioural* model, where psychosis is maintained by environmental contingencies.
4. The *social* model with its emphasis on disorders in role performance.

All medical and psychiatric models tend to change over time, as new concepts are developed and new discoveries are made. Disease entities, such as hypertension or coronary heart disease, are continuously being re-examined, or 'reworked', as new theories of aetiology are advanced and new techniques of diagnosis and treatment are invented. Because of the different models used by clinicians in different specialties, they might perceive and diagnose the *same* episode of ill-health in very different ways, if an ill person consulted with each of them over a period of time.

Nevertheless, despite these variations within the medical model, its predominant approach is still the search for physical evidence of disease, and the use of physical treatments (such as drugs or surgery) in correcting these underlying abnormalities.

'Illness' – the patient's perspective

Cassell[8] uses the word 'illness' to stand for 'what the patient feels when he goes to the doctor', and 'disease' for 'what he has on the way home from the doctor's office. Disease, then, is something an organ has; illness is something a man has.' Illness is the subjective response of the patient, and of those around him, to his being unwell; particularly how he, and they, interpret the origin and significance of this event; how it effects his behaviour, and his relationship with other people; and the various steps he takes to remedy the situation. It not only includes his experience of ill-health, but also the *meaning* he gives to that experience. For example, a person who has suddenly fallen ill might ask themselves: 'Why has it happened to *me*?' or 'Have I done anything wrong to deserve this?' or even, in some societies, 'Has anyone caused me to be ill?' Both the meaning given to his symptoms and his emotional response to them are influenced by his own background and personality, as well as the cultural, social and economic context in which they appear.[9] In other words, the same disease (such as tuberculosis) or symptom (such as pain) may be interpreted completely differently by two patients from different cultures, and in different contexts. And this will also affect their subsequent behaviour and the sorts of treatment they will seek out.

The patient's perspective on ill-health is usually part of a much wider conceptual model used to explain misfortune in general; within this model illness is only a specialized form of adversity. For example, in many societies, *all* forms of misfortune are ascribed to the same range of causes: a high fever, a crop failure, the theft of one's property, a roof collapsing, might all be blamed on witchcraft, or on divine punishment for some moral transgression. In the latter case, they may cause similar emotions of shame or guilt, and call for similar types of treatment, such as prayer or penitence. Illness therefore often shares the psychological, moral and social dimensions associated with other forms of adversity within a particular culture. It is a wider, though more diffuse, concept than 'disease', and should be taken into account in understanding how people interpret their ill-health and how they respond to it.

Becoming 'ill'

Definitions of what constitutes both 'health' and 'illness' vary between individuals, cultural groups and social classes. In most cases, health is seen as more than just an absence of unpleasant symptoms. The World Health Organisation,[10] for example, defined it in 1946 as 'a state of complete physical, mental and social well-being and not merely the absence of disease or infirmity'. In many non-industrialized societies health is conceived of as a balanced *relationship* between man and man, man and nature, and man and the supernatural world. A disturbance of any of these may manifest itself by physical or emotional symptoms. Among Western communities, definitions of health tend to be less all-embracing, but they also include physical, psychological and behavioural aspects. They also vary between social classes. For example, Fox[9] quotes a study of 'Regionville', a town in upper New York State, where members of the highest socioeconomic class usually reported a persistent backache to their physician as an 'abnormal' symptom, while members of the lower socioeconomic class regarded it as 'an inevitable and innocuous part of life and thus as inappropriate for referral to a doctor'. Similarly, in Blaxter and Paterson's study[11] in Aberdeen, working-class mothers did not define their children as ill, even if they had abnormal physical symptoms, provided that they continued to walk around and play normally. This functional definition of health, common among poorer people, is probably based on the (economic) need to keep working, however they feel, as well as on low expectations of medical care. These lay definitions of health can obviously differ from those of the medical profession, as will be described below.

On an individual level, the process of defining oneself as being ill can be based on one's own perceptions, on the perceptions of others, or on both. Defining oneself as being ill usually follows a number of subjective experiences including:

1. Perceived changes in bodily appearance, such as loss of weight, changes in skin colour, or hair falling out.
2. Changes in regular bodily functions, such as urinary frequency, heavy menstrual periods, irregular heart beats.
3. Unusual bodily emissions, such as blood in the urine, sputum or stools.
4. Changes in the functions of limbs, such as paralysis, clumsiness or tremor.
5. Changes in the five major senses, such as deafness, blindness, lack of smell or loss of taste sensation.
6. Unpleasant physical symptoms, such as headache, abdominal pain, fever or shivering.
7. Excessive or unusual emotional states, such as anxiety, depression, nightmares or exaggerated fears.

8. Behavioural changes in relation to others, such as marital or work disharmony.

Most people experience some of these abnormal changes in their daily lives, though usually in a mild form, and this has been demonstrated in several studies. In Dunnell and Cartwright's study,[12] mentioned earlier, 91% of a sample of adults had experienced one or more abnormal symptom in the two weeks preceding the study (although only 16% had consulted a doctor during this time). Having one or more abnormal changes of symptoms may therefore not be enough to label oneself as being ill. For example, in Apple's study[13] of middle-class Americans, abnormal symptoms were only considered as illness if they interfered with the usual daily activities, were recent in onset, and were 'ambiguous' – that is, difficult for a layman to diagnose.

Other people can also define one as being ill, even in the absence of abnormal subjective experiences, by statements such as, 'You look pale today, you must be ill' or 'You've been acting very oddly recently'. In the case of behavioural changes, cultures vary on whether a particular form of behaviour is defined as illness or not. In Guttmacher and Elinson's study,[14] different American ethnic groups in New York City were asked whether certain types of socially deviant behaviour (such as transvestism, homosexuality or getting into fights) were evidence of illness. The Puerto Rican group were found to be less likely to describe these as illness than other groups such as the Irish, Italians, Jews or Blacks. In most cases, though, people are defined as ill when there is agreement between their perceptions of impaired well-being and the perceptions of those around them. In that sense, becoming ill is a *social* process which involves other people besides the patient. Their cooperation is needed for a person to adopt the rights and benefits of the sick role – that is, of the socially acceptable role of an 'ill person'. People who are so defined are able temporarily to avoid their obligations towards the social groups to which they belong, such as family, friends, workmates or religious groups. At the same time, these groups often feel obligated to care for their sick members while they are ill. The sick role therefore provides, as Fox[9] points out, 'a semi-legitimate channel of withdrawal from adult responsibilities and a basis of eligibility for care by others'. In most cases, this role is most potent when validated by a doctor or some other health professional. In general, this care takes place within the popular sector of health care, especially within the family, where patients' symptoms are discussed and evaluated, and decisions made about whether they are ill or not, and if so how they should be treated.

The process of 'becoming ill' involves, therefore, both subjective experiences of physical or emotional changes, and, except in the very isolated, the confirmation of these changes by other people. In order for this confirmation to take place there must be a *consensus* among all concerned about what constitutes both health and abnormal symptoms and signs. There must also be a standardized way in which an ill person can draw attention to these abnormal changes to mobilize care and support. As Lewis[15] puts it, 'in every society there are some conventions about how people should behave when they are ill . . . in most illness there is some interplay of voluntary and involuntary responses in the expression of illness. The patient has some control of the way in which he shows his illness and what he does about it.' Both the presentation of illness, and others' response to it, are largely determined by sociocultural factors. Each culture has its own *language of distress*, which bridges the gap between subjective experiences of impaired well-being and social acknowledgement of them. Cultural factors determine *which* symptoms or signs are perceived as abnormal; they also help to *shape* these diffuse emotional and physical changes into a pattern which is recognizable to both the sufferer and those around him. The resultant pattern of symptoms and signs may be termed an 'illness entity', and represents the first stage of becoming ill.

The explanatory model

Kleinman,[16] of Harvard University, has suggested a useful way of looking at the process by which illness is patterned, interpreted and treated, which he terms the *explanatory model* (EM). This is defined as 'the notions about an episode of sickness and its treatment that are employed by all those engaged in the clinical process'. EMs are held by both patients and practitioners, and they 'offer explanations of sickness and treatment to guide choices among available therapies and therapists and to cast personal and social meaning on the experience of sickness'. In particular, they provide explanations for five aspects of illness:

1. The aetiology of the condition.
2. The timing and mode of onset of symptoms.
3. The pathophysiological processes involved.

4. The natural history and severity of the illness.
5. The appropriate treatments for the condition.

These models are marshalled in response to a *particular* episode of illness, and are not identical to the general beliefs about illness that are held by that society. According to Kleinman, lay EMs tend to be idiosyncratic and changeable, and to be heavily influenced by both personality and cultural factors. They are partly conscious and partly outside of awareness, and are characterized by 'vagueness, multiplicity of meanings, frequent changes, and lack of sharp boundaries between ideas and experience'. He contrasts this with physicians' EMs, which are also marshalled to deal with a particular illness episode, but are mostly based on 'single causal trains of scientific logic'. Explanatory models, therefore, are used by individuals to explain, organize and manage particular episodes of impaired well-being. Consultations with a doctor are actually transactions between the lay and medical EMs of a particular illness. However, explanatory models can be fully understood only by examining the specific *context* in which they are employed, as this usually has a major influence upon them. The context of an EM may include the social and economic organization and dominant ideology (or religion) of the society in which that individual became ill, and in which he or she consulted a doctor. For example, ill people's assessment of how serious an illness is (and how it will affect their lives) may depend not only on how they explain the origin of the condition, but also on whether they are able to afford to be off work, whether they can afford private health insurance, and whether the state will provide them with free health care and disability payments while they remain unfit to work. The social and economic context will also influence the types of treatment they can afford for their illness, and whether this takes place mainly in the popular, folk or professional sectors.

The ways that lay and medical EMs interact in the clinical consultation are influenced not only by the physical context in which they occur (such as a hospital ward or a doctor's office),[17] but also by the social class and gender of the two parties involved. The power invested in clinicians by virtue of their background and training may allow them to mould the patient's EM to make it fit into the medical model of disease, rather than allowing the patient's own perspective on illness to emerge.

Another way of looking at lay explanations of ill-health is to examine the sorts of questions that people ask themselves when they perceive themselves as being ill,[18] and how they weave the answers to these questions into the story or narrative of their ill-health. These questions are:

1. *What has happened?* This includes organizing the symptoms and signs into a recognizable pattern, and giving it a name or identity.
2. *Why has it happened?* This explains the aetiology of the condition.
3. *Why has it happened to me?* This tries to relate the illness to aspects of the patient, such as behaviour, diet, body build, personality or heredity.
4. *Why now?* This concerns the timing of the illness and its mode of onset, sudden or slow.
5. *What would happen to me if nothing were done about it?* This considers its likely course, outcome, prognosis and dangers.
6. *What are its likely effects on other people (family, friends, employers, workmates) if nothing were done about it?* This includes loss of income or of employment, and strain on family relationships.
7. *What should I do about it – or to whom should I turn for further help?* Strategies for treating the condition include self-medication, consultation with friends or family, or going to see a doctor.

For example, a patient suffering from a head cold might answer these questions as: 'I've picked up a cold. It's because I went out into the rain on a cold day, directly after a hot bath, when I was feeling low. If I leave it, it may go down to my chest and make me more ill. Then I might have stay at home for a long time, and lose a lot of money. I'd better go to see the doctor and get some medicine for it.' Before these questions can be asked, or answered, the patients must see their symptoms or signs – such as muscular aches, shivering, or a runny nose – as abnormal, before grouping them into the recognizable pattern of a cold. This implies a fairly widespread belief in the patient's community about what a cold is, and how it can be recognized, though the EM of a particular cold is likely to have personal, idiosyncratic elements. Where many people in a culture or community agree about a pattern of symptoms and signs – and its origin, significance and treatment – it becomes an illness entity or *folk illness*, with a recurring identity. This identity is more loosely defined than medical diseases, and is greatly influenced by the sociocultural context in which it appears.

Folk illnesses

Rubel[19] has defined folk illnesses as 'syndromes from which members of a particular group claim to suffer and for which their culture provides an aetiology, a diagnosis, preventive measures and regimens of healing'. Anthropologists have described dozens of these folk illnesses from around the world, each with its own unique configuration of symptoms, signs and behavioural changes. Some examples are *susto* throughout Latin America, *amok* in Malaysia, *windigo* in north-eastern America, *narahatiye qalb* ('heart distress') in Iran, *koro* in China, *brain fag* in parts of Africa, *tabanka* in Trinidad, *nervios* in Costa Rica and other parts of Latin America, *vapid unmada* in Sri Lanka, *crise de foie* in France, *high blood* in the USA, and *colds* and *chills* in much of the English-speaking world. Each of these is a 'culture-bound syndrome' in the sense that it is a unique disorder, recognized mainly by members of a particular culture. One is dealing with a culture-bound folk illness when, as Rubel puts it, 'symptoms regularly cohere in any specified population, and members of that population respond to such manifestations in similarly patterned ways'.

Folk illnesses are more than specific clusterings of symptoms and physical signs. They also have a range of symbolic meanings – moral, social or psychological – for those who suffer from them. In some cases they link the suffering of the individual to changes in the natural environment, or to the workings of supernatural forces. In other cases, the clinical picture of the illness is a way of expressing, in a culturally standardized way, that the sufferer is involved in social conflicts or disharmony with friends or family.

Case history: 'Heart distress' in Maragheh, Iran

Byron Good[20] has described an example of this type of folk illness, *narahatiye qalb* or 'heart distress', in Maragheh, Iran. This is a complex folk illness which usually manifests itself by physical symptoms – such as 'trembling', 'fluttering' or 'pounding' of the heart – and with feelings of anxiety or unhappiness, also associated with the heart ('My heart is uneasy'). This illness is 'a complex which includes and links together both physical sensations of abnormality in the heart beat and feelings of anxiety, sadness, or anger'. The abnormal heart beat is linked both to unpleasant affective states, and to experiences of social stress. It is more frequent among Iranian women, and expresses some of the strains and conflicts of their lives. Heart distress often follows quarrels or conflict within the family, the deaths of close relatives, pregnancy, childbirth, infertility and the use of the contraceptive pill (which is seen as a threat to fertility and lactation). It is primarily a self-labelled folk illness which expresses a wide range of physical, psychological and social problems at the same time; the label 'heart distress' is 'an image which draws together a network of symbols, situations, motives, feelings and stresses which are rooted in the structural setting in which the people of Maragheh live'. The basic presentation of this illness, however, is in the form of common physical symptoms associated with the heart.

A feature of many folk illnesses is that of *somatization* (see Chapter 10), which Kleinman[21] defines as 'the substitution of somatic preoccupation for dysphoric affect in the form of complaints of physical symptoms and even illness'. That is, unpleasant emotional states (such as depression), or the experience of social stresses, is expressed in the form of physical symptoms. In Taiwan, for example, Kleinman describes how depression is commonly presented in the form of physical symptoms and signs. In Taiwanese culture, mental illness is heavily stigmatized, as is the use of psychotherapy, and therefore stress from family problems or financial difficulties is often expressed by physical symptoms. Although these symptoms do not necessarily appear in a standardized form, they are more easily recognized by Chinese folk healers (who are more familiar with this mode of presenting personal problems and conflicts) than by Western-trained physicians.

Folk illnesses can be 'learnt', in the sense that a child growing up in a particular culture learns how to respond to, and express, a range of physical or emotional symptoms, or social stresses, in a culturally patterned way. Children see relatives or friends suffering from that condition, and gradually learn to identify its characteristic features, both in themselves and in others. Frankenberg[22] notes how people's experience of a particular form of ill-health is also shaped by wider cultural and social forces, such as television, newspapers and novels, as well as by the dominant ideology and social structure of the society in which they live.

A doctor or nurse working in any culture or society should therefore be aware of how folk illnesses are generated, how they are acquired and displayed, and how this may affect their patients' behaviour and the diagnosis of ill-health.

Metaphors of illness

In both the urban and rural areas of modern industrial society, a large number of folk illnesses still persist, many of them largely untouched by the medical model and still rooted in traditional folklore. In addition, certain serious and life-threatening diseases (such as cancer, heart disease or AIDS) have also become 'folk illnesses', though of a particularly powerful type. Often these conditions are linked in the public imagination with traditional beliefs about the moral nature of health, illness and human suffering. These diseases (especially those that are difficult to treat or control) come to symbolize many of the more general anxieties that some people have, such as a fear of the breakdown of ordered society, or of invasion, or of divine punishment. In the minds of many in the population, these diseases become more than just a clinical condition: they become *metaphors* for many of the terrors of daily life.

Susan Sontag[23] has described how, historically, certain serious diseases – especially those whose origin was not understood, and whose treatment was not very successful – became metaphors for all that was 'unnatural', and socially or morally wrong with society.

In the Middle Ages, epidemic diseases such as plague were the metaphors for social disorder, and the breakdown of the social, religious and moral order. In the past two centuries, syphilis, tuberculosis and cancer have all been used as more contemporary 'metaphors for evil'. In the twentieth century particularly, *cancer* has been described (in the media, literature and popular discourse) as if it were a type of unrestrained and chaotic evil force, unique to the modern world, which is composed of 'primitive', 'atavistic', 'chaotic' and 'energetic' cells, who behave completely 'without inhibitions' – and which always destroy the natural order of the body (and of society). According to Sontag, a result of this moral model of cancer is that for many sufferers the disease is 'often experienced as a form of demonic possession – tumours are "malignant" or "benign", like forces – and many terrified cancer patients are disposed to seek out faith healers, to be exorcised'. In the media, too, crime, drug abuse, strikes, immigration and even political dissent have all been described as 'a cancer', a demonic force gradually destroying the very fabric of society.

Thus these metaphors of ill-health – particularly when they attach to such serious conditions as cancer – carry with them a range of symbolic associations which can seriously affect how the sufferers perceive their own condition, and how other people behave towards them. For example, Peters-Golden[24] has described how the stigma associated with breast cancer can cause other people to avoid the sick person, and to withdraw their social support from her. In her study of 100 women with breast cancer, 72% of the sample said that other people treated them differently after they knew the diagnosis; 52% found they were 'avoided' or 'feared', 14% felt they were pitied, and only 3% thought people were nicer to them than they had previously been.

Metaphors of AIDS

One of the most serious diseases of our age is the acquired immune deficiency syndrome (AIDS). According to the World Health Organisation,[25] by 1987, 91 433 cases of the disease had been reported to them from more than 100 countries, and it has also been estimated that several million people worldwide are now HIV seropositive.[26] Like the plague, cancer and tuberculosis before it, AIDS in the popular perception has become a metaphor – or, rather, a cluster of metaphors – and a vehicle for expressing many of the fears and anxieties of modern life.

In the last few years, particularly in the lurid headlines of the popular press, a number of recurrent images or metaphors of AIDS can be identified. These include:

1. AIDS as a *plague* (sometimes even called 'the gay plague'[27]) – an image which echoes those of medieval 'pestilence' or plague mentioned above; that is, of an invisible, spreading destructive force that brings with it chaos, disorder and the breakdown of ordered society, family life and interpersonal relationships.
2. AIDS as an invisible *contagion* – in this image, apparently based on older folk models of infectious diseases, AIDS is seen as an unseen influence transmitted by virtually *any* contact with an infected person, whether this contact is with the body surface, body wastes, or even with the air they breathe. This invisible influence can occur at work, at school, at home or even at church. Like medieval theories of disease,

it is as if the sufferer were surrounded by an infective 'miasma', or cloud of poisonous 'bad air', which causes disease in others nearby. Implicit in this image is the idea that the sexual lifestyles of sufferers from the disease might also be 'contagious' to those around them.

3. AIDS as *moral punishment* – in this image, victims of the disease are usually divided into two groups: those who are 'innocent' (the recipients of blood transfusions, such as haemophiliacs and children, and the spouses of those who are bisexual, or who engage in extramarital sex), and those who are 'guilty' (such as homosexual men, bisexuals, promiscuous people, prostitutes and intravenous drug users).[28] The image of AIDS as 'judgement', 'divine punishment' or 'Nemesis' for a deviant lifestyle – like other forms of 'victim-blaming' (see Chapter 4) – is still prominent in popular press coverage of the disease.

4. AIDS as *invader* – an image which usually includes themes of *xenophobia* and 'foreign invasion', since it often involves prejudices against foreigners and immigrants, especially Africans, Haitians and others, coupled with the fear of a hidden invasion by 'alien AIDS-carriers'.

5. AIDS as *war* – an image linked to the previous one, where AIDS is seen as a war waged on conventional society by 'immoral' lifestyles, promiscuity, foreign influences, and stigmatized minorities (such as gays, prostitutes, immigrants or drug abusers); here, heterosexual victims of the disease have sometimes been depicted as if they were innocent civilian casualties caught up in the crossfire of a war.[29]

6. AIDS as a *primitive* or presocial force or entity – a similar image to that of cancer described above, but characterized more by images of childlike hedonism and unrestrained and unconventional sexuality.

These metaphors, attached in the media and in popular discourse to the very word AIDS, mean that it is no longer only a serious physical disease, but has also become one of the major folk illnesses of our time.

Furthermore, these metaphors have often been used for political purposes, especially to stigmatize even further certain groups in society, such as homosexuals, immigrants and drug abusers. However, from a medical anthropological perspective, these metaphors are dangerous for many reasons – and especially because they may impede any *rational* assessment of the risks of the disease, and how it is to be recognized, controlled, prevented and treated. Watney[30] has noted how the 'moral panic' and prejudice in most media commentary on AIDS makes any rational evaluation of the disease very difficult, since these prejudices 'heavily overdetermine all discussion of the virus'. Cominos et al.[31] also point out that the only way to prevent person-to-person transmission is by education, 'which is only effective if predicated upon in-depth understanding of prevailing knowledge, attitudes and practices related to HIV infection in diverse societies and subgroups'. However, such research on the transmission of AIDS will not be possible if the stigmas and metaphors attached to it make many people unwilling to come forward for diagnosis and treatment.

Another danger of AIDS metaphors is that the media imagery of moral punishment and the over-emphasis on stigmatized subcultures, such as gay men or intravenous drug users, may prevent AIDS patients from getting the compassionate care and medical treatment they deserve. For example, Cassens[27] has described the serious social and psychological consequences that gay men diagnosed as having AIDS often have to suffer, including rejection by family and others. At a time of major psychological stress, they may also have to undergo what I have elsewhere (see Chapter 11) termed a 'social death' of isolation and the withdrawal of social support.

As the example of AIDS illustrates, therefore, under certain circumstances, certain medical *diseases* can also become a form of *folk illness*, and this can seriously impair the management and control of these conditions.

Lay theories of illness causation

As noted above, lay theories about illness are part of wider concepts about the origin of misfortune in general. They are also based on beliefs about the structure and function of the body, and the ways in which it can malfunction. Even if based on scientifically incorrect premises, these lay models frequently have an internal logic and consistency, which often helps the victim of illness 'make sense' of what has happened, and why. In most cultures they are part of a complex body of inherited folklore, which is often influenced by concepts borrowed from the media and from the medical model.

In general, lay theories of illness place the aetiology of ill-health in one of the following sites:

1. Within the individual patient.
2. In the natural world.

3. In the social world.
4. In the supernatural world.

This is illustrated in Figure 5.1 In some cases, illness is ascribed to combinations of causes, or to interactions between these various worlds.

Social and supernatural aetiologies tend to be a feature of some communities in the non-industrialized world, while natural or patient-centred explanations of illness are more

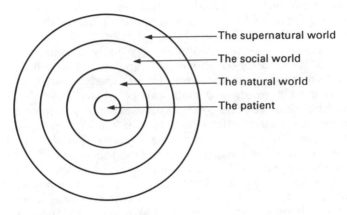

Figure 5.1 Site of illness aetiology

common in the Western industrialized world, though the division is by no means absolute. For example, Chrisman[32] has described eight groups of lay aetiologies that are common among patients in the USA, and most of which are patient centred. They are:

1. Debilitation.
2. Degeneration.
3. Invasion.
4. Imbalance.
5. Stress.
6. Mechanical causes.
7. Environmental irritants.
8. Hereditary proneness.

These and other lay aetiologies will be discussed in more detail below.

The patient

Lay theories that locate the origin of ill-health within the individual deal mainly with malfunctions within the body, sometimes related to changes in diet or behaviour. Here the *responsibility* for illness falls mainly (though not completely) on the patient.[1] This belief is especially common in the Western world (where it is often encouraged by government health education), and where ill-health is increasingly blamed on 'not taking care' of one's diet, dress, hygiene, lifestyle, relationships, smoking and drinking habits, and physical exercise. Ill-health is therefore evidence of such carelessness, and the sufferer should feel guilty for causing it. This applies especially to stigmatized conditions such as obesity, alcoholism, sexually transmitted diseases, and, as mentioned above, to some extent to AIDS. Other more common conditions are also ascribed to incorrect *behaviour*: in the UK, colds and chills can be caused by doing something 'abnormal' such as 'going outdoors when you have a fever', 'sitting in a draught after a hot bath', or 'walking barefoot on a cold floor'. Wrong *diet* can also cause ill-health. For example, as described in Chapter 2, 'low blood' and low blood pressure in the southern USA are thought to result from eating too many acid or astringent foods, such as lemons, vinegar, pickles, olives and sauerkraut, while 'high blood' results from eating too much rich food, especially red meat.[33] In another study,[34] a quarter of the women interviewed believed one should eat differently during menstruation to avoid causing ill-health. For example, sweets were said to keep the menstrual flow going longer, while other foods caused it to stop – resulting in menstrual cramps, sterility, strokes, or 'quick TB'. Similar dietary prohibitions applied to pregnant women. Other examples of personal responsibility for ill health are some traumatic *injuries* (also ascribed to 'carelessness'), or injuries which are clearly self-inflicted, such as unsuccessful attempts at suicide.

Whether people perceive ill-health as resulting from their own behaviour depends on a number of factors. Pill and Stott,[35] in their study of 41 working-class mothers in Cardiff, Wales, found that the extent to which people believed that their health is determined by their own actions (as opposed to 'luck', 'chance' or powerful external forces) correlated with socioeconomic variables such as education and home ownership. Those people who had most economic control over their own lives accepted more responsibility for ill-health causation than those who perceived themselves as socially and economically powerless; in this latter group, illness was believed to result from external forces over which the victim had no control, and for which she felt no responsibility.

Other aetiological factors are believed to lie within the body, but to be outside the victim's conscious control. This includes notions of personal *vulnerability* – psychological, physical or hereditary. Personality factors include the 'type of person one is', especially if one is overanxious or easily worried. In Pill and Stott's study, this is illustrated in quotes such as: 'Well, I think something like you bring on yourself, like nerves or anything like that, it's partly down to you I would think – to what sort of person you are. Like I'm a little bit highly strung, you know.' Physical vulnerability is based on lay notions of *resistance* and *weakness*. Some people in the sample were believed to be more 'resistant' to illness than others: 'I think some people have got a better body resistance than somebody else. I don't really know why – whether it's to do with the blood grouping'.[35] This resistance could be strengthened by proper diet, clothing, tonics and so on, but was often seen as being inherited and constitutional: 'Some people are born resistant to colds and things'. Similarly, 'weakness' can be inherited or acquired; in the UK, some weaknesses are thought to 'run in families' ('all our family have weak chests'), but people who have been severely penetrated by environmental cold may also retain a permanent weakness – or gap in their defences – in that part of their body ('a weakness of the chest'). In Chrisman's[32] classification *debilitation* – a weakness of the body that results from overworking, being 'run-down', a chronic disease or a 'weak spot' in the body was a common lay aetiology. There was also *hereditary proneness*, which is the genetic transmission of a particular illness, quality or trait, which includes 'weakness'. In addition, he describes *degeneration* in the structure or function of body tissues or organs, such as occurs in the process of ageing, and *invasion* which, in the USA, spans the 'individual' and 'natural' zones of aetiology, and where illness is due either to external invasion by a 'germ' or other object, or internal spread from an existing problem, such as cancer. The other common individual aetiologies are *imbalance* – perceived as a state of disequilibrium, excess or depletion, such as 'vitamin deficiency' or 'a lack in the blood' – and *mechanical causes*, such as abnormal functioning of organs or systems ('bad circulation'), damage to parts of the body, 'blockage' of organs or blood vessels, and 'pressure' inside organs or parts of the body.

Explanations for ill-health that are patient centred are

important in determining whether people take responsibility for their health or whether they see the origin, and curing, of illness as lying outside their control.

The natural world

This includes aspects of the natural environment, both living and inanimate, which are thought to cause ill-health. Common in this group are climatic conditions such as excess cold, heat, wind, rain, snow or dampness. In the UK, for example, areas of environmental cold are believed to cause colds or chills if allowed to penetrate the boundary of the skin; cold draughts on the back cause a 'chill on the kidneys', cold rain on the head causes 'a head cold'. In Morocco excess environmental heat, as in sun-stroke, can enter the body and expand the blood vessels to cause a fullness and throbbing in the head – 'the blood has risen to my head'; as in the UK, cold air, cold draughts and getting wet are the cause of colds (*berd*) or chills (*bruda*).[36] Other climatic conditions include natural disasters such as cyclones, tornadoes or severe storms.

I would also include here the supposed influences on health of the moon, sun and planetary bodies, which is a common feature of societies where astrology is practised, although astrological birth signs can also be seen as a form of hereditary proneness to health or illness. Other natural aetiologies include injuries caused by animals or birds, and, at least in the Western world, *infections* caused by micro-organisms. In the UK, infectious fevers are ascribed to penetration of the body by living entities called, interchangeably, 'germs', 'bugs' or 'viruses', which are commonly thought of as being insect-like ('a tummy bug'). In some cases cancer is conceived of as invasion of the body by an external, living 'entity' which then grows and 'eats up' the body from within. Parasitic infestations, such as roundworms or threadworms, also form part of this group, as do accidental injuries, which also originate in the natural world. In Chrisman's classification, *environmental irritants* – such as allergens, pollens, poisons, food additives, smoke, fumes and other forms of pollution – were commonly ascribed causes of illness in the USA.

The social world

Blaming other people for one's ill-health is a common feature of smaller-scale societies, where interpersonal conflicts are frequent.

In some non-industrialized societies, the commonest forms of these are witchcraft, sorcery and the 'evil eye'. In all three, illness (and other forms of misfortune) is ascribed to inter-personal malevolence, whether conscious or unconscious. In *witchcraft* beliefs, which are particularly common in Africa and the Caribbean, certain people (usually women) are believed to possess a mystical power to harm others; as Landy[37] points out, this power is usually an intrinsic one, and is inherited, either genetically, or by membership of a particular kinship group. The witch is usually 'different' from other people, either in appearance or in behaviour; often they are ugly, disabled or socially isolated. They are usually the deviants or outcasts of a society, on whom all the negative, frightening aspects of the culture are projected. Their malevolent power, however, is often unconsciously practised, and not all witches are observ-ably deviant. Anthropologists have pointed out that witchcraft accusations are more common at times of social change, uncertainty and social conflict; competing factions within a society, for example, may accuse each other of causing their misfortunes by practising witchcraft. Under these circum-stances, the identity of the witch may need to be exposed in divinatory ritual, and its negative effect exorcised. Witchcraft beliefs were common in Europe in the Middle Ages; in Britain, illness was often ascribed to a witch's *maleficium*, and thousands of women were condemned as witches in the sixteenth and seventeenth centuries. This belief system has largely dis-appeared, but traces of interpersonal conflicts causing ill-health still persist in the language: 'He broke her heart' or 'She caused him much pain', or in modern psychiatric concepts such as the 'schizophrenogenic mother'.

Sorcery, defined by Landy[37] as 'the power to manipulate and alter natural and supernatural events with the proper magical knowledge and performance of ritual', is different from witchcraft. It is also extremely common in non-Western societies. The sorcerer exerts his or her power consciously, usually for reasons of envy or malice. He causes illness by certain spells, potions or rituals. For example, in a study[38] of health beliefs among low-income Black Americans, ill-health was often ascribed to sorcery – known as voodoo, hoodoo, crossing up, fixing, hexing or witchcraft. Sorcery is often practised among one's social world of friends, family or neighbours, and is often based on envy: as one informant put it, 'Put on a few little clothes and some people get begrudged-hearted'. The daughter of another informant had been 'killed by sorcery' practised by her in-laws, who were 'jealous of her pretty face, attentive husband and nice home'. In other cases, sorcery was used to control the behaviour of others, such as a wife using spells to prevent her husband leaving her. Illnesses that were ascribed to sorcery included a range of gastro-intestinal conditions, as well as general changes such as anorexia or weight loss. Sorcery beliefs of this type usually occur in groups whose lives are characterized by poverty, insecurity, danger, apprehension and a feeling of inadequacy and powerlessness.

The *Evil Eye* as an aetiology of illness has been reported throughout Europe, the Middle East and North Africa. In Italy it is the *mal occhia*, in Hispanic cultures it is *mal de ojo*, in Arabic cultures the *ayn*, in Hebrew the *ayin ha-ra*, in Iran the *cašm-e šur*. It is also known as 'the narrow eye', 'the bad eye', 'the wounding eye', or simply as 'the look'. According to Spooner,[39] it is found in the Middle East among all the communities there, whether Islamic, Jewish, Christian or Zoroastrian. He defines the main features of the Evil Eye as 'it relates to the fear of envy in the eye of the beholder', and says that 'its influence is avoided or counteracted by means of devices calculated to distract its attention, and by practices of sympathetic magic. Jealousy can kill via a look.' It can also cause several types of ill-health. The possessor of the Evil Eye usually harms unintentionally, and is often unaware of his powers and is unable to control them. In their study of Yemen, Underwood and Underwood[40] point out that such a person 'is usually either a stranger or a local person whose social activity, appearance, attitudes or behaviour is to some degree unorthodox or different', especially a person who 'stares' rather than speaks. In this type of society, therefore, either a tourist or a health worker from overseas might be thought of as a source of illness, whatever their good intentions – especially if they were seen staring at a child, and complimenting its appearance, just before it became ill.

The social aetiology of illness also includes physical injuries – such as poisoning or battle wounds – inflicted by other people. In many non-industrialized societies, however, other people usually cause illness by 'magical' means, such as witchcraft, sorcery or the Evil Eye. In modern Western society, lay notions of *stress* (see Chapter 11) also place the origin of ill-health within other people; in this model, illnesses are blamed on conflicts with spouses, children, family, friends, employers or work-mates. For example, 'I usually get a migraine if I have a row with the family', or 'I get ill whenever my boss gives me stress'.

Infections, too, can be blamed on other people, in the sense of 'He gave me his cold' or 'I caught his germ'. In addition, it could be argued that the over-use of litigation, especially in the USA, is analogous to witchcraft accusations, because it displaces the blame for suffering on to the malevolence or carelessness of others. In general, though, the widespread blaming of other individuals for one's own ill-health is more commonly a feature of smaller and pre-industrial societies than the more urban Western societies.

The supernatural world

Here illness is ascribed to the direct actions of supernatural entities, such as *gods, spirits* or *ancestral shades*. In the study of low-income Black Americans, quoted above, illness was often described as a 'reminder' from God for some behavioural lapse, such as neglecting to go to Church regularly, not saying one's prayers, or not thanking God for daily blessings. Illness was a 'whuppin', a divine punishment for sinful behaviour. On this basis, neither home remedies nor a physician were considered useful in treating the condition. A cure involves acknowledgement of sin, sorrow for having committed it and a vow to improve one's behaviour. Here, as Snow puts it, 'Prayer and repentance, not penicillin, cure sin'.[38] Similar approaches that link ill-health to divine disapproval of one's behaviour have also been described among middle-class suburban Americans.

In other societies illness is ascribed to capricious, malevolent 'spirits'. These have been described by Lewis[41] in some African communities where 'disease-bearing spirits' strike unexpectedly, causing a variety of symptoms in their victims. Their invasion is unrelated to the behaviour of the individual, who is therefore considered blameless and worthy of sympathetic help from others. Like 'germs' or 'viruses' in the Western world, these pathogenic spirits reveal their identity by the particular symptoms they cause, and can only be treated by driving them out of the body. A similar form of spirit possession – the *jinn* or *ginn* – is common in the Islamic world; in the Underwoods'[40] description, they are ubiquitous and capricious spirits that are 'semihuman rather than supernatural', and can also cause ill-health. Another form of 'spirit possession' described by Lewis[41] occurs when individuals are invaded, and made ill, by the spirits of their ancestors whom they have offended. This happens when the victim is guilty of immoral, blasphemous or antisocial behaviour. Diagnosis takes place in a divinatory séance, where illness is seen as punishment for these transgressions, and the moral values of the group are reaffirmed. While such supernatural explanations for illness as divine punishment or spirit possession are rare in the industrialized West, the only modern equivalent is blaming ill-health on 'bad luck', 'fate', 'the stars', or 'an act of God'.

In most cases lay theories of illness aetiology (like medical explanations) are *multicausal*; that is, they postulate several causes acting together. This means that individual, natural, social and supernatural causes are not mutually exclusive, but are usually linked together in a particular case. For example, careless or immoral behaviour may predispose to natural illnesses, divine anger or spirit possession, or an ostentatious lifestyle may attract sorcery or the Evil Eye. In any specific case of illness, moreover, lay explanatory models vary in how they explain its aetiology; in Blaxter's[42] study of working-class women in Aberdeen, for example, there was marked variation in how some common conditions were explained. Of the 30 women interviewed, eight attributed 'bronchitis' to environmental factors, two to behaviour, four to heredity, three to 'susceptibility', ten as secondary to other conditions, and three as the consequence of pregnancy or childbirth. While these are seen as discrete categories in Blaxter's study, most explanatory models see illness as multicausal, with elements of several types of aetiology involved in a particular episode of ill-health.

Classification of illness aetiologies

Foster and Anderson[43] have proposed an alternative way of classifying lay illness aetiologies, especially in non-Western societies. They differentiate between *personalistic* and *naturalistic* systems. In the former, illness is due to the purposeful active intervention of an *agent*, such as a supernatural being (a god), a non-human being (ghost, ancestral spirit, capricious spirits), or human being (witch or sorcerer). One could also include modern notions of 'germs' in this category, especially those causing fevers. In naturalistic systems, illness is explained in impersonal, systemic terms; it can be caused by natural forces or by conditions such as cold, wind or damp, or by disequilibrium within the individual or the social environment. Included in this disequilibrium group are systems of illness explanation such as humoral or hot–cold systems in Latin America, Ayurvedic medicine in India, and the *yin–yang* system of traditional

Chinese medicine. The colds and chills caused by environmental cold could also be included here.

Young[44] has classified belief systems about ill-health as either *externalizing* or *internalizing*. Externalizing belief systems concentrate mainly on the aetiology of the illness, which is believed to arise *outside* the sick person's body, especially in the social world. Thus, in trying to identify a cause for the individual's illness, they examine closely the circumstances and social events of the patient's life before falling ill – such as tracing the cause of an illness from a grudge between two people, then to feelings of resentment, then to some pathogenic act (such as witchcraft, or sorcery), which then led to the illness itself. Many of the lay models of illness aetiology from different parts of the world, described in this chapter, can therefore be described as externalizing types of explanations. By contrast, internalizing belief systems concentrate less on aetiological explanations, but more on events that occur (and arise) *inside* the individual's body – and they always emphasize physiological and pathological processes as explanations for how, and why, some people become ill. This is the perspective of the modern, scientific medical model. Its strength lies in its detailed perception of physiological events within the individual body, but its weakness lies in ignoring the social and psychological events that preceded the onset of symptoms – while the reverse is true of the externalizing systems.

Another feature of externalizing explanations for ill-health is that they often take the form of a *narrative* or story about how and why that person became ill. This story may include events from the sufferer's life, and even events that preceded his or her birth (such as 'I inherited my weak chest from my father's family'). As Brody[45] points out, telling such 'stories of sickness' is a way of giving *meaning* to the experience of ill-health, of placing it in the context of the individual's life history, and of relating it to the wider themes of the society and culture in which he or she lives.

In the following case histories, two folk illnesses, one from the USA and one from the UK, are briefly described. In both cases the illness is a cluster of symptoms and signs which are subject to individual and contextual variations.

Case history: 'Hyper-tension' in Seattle, USA

Blumhagen's study,[46] carried out in Seattle at the Veterans Administration Medical Center, was on patients suffering from hypertension. He discovered a lay EM held by many of the patients about their condition, termed 'hyper-tension'. The majority saw their condition as arising from 'stress' or 'tension' in their daily lives (hence hyper-*tension*). In 49% of the sample, chronic 'external stress' such as overworking, unemployment, 'life's stresses and strains' and certain occupations were blamed for the condition; 14% blamed chronic 'internal stress', such as psychological, interpersonal or family problems. Of the total sample 56% thought the condition could be precipitated by 'acute stress', such as anxiety, excitement or anger. In this model, hyper-tension is characterized by subjective symptoms such as nervousness, fear, anxiety, worry, anger, upset, tenseness, overactivity, exhaustion and excitement. It is brought on by stress, which makes the individual susceptible to becoming hyper-tense. In many cases, they did not perceive that hypertension was the same as 'high blood pressure', because their model emphasized the psychosocial origin, and manifestations of the condition. A smaller number saw hyper-tension as resulting from hereditary or physical factors, such as excess salt, water, fatty foods. Overall, though, 72% believed that hyper-tension is 'a physical reflection of past social and environmental stressors, which are exacerbated by current stressful situations', and this allowed them to withdraw from familial, social or work obligations which they saw as sources of tension. They also labelled themselves as hyper-tense, even in the absence of medical evidence for hypertension.

Case history: 'Colds', 'chills' and 'fevers' in London, UK

I have described a set of commonly held beliefs about 'colds', 'chills' and 'fevers' in a London suburb.[47] Colds and chills are caused by the penetration of the natural environment (particularly areas of cold or damp) across the boundary of the skin and into the human body. In general, damp or rain (cold/wet environments) cause cold/wet conditions in the body, such as a 'runny nose' or a 'cold in the head', while cold winds or draughts (cold/dry environments) cause cold/dry conditions such as a feeling of cold, shivering and muscular aches. Once they enter the body, these cold forces can move from place to place – from a 'head cold', for example, down to a 'chest cold'. Chills occur mainly below the belt ('a bladder chill', 'a chill on the kidneys', 'a stomach chill'), and colds above it ('a head cold', 'a cold in the sinuses', 'a cold in the chest'). These conditions are caused by careless behaviour, by putting oneself in a position of risk *vis-á-vis* the natural environment; for example, by 'walking barefoot on a cold floor', 'washing your hair when you don't feel well', or 'sitting in a draught after a hot bath'. Temperatures intermediate between hot and cold, where the former gives way to the latter, such as going outdoors after a hot bath, or else in autumn, where 'hot' summer gives way to 'cold' autumn, are specially conducive to 'catching cold'. Because colds and chills are brought about primarily by one's own behaviour, they provoke little sympathy among other people; individuals are often expected to treat themselves by rest in a warm bed, eating warm food ('Feed a cold, starve a fever') and drinking a hot drink.

By contrast, fevers are caused by 'germs', 'bugs' or 'viruses', which penetrate the body by its orifices (mouth, nose, ears, anus, urethra, nostrils) and then cause a raised temperature and other symptoms. The causative agents are conceived of as invisible, amoral, malign entities which exist in and among people, and which travel between people through the air. Some, like 'tummy bugs', are though of as almost insect-like, though of a very small size. Germs have 'personalities' of symptoms and signs, which reveal themselves over time ('I've got that germ, doctor, you know – the one that gives you the dry cough and the watery eyes'). Unlike victims of colds, the victims of a fever are blameless, and can mobilize a caring community around themselves. The germs responsible for these conditions can be 'flushed out' by fluids (such as cough medicines), starved out by avoiding food, or killed in the body by antibiotics, though in the latter case no differentiation is made between viruses and 'germs'. These lay beliefs about the colds/chills/fevers range of illnesses can affect behaviour, self-treatment and attitudes towards medical treatment.

The doctor–patient consultation

Against this background of lay beliefs about illness, one can view three aspects of the doctor–patient interaction:

1. Why do people decide (or not decide) to consult a doctor when ill?
2. What happens during the consultation?
3. What happens after the consultation?

Reasons for consulting or not consulting a doctor

Several studies have examined the reasons why some ill people consult a doctor, while others with the same complaint do not. Often this is because people cannot afford to pay for medical care, but even when they *can* afford it there is often little correlation between the severity of a physical illness and the decision to seek medical help. In some cases this delay can have serious consequences for the patient's health. Other studies have shown that abnormal symptoms are common in the population, but only a small percentage are brought to the attention of doctors. There are therefore a number of *non*-physiological factors that influence what Zola[48] terms the 'pathways to the doctor'. These include:

1. The availability of medical care.
2. Whether the patient can afford it.
3. The failure, or success, of treatments within the popular or folk sectors.
4. How the patient perceives the problem.
5. How others around them perceive the problem.

In this section, only the last two points, and the relationship between them, will be discussed.

The process of becoming 'ill' has already been described, particularly the definition of some symptoms as 'abnormal' by patients and their families. Zola[48] has pointed out how this definition depends on how common the symptom is in their society, and whether it fits with the major values of that society or group. If the symptom is very common, it may be considered 'normal' (though not necessarily 'good') and therefore be accepted fatalistically; for example, as Zola found, 'tiredness' is often considered to be normal, even though it is sometimes a feature of severe illness. In the study of Regionville mentioned above, backache was considered to be a normal part of life, at least by the lower socioeconomic groups. The second point is that symptoms or signs must fit with a society's view of what constitutes 'illness' for it to gain sympathetic attention and for treatment to be arranged. The same symptom or sign might be interpreted differently, therefore, by different groups of individuals – as illness in one and as normal in another. In both cases, the definition of ill-health depends on the underlying concept of health which, as noted earlier, often includes social, behavioural or emotional elements.

Zola[49] has also examined how this wider definition of health affects patients' decisions to consult a doctor. He interviewed over 200 patients from three ethnic groups – Irish Americans, Italian Americans and Anglo-Saxon Protestant Americans – attending out-patient clinics in two Boston hospitals. The study aimed to find out why they had decided to consult a doctor, and how they communicated their distress to him. It was found that there were two ways of perceiving, and communicating, one's bodily complaints: either 'restricting' or 'generalizing' them. The first was typical of the Irish, the second of the Italians. The Irish focused on a specific physical dysfunction (such as poor eyesight or ptosis) and restricted its effect to their physical functioning. The Italians displayed many more symptoms, and a more 'global malfunctioning' of many aspects of their body – appearance, energy level, emotions and so on. In their perception, the physical symptoms (such as poor eyesight) interfered with their general mode of living, their social relationships, and their occupations.

On this basis, Zola was able to identify five non-physiological 'triggers' to the decision to seek medical aid:

1. An interpersonal crisis.
2. Perceived interference with personal relationships.
3. 'Sanctioning'; that is, one individual takes primary responsibility for the decision to seek medical aid for someone else (the patient).
4. Perceived interference with work or physical functioning.
5. The setting of external time criteria ('If it isn't better in 3 days . . . then I'll take care of it.').

Both 1 and 2 draw attention to the symptom, by signifying that there is 'something wrong' in the patients' daily lives; this pattern was common among the Italians. Pattern 3 was common among the Irish, and also illustrates the social dimensions of illness ('Well I tend to let things go but not my wife, so on the first day of my vacation my wife said, "Why don't you come, why don't you take care of it now?" So I did.'). The 'functional' definition (4) of health was common among both Irish and Anglo-Saxon groups (cf. Blaxter and Paterson[11]). Attitude 5 was common among all the groups.

This study illustrates that the decision to consult a doctor may be related to sociocultural factors, such as wider definitions of health, rather than to the severity of the illness. As Zola points out, in any community unexplained epidemiological differences may be due more to the differential occurrence of these factors, which reflect the 'selectivity and attention which get people and their episodes into medical statistics, rather than to any true difference in the prevalence and incidence of a particular problem or disorder' (see Chapter 12).

Apple[13] has pointed out the dangers of defining a symptom as illness only when it interferes with one's usual activities and is of fairly recent onset. It means that more chronic insidious conditions, such as heart disease, cancer or HIV infection may not be defined as abnormal provided one can carry on with daily life. Other reasons for the delay in seeking medical advice have been studied at the Massachusetts General Hospital in Boston. Hackett et al.[50] there examined the delay between the first sign or symptom of cancer and the search for medical help in 563 patients. Only 33.7% were 'early responders' and consulted within the first 4 weeks, while two-thirds waited over a month; 8% of the sample avoided medical help until they could no longer function independently, and only then did they 'yield to family or community pressure and receive medical help'. The role of emotional factors was important: people who worried more about cancer tended to delay seeking help more than non-worriers and it was hypothesized that the reason for the delay might be to avoid hearing the fatal diagnosis. The label given to the illness also affected the delay; labelling it candidly as cancer led to a quicker response. In general, patients from higher socioeconomic levels delayed a shorter time than those from poorer classes, though 'there is little evidence that cancer education programs per se can be credited for this difference'. In another study, Olin and Hackett[51] studied 32 patients with acute myocardial infarction. Most had explained away their chest pain as resulting from less serious conditions, such as 'indigestion', 'lung trouble', 'pneumonia' or 'ulcer', despite the fact that they were familiar with the symptoms of coronary heart disease. The immediate response was denial, which was 'the consequence of an emotional crisis induced by chest pain and the menacing associations it evokes'. In the majority of cases, only increasing incapacity, or the persuasion of family or friends, led them to seek medical help.

Whether medical care – provided it is available and affordable – is utilized also depends on the perceived aetiology of the condition: whether it is believed to originate in the individual, or in the natural, social or supernatural worlds. Some groups consider that medicine is the better treatment for symptoms than eliminating the cause, especially if it is supernatural. In a study[52] of five ethnic groups in Miami, for example, patients sought symptomatic relief from a medical doctor but expected a folk healer to explain the cause in culturally familiar terms (such as witchcraft), and then to treat it by mystical means.

In all the above cases, a number of non-physiological factors – social, cultural and emotional – influence whether ill people or their families seek medical help or not. These factors also influence how this illness is presented in the doctor–patient consultation.

The presentation of illness

Elsewhere I have described how different sociocultural groups utilize different *languages of distress* in communicating their suffering to others, including to doctors. A clinician who is unable to 'decode' this language, which may be verbal or non-verbal, is in danger of making the wrong diagnosis. For example, in Zola's[49] study the Italian Americans presented their illness in a more voluble, emotional and dramatic way, complaining of many more symptoms, and stressing its effect on their social circumstances, while by contrast the Irish tended to underplay their symptoms. Where *no* organic disease was found, the physicians tended to diagnose the Italians as having neurotic or psychological conditions, such as 'tension headaches', 'functional problems' or 'personality disorder', while the Irish were given a neutral diagnosis such as 'nothing found on tests', without being labelled neurotic. At the same time, the Irish stoicism in the presentation of illness could lead to more serious conditions being missed. Zborowski's[53] findings were similar, in his study of responses to pain by Irish American, Italian American and Jewish American patients in New York; the more emotional the language of distress, the more likely was the patient to be *wrongly* labelled neurotic or over-emotional.

The presentation of illness may also be learnt from doctors, as well as from the media, especially by patients with chronic diseases. They learn to display the 'typical' clinical picture that the doctors are looking for. In my own study[54] a patient who was mistakenly diagnosed as having angina from 'heart trouble' developed psychosomatic chest pain which gradually came to resemble 'real' angina the more contact he had with clinicians, especially cardiologists. This 'symptom choice', in the absence of physical disease, has been described by Mechanic[55] in the case of 'medical students' disease', a form of hypochondria believed to afflict up to 70% of medical students. As they learn about the various diseases, they frequently imagine they are suffering from them, and even develop their 'typical' symptoms and signs. According to Mechanic, the stressful conditions of medical school cause many transient symptoms in the students, and those 'diffuse and ambiguous symptoms regarded as normal in the past may be reconceptualized within the context of newly acquired knowledge of disease'. This may influence the patterning and presentation of their symptomatology. This, then, is an example of a language of distress acquired from the medical profession.

Problems of the doctor–patient consultation

The clinical consultation, as Kleinman[16] has noted, is a transaction between lay and professional explanatory models – though it is also a transaction between two parties separated by differences in power, both social and symbolic. Although the consultation is characterized by ritual and symbolic elements, its manifest functions are:

1. Presentation of 'illness' by the patient, both verbally and non-verbally.
2. Translation of these diffuse symptoms or signs into the named pathological entities of medicine, that is, converting 'illness' into 'disease'.
3. Prescribing a treatment regimen which is acceptable both to doctor and to patient.

Some of its more latent functions, especially in relation to social control, have already been discussed in the previous chapter. For the consultation to be a success, there must be a *consensus* between the two parties about the aetiology, diagnostic label, physiological processes involved, prognosis and optimal treatment for the condition. The search for a consensus – for an agreed interpretation of the patient's condition – has been called 'negotiation' by Stimson and Webb.[56] In this process, each tries to influence the other regarding the outcome of the consultation, the diagnosis given and the treatment prescribed. Patients may try to reduce the seriousness of a diagnosis or the severity of a treatment regimen, for example. In particular, they may strive for diagnoses and treatments that make sense to them in terms of their lay view of ill health, such as the appeal for tonics or vitamins in the UK, which have deep roots in traditional medicine. The consultation is also a *social* process, whereby the ill person acquires the social role of patient, with all the rights and obligations that this entails.

Within the consultation, one can isolate a number of recurring problems that interfere with the development of consensus.

These problems, many of which have already been described, include the following.

Differences in the definition of 'the patient'

Western medicine focuses increasingly on the individual patient and his or her problems,[1] but it may be the *family* – or even the community – who are pathological, and not the individual. An inappropriate focus only on the individual and their symptoms, and ignoring wider social issues, may make both a consensus and a solution to the problem difficult to achieve.

Misinterpretation of patients' 'languages of distress'

These are illustrated in the studies of Zola, Apple, Mechanic and Zborowski. This phenomenon is more likely if doctor and patient come from different cultural or religious backgrounds, or socioeconomic classes.

Incompatibility of explanatory models

Medical and lay models may differ greatly in how they interpret a particular illness episode, especially its aetiology, diagnosis and appropriate treatment. They are based on different understandings of the structure, function and malfunction of the body. They also vary on definitions of health or ill-health, and the forces which may change one state into the other. For example, Western-trained doctors working in a rural setting in the developing world may have difficulty in understanding supernatural or interpersonal explanations of ill-health, or definitions of good health as moral or social 'balance'. The disease perspective of modern medicine, with its emphasis on quantifiable physical data, may ignore the many dimensions of meaning – psychological, moral or social – that characterize the illness perspective of the patient, and those around him. Emotional states such as guilt, shame, remorse or fear on the patient's part may not be taken into account by the doctor who concentrates only on the diagnosis and treatment of physical dysfunction.

Disease without illness

This is a common phenomenon in modern medicine, with its emphasis on the use of diagnostic technology. Physical abnormalities of the body are found, often on the cellular or chemical level, but the patient does not feel ill. Examples of this are hypertension, raised blood cholesterol, cervical carcinoma-in-situ, or HIV infection, which are found on routine health screening programmes. Patients who are asymptomatic may not make use of these programmes, or may refuse treatment if an abnormality is found ('But I don't *feel* unwell'). This may also explain much of the reported non-compliance with prescribed medication; for example, patients prescribed a 1-week course of antibiotics may stop taking them after 2 or 3 days because they no longer feel 'ill'.

Illness without disease

Here the patients feel that 'something is wrong' in their life – physically, emotionally or socially – but despite their subjective state they are told, after a physical examination, that 'there is nothing wrong with you'. However, in many cases, they still continue to feel unwell or unhappy. Included in this group are the many unpleasant emotions or physical sensations for which no physical cause can be found – many of them arising from the stress of everyday life; the various psychosomatic disorders (such as irritable colon, spasmodic torticollis, hyperventilation syndrome or Da Costa's syndrome); hypochondria (such as medical students' disease); and the wide range of folk illnesses (such as spirit possession, *susto* or 'high blood'). In each of these cases the 'illness' plays an important part in the patient's life, and reassurance that nothing is wrong physically may not be enough to treat it, as illustrated in the following case history.

Case history: Illness without disease

Balint[57] describes the case of Mr U., aged 35, a skilled workman who was partly disabled following polio in childhood. Nevertheless he had managed to work, 'over-compensating his physical shortcomings by high efficiency'. One day he received a severe electric shock at work, and was knocked unconscious; no organic damage was found at the hospital, and he was discharged. He then consulted his family doctor for 'pains' in all parts of his body, which were getting worse and worse, and 'he thought that something had happened to him through the electric shock'. Despite exhaustive tests, no physical abnormality was found, but Mr U. still experienced his symptoms: 'They seem to think I am imagining things: I know what I've got.' He still felt definitely ill and wanted 'to know what condition he could have causing all these pains'. Despite more hospital tests that were negative, he still felt himself to be ill. In Balint's view he was 'proposing an illness' to the doctor, but this was consistently rejected; the doctor's emphasis was not on the patient's pains, anxieties, fears and hopes for sympathy and understanding, but on the exclusion of an underlying physical abnormality.

Problems of terminology

Clinical consultations are usually conducted in a mixture of everyday language and medical jargon. This is largely because the language of medicine itself has become more and more technical and esoteric over the past century or so,[58] and increasingly incomprehensible to the lay public. Where medical terms *are* used by either party, there is often a danger of mutual misunderstanding; the same term, for example, may have entirely different meanings for doctor and patient. Boyle[59] studied the differences between doctors' and patients' interpretation of common medical terms, such as stomach, heartburn, palpitation, flatulence or lungs (see Chapter 2). He found marked variations between the two groups, which could have important clinical implications, especially since many consultations include questions such as, 'Do you have pain in your stomach?' (which 58.8% of the patients thought occupied their entire abdominal cavity). A study by Pearson and Dudley[60] had similar findings, with misunderstanding of terms like gallbladder, stomach or liver. They point out that patients awaiting cholecystectomy may become extremely anxious if, like some of the sample, they believe that the gallbladder is concerned with the storage of urine. Similarly, in Blumhagen's study, lay beliefs about the meaning of hyper-tension were different from medical definitions of hypertension. In the study of lay beliefs about germs and viruses quoted above, these bore little relation to their description in microbiology; both were considered vulnerable to antibiotics, and these drugs were demanded even if the diagnosis was 'a viral infection'. The use of the same terminology by doctor and patient is not, therefore, a guarantee of mutual understanding; the terms, and their significance, may be conceptualized by both parties in entirely different ways.

Patients' use of specialized folk terminology may also confuse the clinician: statements such as 'I have been hexed' or 'a spirit has made me ill' may be incomprehensible to the doctor, unless he is aware of lay theories of illness causation. The same applies to self-labelled folk illnesses, such as *susto*, 'heart distress' or 'brain fag', especially where the clinician originates in a different culture.

Questions in the consultation that are designed to uncover emotional distress may also involve problems of terminology. For example, Leff,[61] in a study in London, compared psychiatrists' and patients' concepts of unpleasant emotions. It was found that the psychiatrists clearly differentiated between anxiety, depression and irritability as discrete types of emotional distress, while the patients saw them as closely overlapping. To the patients, somatic symptoms such as palpitations, excessive perspiration or shakiness were considered to be as characteristic of depression as of anxiety. This would clearly influence how patients responded to specific questions such as 'Do you feel depressed?' or 'Do you feel anxious?' Again, ignorance of how patients conceptualize and label ill-health can lead to the misinterpretation of symptoms during the consultation.

Problems of treatment

For medical treatment to be acceptable to patients, it must make sense in terms of their explanatory models. Consensus here about the form and purpose of treatment are as important as consensus in diagnostic labelling. This is particularly important if the prescribed treatment involves unpleasant physical sensations, or side-effects – that is, where it induces a form of temporary 'illness'. This is the case in surgery, injections, biopsies, radiotherapy, chemotherapy, and certain diagnostic tests such as sigmoidoscopy. Prescribed medication may not be taken if it is perceived to cause illness, or – as in the case of asymptomatic hypertension – if the patient does not feel at all ill. If relatives or friends have had side-effects from the same drug, it may also not be taken. Another problem, mentioned elsewhere, is that self-medication is common, often in conjunction with the use of prescribed drugs; both may be used by patients in ways that make sense to them in terms of their lay view of ill-health. The phenomenon of non-compliance has been estimated, in the UK, as 30% or more.[62] In one study by Waters et al.,[63] out of 1611 prescriptions issued by general practitioners, 7% were not even presented to pharmacists. The misuse of prescribed medication, based on specific lay perspectives on medical treatment, has been described by Harwood[64] among a group of Puerto Ricans in New York City (see Chapter 3), who divided all illnesses, foods and medicines into 'hot', 'cold' and sometimes 'cool'. Penicillin was regarded as a 'hot' drug, and was appropriate for prophylactic treatment in rheumatic heart disease (a 'cold' illness); if, however, the patient experienced diarrhoea or constipation (hot conditions), he would immediately break off penicillin treatment. In pregnancy, 'hot' foods or medications were avoided, lest they caused 'hot' illnesses, such as rashes or red skin, in the baby; because iron supplements or vitamins were 'hot', they might also be refused. Similar avoidance of 'hot' foods or medications during pregnancy have been found in other communities, in different parts of the world.

The success of a treatment or medication is often measured in different ways by doctor and patient. The disappearance of an identifiable disease may not be accompanied by the disappearance of illness, though this situation can be reversed. For example, Cay et al.[65] examined patients' assessment of the results of surgery for peptic ulcers, and compared these with the surgeons' assessments. They found marked discrepancies in these two perspectives. Doctor-determined criteria of success, such as acid reduction, absence of diarrhoea, freedom from recurrence or completeness of antrectomy or vagotomy, differed from those of patients who used psychosocial criteria such as effect on family life, social life, work, sex and sleeping habits. A success in the eyes of a surgeon may be a failure in the eyes of the patient, if the operation interferes with any of these aspects of the 'quality of life'. That is, 'a bad result . . . is determined more by psychosocial than physical evidence of failure'. Conversely, operations which the surgeons regarded as failures – due to residual symptoms of diarrhoea, for example – were regarded by patients as a success, and the residual symptoms 'a price worth paying' for the absence of severe and unpredictable ulcer symptoms. In both cases one can hypothesize an underlying functional definition of health, against which the success of the operation was judged.

The role of context

A final area of problems in the doctor–patient consultation is the role played by the *context* of that consultation.[17] There are two aspects to this context, both of which play a part in the consultation:

1. An *internal context* of the prior experience, expectations, cultural assumptions, explanatory models, and prejudices (based on social, gender, religious or racial criteria) that each party brings to the clinical encounter.
2. An *external context* which includes the actual setting in which the encounter takes place (such as a hospital, clinic or doctor's office) and the wider social influences acting upon the two parties – such as the dominant ideology, religion or economic system of the society – and which in turn helps to define who has power in the consultation, and who does not.

The sum of these two types of contexts can greatly influence the types of communication possible between doctor and patient, because they help determine what is said in the consultation, how it is said, and how it is heard and interpreted.[66]

The doctor–patient relationship: strategies for improvement

In this chapter I have outlined some of the differences in medical and lay perspectives on ill-health – between models of 'disease' and those of 'illness' – and some of the problems that this raises in the consultation. Four main strategies can be suggested to deal with these problems:

1. Understanding illness.
2. Improving communication.
3. Treating illness *and* disease.
4. Assessing the role of context.

Understanding 'illness'

As well as searching for 'disease', the clinician should try to discover how patients, and those around them, view the origin, significance and prognosis of the condition, and also how it affects other aspects of their lives – such as income or social relationships. The patients' emotional reactions to ill-health (such as guilt, fear, shame, anger, uncertainty) are all as relevant to the clinical encounter as physiological data. Patients' explanatory models should be elicited, by obtaining the answers to the seven questions listed above. Information should also be gathered about patients' cultural, religious and social background, economic status, previous experience of ill-health, and, if possible, view of misfortune in general, to put their explanations for ill-health in context.

Improving communication

The clinician should acquire a knowledge of the specific language of distress utilized by the patient, especially the presentation of culturally specific folk illnesses. There should also be an awareness of the problems of terminology mentioned above, especially the misinterpretation of medical terms by the patient. The clinician's diagnosis and treatment must *make sense* to the patient, in terms of their lay view of ill-health, and should acknowledge and respect the patient's experience and interpretation of his or her own condition. As Mechanic puts it, 'the efficacy of the doctor's interpretations of his patient's problems will depend on the extent to which they are credible in terms of the patient's experiences and the extent to which he anticipates the patient's reactions to symptoms and treatment.' The clinician should always reflect on the role of his or her *own* social background, culture, economic status, religion, education, gender, personal prejudices, and professional power in either improving, or reducing, both doctor–patient communication and the provision of effective health care.

Treating 'illness' and 'disease'

Medical treatment should never deal only with physical abnormalities or malfunctions; the many dimensions of 'illness' – emotional, social, behavioural, religious – should be treated by adequate explanation and reassurance in terms that make sense to the patient. Where necessary, treatment may have to be shared with a psychotherapist, counsellor or priest, or with a social worker, self-help group, housing or employment agency, or community organization – or even, in some settings, with a culturally sanctioned folk healer. In this way, *all* dimensions of the patient's 'illness' can be treated, as well as any physical 'disease'.

Assessing the role of context

To understand any doctor–patient interaction, the role of both internal and external contexts described above should always be assessed. It is particularly important to understand those external contexts, such as social and economic factors (including poverty or unemployment), that may contribute to the origin, presentation and prognosis of ill-health. A consideration of context also helps the clinician decide *who* is the real patient, and whether the focus of diagnosis and treatment should be on the sick individual,. their family, their community, or the society in which they live.

Recommended reading

Disease *versus* Illness

Eisenberg, L. (1977) Disease and illness: distinctions between professional and popular ideas of sickness. *Cult. Med. Psychiatry* **1**, 9–23

Kleinman, A. (1980) *Patients and Healers in the Context of Culture*. Berkeley: University of California Press. See Chapters 3 and 4 for a discussion of lay and practitioner explanatory models.

Lock, M. and Gordon, D. (eds). (1988) *Biomedicine Examined.*Dordrecht: Kluwer. A collection of essays on the culture and ideology of modern medicine.

Lay health beliefs

Currer, C. and Stacey, M. (eds). (1986) *Concepts of Health, Illness and Disease.* Leamington Spa: Berg Publishers. A collection of key essays on lay health beliefs.

Foster, G. M. and Anderson B. G. (1978) *Medical Anthropology*. New York: Wiley. See Chapter 4 on Ethnomedicine.

Helman, C. G. (1978) 'Feed a cold, starve a fever': folk models of infection in an English suburban community, and their relation to medical treatment. *Cult. Med. Psychiatry* **2**, 107–137

Chapter 6

Gender and reproduction

All human societies divide their populations into two social categories, which they call 'Male' and 'Female'.

Each of these categories is based on a series of assumptions – drawn from the culture in which they occur – about the different attributes, beliefs and behaviours characteristic of the individuals included within that category.

Although this binary division of humanity into two genders is universal, on closer examination one can see that it is a rather more complex phenomenon, with many variations reported in how 'male' and 'female' behaviour is defined in different cultural groups. To illustrate this point, the following chapter will examine two separate, though interrelated, subjects: anthropological research into gender, and its relationship to health and health care; and pregnancy and childbirth in cross-cultural perspective.

Gender

The nature *versus* nurture controversy

One of the basic debates of social thought, especially for the past century or so, has been the 'nature' *versus* 'nurture' controversy – which in anthropology has been the debate between the ideas of 'nature' and those of 'culture'. In summary, this nature/nurture debate centred on whether human behaviour and the human mind (including its intelligence and personality) – as well as perceived differences between human groups (such as ethnic or religious groups, social classes or genders) – were all due to *nature* or to *nurture*. 'Nature' was conceptualized as rooted in biology, and as something fixed, universal and immutable, while 'nurture' was seen as the influence of the environment (both social and cultural) and therefore was more changeable, and more dependent on local contexts. This conceptual division had all sorts of political and social implications; taking the strict 'nature' line, for example, could

127

mean that one group of people (or one gender) were regarded as 'biologically' inferior to another, and that this could never be altered, no matter what environmental influences were brought to bear upon them. Within the last century this approach has often been used as a justification for the persecution, colonization or exploitation of various groups of people in different parts of the world.

Today this type of debate has largely receded, at least in academic circles, and most anthropologists would reject both extreme biological determinism *and* extreme environmental determinism. In explaining human behaviour they would look instead at the complex *interaction* – within a specific environment – between culture, ecology and social structure, and the psychobiological nature of human beings.[1]

The echoes of the nature/nurture debate still remain in contemporary discussions of gender. Here gender is often described as if it were the result of either 'nature' *or* of 'culture' (that is, of 'nurture'). Feminist anthropologists[2] have pointed out that, in Western thought particularly, women and their sexuality have often been seen as 'less cultural' than men, and equated instead with 'nature' (uncontrolled, dangerous, polluting) rather than with the 'culture' (controlled, creative, ordered) of the male world. They have argued that this conceptual division of 'nature' from 'culture' (and the implied opposition between the two) is in itself artificial, a false dichotomy that represents a specifically Western and culture-bound way of looking at human behaviour. Furthermore, this way of thinking, and the conceptual division of the world into these two value-laden categories, is not found to the same extent elsewhere in the world.

They have also pointed out the social implications of this division, for in Western thought 'culture' is usually seen as superior, and more human, than 'nature'. At its most extreme – especially in the nineteenth century – this model provided a justification for the superiority of men, for it saw female 'nature' as something to be conquered, transformed, and then made productive by the forces of male 'culture'.

In looking at sexual identity, though, it is reasonable to say that both biological *and* environmental influences play some part in the definition of any individual's gender. In all societies, men and women have different body shapes, and different physiological cycles; women menstruate, give birth and lactate, while men do not. However, it is the *cultural meanings* that are given to those physiological events, and how these in turn influence people's behaviour, and even the social, political and economic system of the society, that is of chief interest to the modern anthropologist.

Components of gender

The gender of a particular individual can best be understood as the result of a complex combination of a number of elements. These include:

1. *Genetic gender*, based on genotype, and the combinations of the two sex chromosomes, X and Y (XX = female and XY = male).
2. *Somatic gender*, based on phenotype, especially physical appearance, and the development of secondary sex characteristics (external genitalia, breasts, voice and distribution of body fat and hair).
3. *Psychological gender*, based on the person's own self-perception and behaviour.
4. *Social gender*, based on the wider cultural categories of male and female, which define how that individual is perceived by society, how he or she must look, think, feel, dress, act, and perceive the world that they live in.

However, at each of these levels there are areas of anomaly and ambiguity in this neat binary division of humankind. At the genetic level, for example, the division of the population into either XX or XY can be altered where certain abnormalities of the sex chromosomes occur, such as in Turner's syndrome (XO), Klinefelter's syndrome (XXY), Y polysomy (XYY), or even true hermaphroditism (XX/XY).[3] At the somatic level, abnormalities of hormonal development can lead to secondary sex characteristics that are at variance with genetic gender. Examples include both male and female *pseudohermaphroditism*, where an individual has the genetic constitution and gonads of one sex, but the external genitalia of the other.[3] People may also have both genotype and phenotype of a biological male, be defined as male by the wider society, and yet behave, dress and perceive themselves as essentially *female* – as in the case of some transexuals.

Of all aspects of gender identity, *social* gender is the one most flexible, and most influenced by social and cultural environment. Anthropologists who have studied the two categories of male and female in many societies throughout the world have found a great many variations in the scope and content of each of these categories. That is, they have found that behaviour considered appropriately male (or female) in one group may often be considered more female (or male) in another.

Gender cultures

Until comparatively recently, most of the fieldwork carried out by male anthropologists paid little attention to the 'women's worlds' of the societies that they studied.[4] Where the male and female worlds were very separate, they had virtually no access to the inner secrets of the women's worlds, especially to their beliefs and practices relating to sexuality, pregnancy, childbirth and menstruation. In recent years, however, a large number of ethnographies have been done, especially by female anthropologists, which have corrected this earlier imbalance. One of the features of this new wave of research is to highlight the role of nurture, or social and cultural influences, on the definitions of gender in human societies.

In all societies, the division of the social world into male and female categories means that boys and girls are socialized in very different ways. They are educated to have different expectations of life, and to develop emotionally and intellectually in particular ways, and are subject in their daily lives to different norms of dress and behaviour. Whatever the contribution of biology to human behaviour, it is clear that *culture* also contributes a set of guidelines – both explicit and implicit – which are acquired from infancy onwards, and which tell the individual how to perceive, think, feel and act as either a male or a female member of that society.

One can describe these two sets of guidelines, within a particular society, as the *gender cultures* of that society. In some parts of the world, especially in less industrialized countries, these gender cultures may be so different from one another that one could even describe men and women in that society as living like 'two nations under one flag'.

As an example of this, in many societies in New Guinea, men's and women's worlds are so polarized that they actually live in separate houses, in different parts of the village, and in Keesing's[5] words, 'have sexual relations infrequently in an atmosphere of tension and danger'. In some of these societies, where homosexuality is institutionalized, this adds further to the polarization of the two sexes.

In another example, Goddard[6] has described the different

male and female worlds in the city of Naples, Italy, especially in
relation to sexual behaviour, and to the cultural values of
'honour' and 'shame'. Very different norms, and a moral double
standard, operate for each of the sexes. For example, 'healthy',
'normal' men are expected to have many premarital and
extramarital affairs as proof of their 'masculinity', while women
are barred from either. Men are expected to actively defend their
own and their family's honour, while women's honour lies in
preserving their purity and chastity. Men's honour can be
damaged (and be replaced by shame) if the honour of their
womenfolk is compromised in any way. But, as in other
cultures, there is an ambivalence in the men's attitudes towards
women, who in this Mediterranean community are seen as
'either dangerously vulnerable or eminently available and
seducible'. Dunk[7] has described a similar picture among Greek
villagers living in Montreal. Despite local variations, there is a
general assumption in rural Greece that men's role is to protect
the family honour through their self-respect or sense of honour
(*philotimo*), while women's sexual modesty or shame (*dropi*)
must be protected through their carefully controlled behaviour.
In order to protect their *dropi*, women must exert considerable
self-control both in private and in public. Family honour and
social worth are particularly important, and are constantly being
scrutinized by other families. Shepherd[8] describes a similar
division of norms among Muslim Swahilis in Mombasa, Kenya.
Women are thought (by men) to be 'sexually enthusiastic and
sexually irresponsible, given the opportunity'. They are
expected to be dependent on men, but at the same time the men
also fear the polluting power of their menstrual blood. By
contrast, men are expected to support – and therefore control –
both women and children. This control is considered most
efffective when exerted over the virginity of their unmarried
daughters, but less effective when dealing with the faithfulness
of their wives. For a young girl in that community, marriage and
its consummation are 'the only pathway to female adulthood'.
  In each of the cases quoted above – as elsewhere in the world
– the division of human society into two gender cultures is one
of the basic elements of social structure, and an important part
of the symbolic system of any particular society. However, part
of this binary structure expresses the ambivalence with which
some men regard the women of their community: at times as
nurturant mothers or healers (see Chapter 4), while at other
times as malevolent witches (see Chapter 5), or as dangerous
sources of menstrual pollution (see Chapter 2).

Variations in gender culture

Gender roles, however, are by no means fixed, and they can often change and develop, especially under the influence of urbanization and industrialization. In industrial societies, as Ember and Ember[9] have noted, 'when machines replace human strength and when women can assign child care to others, strict division of labor by sex begins to disappear'.

Although there are always certain constancies cross-culturally in the gender divisions of labour,[4,9] there is also considerable evidence from anthropological research of the wide variation in gender cultures in different parts of the world. That is, what may be seen as typical of the behaviour of one gender in a particular society may not be regarded as such in the next. For example, in some societies women have only a domestic role, and are restricted to the home and never allowed to work outside it (such as the *purdah* system in many Islamic societies[9]), while in other societies women play a major role in the wider economic system. In some industrial societies they are major wage earners – in the USA, for example, more than 50% of married women now work outside the home[9] – while in many peasant societies, as well as maintaining their domestic role, women are also involved in the raising of livestock; in the planting, cultivation, and harvesting of crops; and in the production of clothes, pottery and various handicrafts for market.

Some anthropologists have suggested that the subordination of women (especially their relegation to the 'domestic' rather than the 'public' sphere of life) is a universal phenomenon, and common to all human societies.[10] However, other anthropologists have argued against this concept, and have pointed out that the situation is much more complex, and that each case must be evaluated differently. For one thing, in all societies men envy the biological powers of women to create life, to bring it to birth, and to sustain it with breast milk[4] – especially as this power is reinforced by the rites and religion of almost all societies. Furthermore, in many traditional societies, women – especially older married women with children – wield great personal, symbolic and economic power, have considerable autonomy, and are sometimes key power brokers within that society. As Keesing[4] points out, 'women's power exercised behind the scenes may in some sense be more genuine than men's power enacted on centre stage', which in turn may merely be 'empty posturing and pageantry'.

Later in this chapter, I will be describing some of the relationships between the various gender cultures and health. If one excludes the role of the physiological differences between the sexes, it is possible to see how each of the two gender cultures may – depending on the context – be either *protective* of health or *pathogenic*. That is, the beliefs and behaviours characteristic of a particular gender culture may contribute to the cause, presentation and recognition of various forms of ill-health.

Gender cultures and sexual behaviour

Although gender cultures lay down norms of sexual behaviour for each of the sexes, there are many variations cross-culturally in what those norms are. For example, ethnographic studies indicate that there is much variation between societies in the degree of heterosexual activity permitted before marriage, outside marriage, and even within marriage itself.

As an example of this, studies quoted by Ember and Ember[9] indicate that extramarital sex occurs in many societies, and that in an estimated 69% of the world's societies the men commonly have extramarital sex, and in about 57% the women commonly do. Significantly, although 54% of societies *say* they allow extramarital sex for men, only 11% say they allow it for women.

Patterns of sexual behaviour are important in the transmission of several diseases. Where promiscuity and extramarital sex is common within a society, there is a greater likelihood of the spread of sexually transmitted disease (such as gonorrhoea, syphilis and herpes genitalis), as well as of hepatitis B and possibly cervical cancer (see Chapter 12). A strict 'double standard' of extramarital sexual behaviour, especially with frequent recourse to prostitutes, may also contribute to the persistence, and spread, of these diseases. In this case, the prostitutes may act as reservoirs of the infection within the community. The recent epidemic of the acquired immune deficiency syndrome (AIDS) has led to an increased emphasis by health education authorities on the importance of limiting promiscuous sexual behaviour, among both heterosexuals and homosexuals.

Membership of a particular gender culture does not always coincide with sexual behaviour. For example, there are wide variations world-wide in whether societies are tolerant of some forms of sexual behaviour – such as homosexuality (both male and female) – which transgress the usual norms of a gender culture. In some societies homosexuality is completely forbidden, but in others it is accepted, or else limited to certain times and to certain individuals. Among the Etoro people of New Guinea, for example, heterosexuality was prohibited for as many as 260 days a year, while homosexuality 'is not prohibited at any time and is believed to make crops flourish and boys become strong'.[9] Shepherd[8] has described male and female homosexuality among the Swahili in Mombasa, Kenya, where the rigid gender boundaries were often transgressed by the institution of homosexuality and transvestism. Both male and female homosexuality were common, and were tacitly tolerated. Homosexuality among teenaged boys was particularly common, although most of them would later have heterosexual relations and eventually get married. She points out that this homosexual behaviour does not weaken the rigid conceptual divisions between men and women because whatever their sexual practices, 'their biological *sex* is much more important than their *behaviour* as a determinant of gender'. She contrasts this with modern Britain and the USA, where behaviour is more important in defining one's gender, and male behaviour that transgresses gender rules is often described as 'womanish' or 'effeminate'.

Caplan[11] has argued that where the desire for fertility and childbearing is high, sexuality and fertility are hardly separated from each other conceptually, and – as described above – it is the *biological* sex of individuals which is most important in defining their gender, whatever their sexual behaviour. Where the desire for many children is less (as in the modern, urban Western world), and where contraception is more easily available, sex becomes gradually divorced from fertility, and sexual practices that do not lead to pregnancy – such as homosexuality – are more tolerated; 'gender' in these modern societies is therefore defined less by biological criteria, and more by social and sexual behaviour. It has also been suggested[9] that societies more tolerant of homosexuality are those with population pressure – that is, too many people for their resources – where an increase in population from heterosexual sex is therefore less desirable.

Gender cultures and health care

As described earlier in this book, in almost every culture most primary health care takes place within the family, and in the *popular* sector the main providers of health care are usually women – often mothers and grandmothers. Also within the popular sector, women have often organized themselves into *healing* cults, circles or churches, which act as either self-help groups for their members (such as the Dertleşmek, or 'sharing of sorrow', groups described among Turkish immigrants to Belgium[12]) or groups that combine self-help with the healing of outsiders – such as the *zar* possession cults in Africa, described by Lewis[13], or the churches and cults practising ritual healing in the middle-class suburbs of the USA.[14] Within the *folk* sector, women have always played a central role, from the village 'wise woman' and the several types of female medium or spiritual healer in Britain – to the many female folk healers in the non-industrialized world and the traditional birth attendants (TBAs) who still provide the majority of the obstetric care in those countries.

Within the *professional* sector of modern medicine, however, although the majority of health care professionals (nurses and midwives) are still female, the higher paid and higher prestige jobs are usually held by male physicians. As described in Chapter 4, the medical profession is always, to some extent, an expression of the dominant social ideology and economic system of the society, including its division into social strata and its sexual division of labour. Thus medicine, until quite recently, was a predominately male profession in most Western countries. For example, in the UK in 1901 there were only 212 female doctors out of a total of 36 000 registered medical practitioners.[15] Medicine remained a predominately male profession until the 1970s, since when more women have been admitted into medical schools, until by 1985 about 23% of all British registered medical practitioners were women.[16] Within the National Health Service (NHS) about 75% of personnel are women, but these are mostly found in its lower echelons, as nurses, ancillary workers, caterers and cleaners.[16] Most of the administrators and most of the doctors are men. For example, figures from England in 1981 show that 83% of general practitioners were men and 17% women, while 89% of hospital consultants (specialists) and 75% of junior hospital doctors were men.[17]

The nursing profession

The nursing profession (including midwives) is the largest group of health professionals within the British NHS, and makes up 43% of its total personnel.[17]

Most nurses work within the hospital sector, where (like most other institutions in Western society) many of the basic gender divisions of the wider culture are recreated. Gamarnikow[18] has argued that the relation of doctors to nurses still mirrors the gender divisions of the Victorian family in the days when Florence Nightingale developed her model of nursing. This means that, within the hospital structure, the equation is still doctor = father, nurse = mother, and patient = child. In terms of power relationships in the provision of health care, the nurse's sphere is separate, but still subordinate to that of the male doctor.

This view is supported by much of the family imagery still used in the UK hospital structure, where the various ranks of the nursing profession were designated as either 'nurses', 'sisters' or 'matrons'. Also, a nurse's job – like that of the mother of a young infant – still involves intimate contact with the patient's body (particularly with its surface), and with its various waste products. By contrast, doctors – who spend relatively little time in the company of patients, and have virtually no contact with their bodily wastes – have a specialized knowledge mainly of the inner biological secrets and workings of their patients' bodies. Because gender divisions of labour within the medical profession still persist, despite major social changes this century, two 'anomalous' types of health professional are gradually becoming more common: the ambiguous roles of the 'male nurse' and the 'lady doctor'.

Stacey[15] has described how the nursing profession in the UK grew out of religious orders, and that when hospitals were established in the eighteenth and nineteenth centuries, nurses were incorporated largely to do the domestic work and watch over the sick. From the nineteenth century onwards, nursing gradually emerged as a profession in its own right, but still remained subordinate to the medical profession. The College of Nursing was founded in 1916, a Register of nurses was established in 1918, and the 1943 Nurses Act established a Roll of nurses, in addition to the Register. Since then training within the nursing profession has become increasingly specialized, and in both Europe and the USA many nurses now have postgraduate training within a range of specialties and subspecialties. Nursing is now well established as an independent health profession in its own right.

Case history: Advertisements in medical and nursing journals in the USA

Krantzler[19] has analysed advertisements in medical and nursing journals in the USA. She points out how in recent years these advertisements have shown a gradual reduction of the traditional medical symbols used by doctors (such as the white coat and stethoscope). Instead, this symbolic display of science in action is now more frequently seen in *nursing* journals, and now it is nurses who are more frequently shown using the healing symbols previously associated only with physicians. Nurses are frequently still associated with the older key symbols of nursing – the white uniform and cap – but increasingly these advertisements suggest that nursing symbols and behaviour have come to mimic those of physicians. Krantzler speculates that this 'reflects the desire not merely for respectability but for professional status'. In these nursing advertisements, male physicians now tend to be peripheral, and 'nurses are shown alone, with other nurses or with patients'. She notes that, in the USA, this 'direct relationship with a client, unmitigated by a third party, is an important symbol of professionalization'.

Littlewood[20] has suggested that, although nursing education still takes place within a biomedical framework, nurses are much better placed than physicians to understand – and to deal with – the problems of 'illness', as well as 'disease' (see Chapter 5). She notes the crucial role of nursing in assessing and managing chronic illnesses, disability, pregnancy and the health problems of the elderly. In each of these cases the 'quick fix' of the medical model is either inappropriate or of little benefit. In the case of the chronically sick and disabled – who in this society are marginal people 'with discredited social identities' – nursing can have a major impact on the quality of life, and in understanding the *meanings* patients give to their life and suffering. She therefore sees the nurse as the health professional best placed to 'negotiate between the goals of the doctor. . . and the goals of the patient'.

'Medicalization'

In recent years, the concept of *medicalization* has been put forward by critics of modern medicine, such as Illich,[21] as well as by many medical sociologists. Gabe and Calnan[22] define medicalization as 'the way in which the jurisdiction of modern medicine has expanded in recent years and now encompasses many problems that formerly were not defined as medical entities'. This now includes a wide variety of phenomena, such as many of the normal phases of the female life-cycle (menstruation, pregnancy, childbirth and menopause), as well as old age, unhappiness, loneliness, and social isolation, and the results of wider social problems, such as poverty or unemployment.

There are many explanations for medicalization. Many medical sociologists have argued that modern medicine is increasingly used as an agent of social control (especially over the lives of women)[24] – making people dependent on the medical profession, and on its links with the pharmaceutical and other industries.[21] It has also been seen as a way of controlling socially deviant behaviour, by defining those who do not conform to social norms as 'ill' or 'mad', rather than as 'evil' or 'bad'. Perhaps most importantly, the decline of a religious world-view, and the gradual replacement of 'health' as a moral model of the universe, have meant the spread of medical explanations into areas of life, and its misfortunes, which it was never designed to deal with. Now, for example, the notion of an 'unhealthy lifestyle' leading to ill-health has replaced the earlier religious concepts of 'sinful behaviour' leading to divine retribution. This process has probably been aided by the undoubted successes of technology and science (including medical science) in improving the expectation and quality of life in many other ways. Medicalization is probably also more likely if the body is conceptualized as a machine, and one that is only viewed stripped of its social and cultural context (see Chapter 2). A final possible reason for the growth of medicalization was suggested earlier, in the discussion of the nature/nurture controversy: if some men still see women and their physiology as representative of 'nature' – that which is uncontrolled, unpredictable and dangerously polluting – then medical rituals and medical technology become a way of 'taming' the uncontrolled (especially in the age of feminism) and of making it more 'cultural' in the process.

In discussing cases described by some sociologists and anthropologists as examples of medicalization, this section will focus on:

1. Aspects of the life stresses of women, and their relation to psychotropic drug prescribing.
2. Aspects of female physiology and life-cycle such as menstruation and menopause and, later in this chapter, childbirth.

Women and psychotropic drug prescribing.

The widespread use of psychotropic drugs in the industrialized world as a solution to personal and social problems will be discussed in Chapter 8. However, studies in several Western countries have all indicated that women are prescribed psychotropics roughly *twice* as often as men.[24] The reasons why doctors prescribe more of these drugs for women than for men are complex, but they include the influence of the advertisements from the pharmaceutical industry, promoting these drugs as solutions for women's life stresses and role conflicts. In contrast, *alcohol*, not psychotropic drugs, seems to be the main 'chemical comforter' used by men in many societies.

Case history: Psychotropic drug advertisements in the UK

Stimson[25] has studied advertisements for psychotropic drugs in British medical journals. He has found that their images of women outnumbered those of men by 15 to 1. In the advertisements, women's place in society was predominately shown 'as one which generated stress, anxiety, and emotional problems'. Images of the tired and tearful 'harassed housewife' in a cluttered kitchen, surrounded by crying children, were common. According to Stimson, these advertisements reveal that women's role problems and conflicts are increasingly defined only in medical terms, and the message is that 'certain life events put people in a position where the prescription of a drug might be appropriate'. Furthermore, the descriptions of the drug always show the individual adapting to the situation with the aid of medical help, rather than by changing the situation itself.

This medicalization of the stress and anxieties of some women's lives is part of a wider medicalization of social and personal problems such as bereavement, loneliness, divorce, political upheaval, poverty and unemployment. It is also part of the growing trend towards 'chemical coping', and the search for a stressless and painless utopia, as a modern way of life.

In looking at the concept of medicalization put forward by many critics of modern medicine, it should always be remembered that many women have not seen this process as necessarily a bad thing.[22] Instead they have welcomed the development of medical treatment for the premenstrual syndrome, dysmenorrhoea, menopausal symptoms, and for some of the pain and difficulties of childbirth.

Menstruation

Menstruation is a normal part of female physiology, from the menarche until the menopause. Nevertheless, it is often a process surrounded by a variety of taboos and special behaviours, designed symbolically to *protect* the menstruating woman from harm during this vulnerable period, and also to protect men from the dangerous polluting power of her menstrual blood.

Women in Western industrial countries, especially in urban areas, have very different experiences of menstruation than do women in many developing countries. In developing countries, especially in rural areas, menstrual periods are relatively uncommon for a number of reasons – just as they were last century in the Western world. This is because of a number of major changes in women's lives that have occurred in the industrialized countries over the past century, including: a fall in the birth rate, a reduction in the average number of pregnancies per woman, a lowering of the age of menarche, a decline in infant and maternal mortality, increased life expectancy, and therefore a greater proportion of women who live to the menopausal age.[26] In the 1890s, the average British working-class woman spent 15 years in a state of pregnancy and in nursing a child for the first year of life, while the time so spent today would be only four years,[26] so that many more years of menstruation are likely. In the devloping world, two other factors may also contribute to amenorrhoea, or to infrequent periods: firstly, prolonged breast feeding after birth, which is common in many of those countries, and which can cause amenorrhoea, and secondly inadequate nutrition, which may have the same effect.

In recent years, one aspect of menstruation – the *premenstrual syndrome* (PMS) – has increasingly been seen, not as a physiological phenomenon, but as a problem of pathology and hormonal deficiency. Dalton,[27] for example, has described PMS as 'the commonest endocrine disorder', and one which is due to a deficiency of progesterone. This contrasts with the menopause, which has also been defined by some clinicians as a deficiency disease, though this time of oestrogen (see below). Gottlieb[28] has described the symbolic nature of PMS in contemporary American culture. She sees the negative moods (such as irritability and hostility) that define PMS as the opposite of what is normally expected of women in the USA, a form of symbolic inversion of the idealized behaviour expected of them the rest of the month (to be always 'nice', 'quiet', kind, selfless, and compassionate to others). Women are permitted, and even encouraged, to oscillate between these two extremes of personality, within certain times of the month. According to Gottlieb, many American women have internalized this split model of feminine behaviour. However, their monthly 'ritual of reversal' of these values has a largely conservative effect, as it turns women's experience against themselves, because they 'in effect choose, however unconsciously, to voice their complaints at a time when they know their complaints will be rejected as illegitimate'.

Menopause

Like regular and frequent menstrual periods, the menopause is more a feature of more modern, industrialized societies, where women have a longer life expectancy and most now live to the menopausal age.

Lock[29] has pointed out significant changes in the way menopause has been defined over the past century or so by Western medicine; in the nineteenth century, for example, menopause was thought to *cause* disease, but since the mid-twentieth century it has itself been redefined *as* a 'disease'. Thus a normal feature of the female life-cycle has increasingly become medicalized, although there are often important differences between lay and medical models of menopause.

Kaufert and Gilbert[30] have noted that the biomedical definition of menopause as primarily an *endocrine* disorder (oestrogen deficiency) often leads to the defining as 'menopausal' of only those symptoms which can be attributed to an oestrogen deficiency (such as hot flushes, night sweats, osteoporosis and atrophic vaginitis), while ignoring those symptoms (especially social or psychological ones) which are not easily corrected by hormone replacement therapy (HRT). A further problem of seeing menopause as primarily a medical condition is that once it is defined as a hormonal deficiency disease it can be diagnosed only by a physician and by laboratory tests, treatment can be prescribed only by a physician, and thus it often becomes 'a permanent condition to be permanently managed' by the medical system.

However, as Lock[29] points out, the medical model itself is not uniform, and there is much dispute within the medical literature on the defining symptoms and appropriate treatment of the menopause, as well as on the relation of oestrogen deficiency to both symptoms and other pathological changes (such as osteoporosis). There is also disagreement about other, more vague, menopausal symptoms – such as irritability, depression, tiredness, headaches, dizziness, and loss of libido – and whether these are due to a hormonal deficiency or not. There is of course a physiological change – the end of the menses and of fertility – which occurs at this time. However, this also coincides with a series of *sociocultural* events in the woman's life (hence it is often called a 'change of life'), which are often associated with other social transitions – such as retirement, children leaving home (the 'empty nest syndrome') or ill-health – which may also be responsible for some of the symptoms associated with menopause.

In her own study, carried out in Montreal, Canada, Lock[29] found that the medical management of menopausal symptoms was often very variable, and, while some doctors always prescribed HRT, others hardly ever did. In some cases, the decision to prescribe HRT seemed to be determined by the context in which consultation took place, as well as by the personality, training, age, sex and experience of the clinician, and the social and cultural attributes of the patient herself. Similar findings, also from Canada, are illustrated in the following case history.

Case history: Medicalization of the menopause in Manitoba, Canada

Kaufert and Gilbert[30] studied 2500 women in Manitoba, Canada, aged between 40 and 59. Of these, 37% were premenopausal, 14% perimenopausal, and 30% were postmenopausal; 19% had previously had a hysterectomy. They found that in this sample of women menopause was much less medicalized than anticipated. Overall, just under half the women said they had never discussed their menopausal status with a physician. They concluded that, in the sample, 'the experience of menopause was not a highly medicalized process and was one in which some women involved their physicians not at all. This was unlike childbirth, which is highly medicalized in Canada: childbirth is a publicly visible process with little choice over whether to disclose it, unlike menopause.' In Canada, the 'culture of pregnancy' usually includes seeing a physician, and as in the USA nearly all births involve some form of medical intervention. However, North American society attaches a relatively light weight to menopause, as compared with childbirth, and this may explain why it has only been partially medicalized.

In the case of both the premenstrual syndrome and menopause, it can be argued that two of the natural physiological events of women's lives have been redefined by some clinicians as 'endocrine deficiencies' or 'diseases'. This medicalization means that some women have become more dependent on the medical profession and its treatments than their mothers ever were. However, as mentioned earlier, many women have also welcomed the development of medical treatments that have relieved the unpleasant symptoms of both menstruation and menopause.

Gender cultures and health

The gender roles prescribed by a particular gender culture may – like other cultural beliefs and behaviours – be either protective of health or pathogenic, depending on the context. In this section I will briefly describe how being allocated at birth to the social category of either 'male' or 'female' may, under some circumstances, have a negative effect on an individual's health. One may term those conditions where the beliefs, expectations and behaviours inherent in a particular gender culture can be said to contribute towards ill-health *diseases of social gender*.

Diseases of male social gender

Several aspects of male gender culture can be said to contribute to men's ill-health, or to the risks of such ill-health developing. For example, in comparison with women, men are encouraged to drink more alcohol, to smoke more cigarettes, to be more competitive, and to take more risks in their daily lives. In almost all cultures, both warfare and hunting are exclusive male pursuits, and men's health – particularly that of younger men – is often put at risk by the dangerous and competitive sports, bodily mutilations, rituals of initiation, and public trials of manhood and 'machismo' characteristic of so many cultures.

In the face of suffering and pain, men are usually expected to have an unemotional 'language of distress', to be stoical and uncomplaining, and thus to have a high threshold for consultation with a doctor or other health professional (especially if they too are male). In many cases this stoicism may be counterproductive to health, for it may lead some men to ignore early symptoms of serious disease, or to the doctor's underestimating the seriousness of the disease. Another example of the relation of male gender cultures to ill-health is the type A behaviour pattern (TABP), which is described in more detail in Chapter 11. This is a type of competitive, ambitious and time-obsessed behaviour which has been found to increase the risk of coronary heart disease (CHD) in some individuals. Waldron[31] has explained the fact that death rates in the USA from CHD are twice as high for men as for women, as due partly to cultural factors – espcially different American child-rearing practices. Competitiveness, ambition and other features of TABP are more likely to be encouraged and rewarded in men than in women. Men are expected to succeed in the occupational sphere, while women are expected to succeed in the domestic sphere, and each sphere requires different behavioural adaptations if success is to be achieved. Later in life, this type of socialization may be protective of women, but not of men, in contributing to the development of CHD.

Diseases of female social gender

Some of these have already been discussed in Chapter 2, in the context of the many alterations of body image that occur world-wide, especially among women. In the Western world these include mammoplasty, rhinoplasty and other forms of plastic surgery – all of which carry with them the risks inherent in surgery and anaesthesia, as well as the possibility of post-operative infection. Other more exotic changes in the body surface and appearance, such as foot-binding, scarification, tattooing and lip-piercing, all carry with them clear risks to health. More recent fashions of clothing and body adornment can also be damaging to health: for example, orthopaedic problems may result from wearing platform heels and high-heeled shoes, and contact dermatitis or urticaria can follow the use of cosmetics, bath salts, deodorants and hair dyes. Furthermore, major changes in body shape to conform to current cultural images of female beauty may lead to food fads and diet fads, which can be dangerous for nutrition and health. In some individuals, the cultural emphasis on female slimness may even contribute to the development of anorexia nervosa. It may also lead to depression and a poor self-image among those women with obesity, or those whose bodies do not conform to the current cultural images of female beauty.

In contrast to men, women are socialized to have a low threshold for consultation with a doctor, and to display a more emotional language of distress – such as the various forms of 'nerves' described by anthropologists in different parts of the world.[32] This in turn may lead to a misdiagnosis of 'hysteria' or 'hypochondria' by male clinicians,[33] to the medicalization of their life events and physiological changes, and to the unnecessary use of drug therapy (especially psychotropic drugs). On the other hand, frequent consultations with a doctor may sometimes aid in the early recognition of certain diseases.

Finally, in modern industrial societies, many women are increasingly the focus of contradictory influences from their gender culture. On the one hand their domestic role is emphasized, and they are expected to remain at home with their families, but on the other hand they are expected at the same time to follow careers, and to contribute to the wider economy. These role conflicts have greatly increased the stresses in the lives of many modern women.

Reproduction and childbirth

Anthropologists have reported widespread differences in the perceptions of conception, pregnancy and birth among different cultural groups. Hahn and Muecke[34] call these inherited belief systems the *birth culture* of a particular society, and say that it 'informs members of a society about the nature of conception, the proper conditions of procreation and childbearing, the workings of pregnancy and labor, and the rules and rationales of pre- and postnatal behaviour'.

Anthropologists have described many of these birth cultures, from both industrial and non-industrialized worlds. In modern middle-class Europe and the USA, for example, pregnancy and birth – like menopause and menstruation – have increasingly been seen as *medical* conditions, and thus the proper subjects for medical diagnosis and treatment.

Western birth culture

In all cultures, women giving birth are assisted during the labour by one or more other persons. These people may be female relatives or friends, a traditional midwife or birth attendant, or – in a hospital setting – a medically qualified obstetrician.

Stacey[35] has described how in the UK midwifery was an exclusively female profession until the seventeenth century, when a few 'men-midwives' or *accoucheurs* began to appear. Much of the knowledge of the traditional midwives came from their own experience of pregnancy and childbirth. Although many physicians were opposed to the idea, during the latter half of the nineteenth century midwives were gradually incorporated into the medical system, although they were allowed to attend only 'normal' births. Their position as practitioners in their own right was eventually formalized in the Midwives Act of 1902, but they still remained subordinate to the medically qualified obstetricians. According to Leavitt,[36] a similar process has taken place in the USA. Before 1880, women giving birth were aided mainly by female relatives and birth attendants. Only occasionally were doctors called in to help with difficult labours, but even then the power to make decisions about the birth remained with the woman, her family and friends. From 1880 to 1920, however, although most births still took place at home, the medical profession gradually increased its authority over the birth process, and how it was to be managed. By the 1930s, for the first time, childbirth took place more often in hospital than at home. In this new hospital setting, control over the management of the birth process became almost exclusively a medical matter.

The growth of hospital obstetrics

In 1959 one in three of all births in the UK took place at home or in a nursing home, while today 99% of births take place in an NHS Hospital.[17] In the USA, too, approximately 98% of births take place in a hospital setting.[36] The decline of home deliveries in the UK, and the gradual shifting of childbirth into a hospital environment, is shown by the changes in the numbers of hospital midwives, and those still working in the community: between 1974 and 1980 hospital midwives increased from 15 002 to 17 163, while the number of community midwives actually declined from 4237 to 2773.[17]

In the past half-century or so, modern obstetrics has achieved notable successes in reducing both maternal and neonatal mortality and morbidity, in preserving the lives of premature infants, in diagnosing congenital abnormalities *in utero*, and in successfully treating infertility with *in vitro* fertilization (IVF) and other techniques. However, for all its technical success, the birth culture of Western society – like other aspects of modern medicine – has been criticized by many women on a number of counts. These include:

1. Its over-emphasis on the *physiological*, rather than the psychosocial, aspects of pregnancy and birth.
2. Its tendency to medicalize a normal biological event, turning it into a medical problem, and thus converting the pregnant woman into a passive and dependent 'patient'.

In particular – like the distinction between disease and illness described in the previous chapter – medicine has been criticized for ignoring the *meanings* that women give to both their pregnancy and their childbirth experiences.

This over-emphasis on birth as a technical problem often seems to imply a plumbing model of the woman's body, as described in Chapter 2. In the minds of some obstetricians, birth seems to be seen as merely the technical problem of getting a living object (the baby) from one tube (the uterus), down another (the birth canal), and then out into the hands of the physician.

The origins of Western birth culture

What are the origins of the birth culture of modern Western obstetrics? Davis-Floyd[37] traces it to the seventeenth century image, developed by Descartes, Bacon and Hobbes, of a mechanistic universe, following predictable laws, which could be discovered by science, and controlled by technology. The Cartesian model of mind–body dualism led to the metaphor of the body-as-machine, and the conceptual divorce of body from soul removed the body from the purview of religion, and placed it firmly in the hands of science. She argues further that Christian theology held that women were inferior to men, and closer to nature. Consequently, the men who established the idea of body-as-machine also firmly established the male body as the prototype of this machine; insofar as the female body deviated from the male standard, it was regarded as inherently abnormal, defective, dangerously unpredictable and under the influence of nature, and in need of constant manipulation by men. The demise of midwifery, and the growth of the metaphor of the female body as 'a defective machine, formed the philosophical basis for modern obstetrics. A further feature, especially in American obstetrics, is the hospital as a high-tech factory, dedicated to the production of perfect babies: 'the most desirable end product of the birth process is the new social member, the baby; the new mother is a secondary by-product'.

Furthermore, the conceptual separation of mother and infant is basic to the technological model of birth. The baby is removed from the mother, handed to a nurse who inspects, tests, bathes, diapers and wraps the infant, and administers a vitamin K injection and antibiotic eye drops then – having been 'properly encultered' or 'baptised' into the world of technology, it is handed back to its mother for a short time, and then placed in a plastic bassinet for four hours of observation, before being returned to its mother. To Davis-Floyd, therefore, 'the mother's womb is replaced, not by her arms but by the plastic womb of culture'. This separation is further intensified by assigning a separate doctor – the paediatrician or neonatologist – to the newborn infant.

She describes how, during the birth itself, the mother lies surrounded by medical technology: by external and internal fetal monitors, intravenous drips, charts and instruments. To the woman 'her entire visual field is conveying one overwhelming perceptual message about our culture's deepest values and beliefs: technology is supreme, and you are utterly dependent on it and on the institutions and individuals who control and dispense it'. This impression is strengthened by the frequent use of episiotomies, which 'transforms even the most natural of childbirths into a surgical procedure'.

The medicalization of birth

As Davis-Floyd[37] describes, medicine (including obstetrics) has increasingly defined health and ill-health mainly in terms of physiological dysfunction (see Chapter 5); as it has done so, the gap between lay and obstetrical birth cultures seems to have widened considerably, and the possibility of a culture clash between them seems more likely than before. This is especially true in many parts of the industrialized world, where some women have expressed considerable dissatisfaction with some aspects of the medical management of birth.

For example, Graham and Oakley[38] have described some of the fundamental differences between doctors' and mothers' perspectives on childbearing, particularly whether it is a 'natural' or a 'medical' process. This conflict is part of the wider differences in perspective inherent in all doctor–patient interactions. The medical view of pregnancy abstracts it from the rest of the woman's life experience and treats it as an isolated medical event. The patient enters medical care at onset of pregnancy, and leaves medical care after giving birth. For the mother, on the other hand, it is integrated with *other* aspects of her life, because she acquires (with a first birth) a new social role, as well as profound changes in her financial situation, status, housing situation, and personal relationships. There are also differences in how she and the obstetrician assess the quality of the childbearing experience, how they measure a successful outcome, and how they decide who should control the method and pace of the birth itself. Thus there is an inherent clash between the obstetricians – clinicians (usually men) who have a specialized knowledge of childbirth – and the mothers, whose expertise 'stems not primarily from medical science but rather from a woman's capacity to sense and respond to the sensations of her body'.

As well as having a technical effect, many of the procedures of modern obstetrics can also be described as 'rituals of social transition' or *rites de passage*, which will be described in Chapter 9. For the purposes of this section, however, it is important to note that in all human societies pregnancy and childbirth are more than just biological events. They are also part of an important *transition* of the woman from the social status of 'woman' to that of 'mother'. As with all social transitions, during the dangerous journey from one status to another, the individual must be *protected* from harm by the observance of certain rituals and behaviour. In many of these transitions the person concerned goes through a temporary period of withdrawal from ordinary life, before being 'reborn' into their new social status; as Kitzinger[39] observes, the initiate often 'goes through an act of infantilization, in which he or she is reduced to the state of a small, dependent, submissive child', and 'it is as if only by going back to the beginning can rebirth take place'. However, as Davis-Floyd[37] has argued above, many of the rituals of obstetrics are also ways of transmitting some of society's most basic values to the woman undergoing childbirth. These values include her powerlessness in the face of patriarchy, the 'defectiveness' of her female body, the need of medicine to control her natural processes, her dependence on science and technology, and the enduring importance of institutions and machines over individual beliefs and meanings. This type of cultural 'message' is more likely to be transmitted to the new mother in the impersonal atmosphere of a hospital obstetric unit than when the birth takes place in the familiar atmosphere of the home. As Kitzinger[39] has put it, 'in large centralized, hierarchical institutions existing outside and apart from the family there is a special likelihood of these rituals being used to reinforce the existing system and maintain the power structure'.

Non-Western birth cultures

Hahn and Muecke[34] have described the discrepancies between the birth culture of middle-class USA, and those of some of the social and ethnic groups in that country, such as working-class blacks, Mexican Americans, Chinese and the Hmong (from Laos). In each case, some of the basic assumptions of white middle-class obstetricians – for example, that the husband is likely to be present at the birth – may not be shared by the members of those groups. Among some traditional Chinese groups, for example, women and their bodily products are regarded as dangerous and polluting for men, who therefore avoid the scene of birth and any contact with the woman in the month following the birth. As with other traditional groups, female obstetricians and birth attendants may be preferred to males.

In many cultures in the non-industrialized world, giving birth in the lithotomy or supine position favoured by Western obstetrics is not at all common. In her review of the literature on the subject, MacCormack[40] states that 'throughout the world, in Latin America, northern Thailand, India, Sri Lanka and West Africa, women either stand, squat or sit reclining against something or someone in the latter stages of labour'. In the second stage of labour, the midwife is often seated on the floor in front of the labouring woman. With breach or transverse presentation, traditional birth attendants are often skilled at manipulating the baby into the cephalic position by external version.

Reviewing the literature covering Vietnam, Thailand, Burma, India, East and West Africa, Jamaica, Guatemala and Brazil, MacCormack[40] points out that, unlike in Western obstetrical practice, the umbilical cord is usually cut *after* the placenta is expelled, and not before. In some areas, dung is rubbed into the infant's umbilicus to stop bleeding, and this can increase the risk of neonatal tetanus.[40]

After the birth, women in most cultures observe a special postpartum rest period, during which they have to follow certain dietary and other taboos, and are cared for mainly by other women. This period of rest and seclusion usually lasts between 20 and 40 days. Among Tamils in Sri Lanka, for example, the period of 'childbirth pollution' is 31 days, followed by special rituals which purify the house, as well as a ritual bath for the mother and the shaving of the child's head.[41] Pillsbury [42] describes how in rural Chinese communities, in both the People's Republic of China and Taiwan, 'doing the month' involves one full month of postpartum convalescence, during which time the woman is confined to her home, is looked after by relatives, and has to eat a special diet and observe special taboos. She points out how, in contrast, the 'lying in' period of Western birth culture has given way to the 'puerperium', which does not have the same symbolic importance and 'no longer connotes the specificity of behaviour that continues to character-ize "doing the month"'. A further important aspect of the post-partum period is that many cultures prohibit sexual relations between husband and wife for a period of time after the birth. In some cases, this may last for several months; among many traditional Chinese in the USA, for example, sexual contact is sometimes proscribed for anything up to 100 days after the birth.[34]

Traditional birth attendants

In contrast with the modern, technological model of birth, most births world-wide – especially in rural areas of the developing world – are delivered in a very different way, usually by female birth attendants, such as the *parteras* of Mexico, the *comadronas* of Puerto Rico, or the *nanas* of Jamaica.

In 1978 a report of the World Health Organisation[43] supported the further training of TBAs, who already deliver about two-thirds of the world's babies. TBAs are found in almost every village and in many urban neighbourhoods throughout Africa, Asia and Latin America. The WHO's aim is to increase their numbers and further training, and also consultation with them, and eventually to integrate them into the overall health programmes in developing countries, but ensuring at the same time the 'continuation of the traditional art' and a respect for their roots in traditional cultures.

In countries where TBAs are recognized by the authorities, including in Ghana, Indonesia, Malaysia, Pakistan, the Philippines, Sudan and Thailand, considerable numbers have been trained and used in basic health services during the last 30 years. In Africa and rural India, an estimated 80% of women are assisted during birth by TBAs. Worldwide, the WHO estimates that about 60–80% of women are attended by TBAs.[44]

Despite their lack of formal training, TBAs therefore offer the possibility of non-technological birth care in many parts of the non-industrialized world.

Case history: The *nana* in Jamaica

Kitzinger[39] has described an example of a traditional. birth attendant, the *nana* or folk midwife of Jamaica. She estimates that about 25% of Jamaican babies, especially in rural areas, are delivered by a *nana*. Because these women are not legally recognized by the state, most of these births are registered as 'born unattended' or 'delivered by mother' (or by a friend or relative). In the villages, the *nana* is a person of high standing and great authority, 'a key figure in the cohesion of women in Jamaican rural communities'. Together with the village schoolteacher and the postmistress, she forms 'the political centre' or core of the social networks that tie the community together. *Nanas* are familiar figures, deeply rooted in their communities, and are often called upon for help in a variety of family crises. The midwifery skills of the *nana* are handed down within families, from mother to daughter. *Nanas* are always mothers themselves, for 'to be a *nana* is really an extension of the mothering role, so all *nanas* are mothers who are seen to be successful in their role'. They see their role as shepherding the women safely from conception to birth, by facilitating their natural processes, and in doing so assisting in the drama of 'the rebirth of a woman as a mother'. Their care usually continues from pregnancy until the 9th day after the birth. The *nanas* supervise all the many rituals and taboos of pregnancy and birth (see Chapter 9), which mark the woman's transition from pregnancy to motherhood, and which help to give *meaning* to her experience by placing it in the context of the wider cultural values of her religion and community. Kitzinger contrasts this intimate, culturally familiar approach with the Western-style, technological birth procedures used in many Jamaican hospitals, where nurses and midwives value 'efficiency, speed of delivery of the patient, hospital routines concerning hygiene and order, and the suppression of emotional factors in childbirth so that they can get on with the work in an organized way, and treat the greatest number of patients in the shortest possible time'.

According to Kitzinger, the Jamaican *nanas* – who do things in 'the old time way' – tend to be derided both by the medical profession and by the educated middle-class as inefficient, harmful to health, and as echoes of a past of slavery and subjugation. However, she points out that the *nanas* are very experienced in the techniques of midwifery, are keen to learn more from modern obstetrics, and are quick to call in a trained midwife – or send the woman straight to hospital – if anything goes wrong with the birth. Many rural women now use *nanas* during pregnancy and the first stage of labour, and then transfer to a qualified midwife for the birth itself.

Fertility and infertility

Fertility is a universal human concern, as is anguish over infertility, whatever its cause. Most cultures include a series of rituals or prayers or special precautions to help a woman successfully conceive and to carry her through to a safe delivery. Where a woman fails to conceive, a wide variety of cultural explanations usually comes into play to explain her infertility, and how to deal with it. As described in the previous chapter, such lay explanations for misfortune usually lay the blame either on the individual's behaviour, or on the natural world, or on the malevolence of other people, or on supernatural forces or gods.

Concepts of fertility and infertility are also partly dependent on how people conceptualize the inner workings of their bodies, and the processes of conception and birth. For example, Cosminsky[45] has described how, in a Guatemalan village, some of the traditional midwives believed that infertility was caused by a 'cold womb', which was not 'hot' enough to receive the semen. One form of treatment was to administer 'hot' herbal teas, and to 'warm the womb' in a special sweatbath. If, however, the villagers believed that the sterility was caused by divine intervention, the midwife was not expected to cure it.

In small-scale societies particularly, a 'barren woman' is often a marginalized figure, and seen as someone both personally unfulfilled and socially incomplete. In most traditional societies, blame for the infertility is usually placed on the *woman*. For example, according to McGilvray,[41] among Tamils in Sri Lanka and throughout most of South Asia, infertility is seen as primarily a problem with the woman, and not the man. Sometimes a supernatural cause for the infertility was suggested, but rarely was the potency of her husband questioned, and in the town that she studied most of the men would never acknowledge the possibility of their being sterile.

However, such definitions of who is responsible for the infertility are not static, and they often undergo significant changes during Westernization, migration, urbanization, and other major social changes.

Contraception, abortion and infanticide

Different attitudes to contraception, abortion and infanticide, all of which can be seen as forms of population control, seem to vary widely between cultures. Part of the reason for a society practising infanticide, for example, may be the size of the population, its food supply, and the particular ecological niche that it occupies. In some cases, the infants of one gender may be killed, but not the other – as in the case of the Tenetehara, a Brazilian Indian tribe, who believed that a woman should have three children, but not all of the same sex; if she had two daughters (or two sons) and gave birth to a third, the baby would be killed (see Chapter 12). Overall, as Keesing[46] notes, in the past 'there is little doubt that peoples with finite space and resources in many parts of the world practised infanticide, of both sexes or of females, so as to restrict population numbers.' The particular population policy of a culture may include a widespread tolerance of abortion, acceptance of abortion under certain limited circumstances, or strict taboos against it at any stage of pregnancy, or for any reason. In the Western world the debate on abortion centres both on whether the woman is entitled to control over her own body and fertility, and also on whether the fetus is regarded as a 'person' – with the same rights as other members of the society – or merely as an organ or collection of cells.

Males and pregnancy

Although pregnancy and childbirth are female events, both physically and socially, most men are deeply involved in the birth of their children. In many cultures this emotional involvement is recognized by a series of rituals that the man must carry out during his wife's pregnancy, birth and post-partum period.

Heggenhougen[47] has reviewed much of the literature on the role of fathers in the birth of their children. He points out that in most modern, middle-class Western industrial cultures, the husband has only a minimal role to play – usually that of anxious spectator – in the birth of his child. Overall, the majority of human cultures exclude men from the scene of birth. However, this is not true of certain Native American, Eskimo, African and Maori groups. Where the father is present at the birth, his presence is almost always functional, and the role and rituals that are prescribed for him are believed to be integral to the actual birth process. He has certain tasks to perform, which are designed to protect mother and child, and make the delivery easier – and which may be termed the *ritual couvade*. In many non-industrialized cultures, he is expected to follow certain strict taboos; in Java the husband follows many of the same taboos as his wife, and supports her during labour, and this is also found in some Guatemalan communities, among the Catiguan villagers of the Philippines, and in parts of northern Europe. In the Lan Tsu Miao tribe of Kweichew, South China, the husband not only takes to his bed during his wife's labour, but takes care of and 'mothers' the baby. In the Buka, Ashanti and Chickchee tribes, men performed rituals to fool evil spirits, and attract their attention until the child is safely born. Among the Arapesh people of New Guinea, the verb 'to bear a child' is used indiscriminately for either man or woman, and child-bearing is believed to be as heavy a drain on the man as on the woman. Among the Hopi Indians of the USA and the Chiriguano Indians of Paraguay, both husband and the last-born child go into couvade during the wife's pregnancy. In the modern Western world, largely under the influence of the women's movement and the trend towards natural childbirth, men tend to be more involved in their partners' pregnancies, and are often present at the actual birth, but they lack the protection of a ritually prescribed role (see Chapter 9), characteristic of more traditional societies.

In many cultures, especially those where the ritual couvade is not practised, men have often been reported as suffering from physical and/or psychological symptoms during their wife's pregnancy, birth and postpartum period. This is known as the *couvade syndrome* (from the Basque word *couver*, to brood or hatch), and has been reported from many parts of the world. According to Heggenhougen,[47] one can view this syndrome as 'a subconscious form of participation or perhaps even competition, with the wife', while ritual couvade is 'a conscious participation, though it may have a subconscious base'.

A contemporary illustration of this syndrome, from the USA, is described in the following case history.

Case history: Couvade syndrome in Rochester, New York

Lipkin and Lamb[48] carried out a study on the couvade syndrome in Rochester, New York. They defined this syndrome as the occurrence of new physical or psychological symptoms in the mates of pregnant women, for which they sought medical care, and which were not otherwise objectively explained. In their study of 267 mates of postpartum women, 60 (22.5%) of the men were found to have suffered from this syndrome. This translates to a prevalence rate of 225 of 1000 husbands at risk due to their wife's pregnancy. Many of their symptoms were vague and non-specific – such as 'feeling rundown', 'feeling lowdown', and 'weakness' – as well as more 'pregnant' symptoms such as backache, genital burning, water retention (not confirmed on physical examinations), retrosternal burning, groin pain, dizziness, and abdominal cramps. One patient complained of a chest pain that felt like 'something was pushing out'.

Whatever the cause, the evidence is that men are physically, as well as emotionally, involved in the birth of their children, and clinicians should be aware of the possibility of unexplained symptoms – both physical and psychological – in many expectant fathers.

Recommended reading

Ember, C.R. and Ember, M. (1985) *Cultural Anthropology*. Englewood Cliffs, NJ: Prentice-Hall. See Chapter 9, Sex and culture.
Hahn, R.A. and Muecke, M.A. (1987) The anthropology of birth in five US ethnic populations: implications for obstetrical practice. *Curr. Probl. Obstet. Gynecol. Fertil.* **10**, 133–171. A survey of the birth cultures of five groups of Americans: middle-class whites, working-class blacks, Mexicans, Chinese and Hmong.

Heggenhougen, H.K. (1980) Fathers and childbirth: an anthropological perspective. *J. Nurse Midwifery* **25**, 21–26

Keesing, R. (1981) *Cultural Anthropology*. New York: Holt, Rinehart and Winston. See Chapter 14, Worlds of women, worlds of men.

MacCormack, C.P. (ed.) (1982) *Ethnography of Fertility and Birth*. London: Tavistock. A survey of birth cultures from Africa, Asia, Latin America and the Caribbean.

Chapter 7

Pain and culture

Pain, in one form or another, is an inseparable part of everyday life. It is probably also the commonest symptom encountered in clinical practice[1] – a feature of many normal physiological changes such as pregnancy, childbirth or menstruation, as well as of injury and disease. Many forms of healing or diagnosis also involve some form of pain: for example, surgical operations, injections, biopsies or venesection. But in each of these situations there is more to pain than merely a neurophysiological event; there are social, psychological and cultural factors associated with it that also need to be considered. In this chapter I will be examining some of these factors to illustrate the following propositions:

1. Not all social or cultural groups may respond to pain in the same way.
2. How people perceive and respond to pain, both in themselves and in others, can be largely influenced by their cultural background.
3. How, and whether, people *communicate* their pain to health professionals and to others can also be influenced by social and cultural factors.

Pain behaviour

From a physiological perspective pain can be thought of as what Weinman[2] terms 'a type of signalling device for drawing attention to tissue damage or to physiological malfunction'. Pain arises when a nerve or nerve ending is affected by a noxious stimulus, either from within the body or from outside it. It is therefore of crucial importance for the protection and survival of the body in an environment full of potential dangers. Because of this biological role, it is sometimes assumed that pain is culture-free, in the sense of being a universal biological reaction to a specific type of stimulus, such as a sharp object or extremes of hot or cold. However, anthropologists differentiate between two forms of this reaction:

1. An *involuntary*, instinctual reaction, such as pulling away from the sharp object.
2. A *voluntary* reaction, such as:
   (a) removing the source of pain and taking action oneself to treat the symptom (by taking an aspirin, for example)
   (b) asking another person for help in relieving the symptom.

Voluntary reactions to pain that involve other people are particularly influenced by social and cultural factors, and will be described below in more detail, with examples.

As Engel[3] puts it, pain has two components: 'the original sensation, and the reaction to the sensation'. This reaction, whether voluntary or not, has been called *pain behaviour* by Fabrega and Tyma,[4] and includes certain changes in facial expression, grimaces and changes in demeanour or activity, as well as certain sounds made by the victim, or words used to describe his condition or appeal for help. It is possible, though, to exhibit pain behaviour in the absence of a painful stimulus or, conversely, *not* to exhibit such behaviour, despite the presence of the painful stimulus. To clarify this point, it is useful to identify two types of pain behaviour, or reactions to pain: *private* pain and *public* pain.

Private pain

As Engel[3] points out, pain is 'private data'; that is, for us to know whether a person is in pain we are dependent on that person signalling that fact to us, either verbally or non-verbally. When that happens, the private experience and perception of pain become a social, public event; private pain becomes public pain. Under some circumstances, however, the pain may remain private: there may be no outward clue or sign that the person is experiencing pain. This type of behaviour is common among societies that value stoicism and fortitude, such as the Anglo-Saxon 'stiff upper lip' in the presence of hardship. It is more likely to be expected of men, particularly younger men or warriors. In some cultures the ability to bear pain without flinching – that is, without displaying pain behaviour – may be one of the signs of manhood, and part of initiation rituals marking the transition from boy to man. Among the Cheyenne Indians of the Great Plains, for example, young men who wanted to display their manhood and gain social prestige would undergo ritual self-torture in the Sun Dance ceremony – such as suspending themselves from a pole by hooks passed through the skin of their chests, and accepting the pain without complaint.[5] Other, less dramatic forms of a lack of pain behaviour occur in those who are semi-conscious, paralysed, or too young to articulate their distress, or in situations where such behaviour is unlikely to bring a sympathetic response from other people. Therefore, an absence of pain behaviour does not necessarily mean the absence of 'private pain'.

Public pain

Pain behaviour, especially its voluntary aspects, is influenced by social, cultural and psychological factors. These determine *whether* private pain will be translated into pain behaviour, and the *form* that this behaviour takes, and the social settings in which it occurs.

Part of the decision of whether to translate private into public pain depends on the person's interpretation of the *significance* of the pain; whether, for example, it is seen as 'normal' or 'abnormal' pain – the latter being more likely to be brought to the attention of others. An example of 'normal' pain is dysmenorrhoea. In two studies quoted by Zola,[6] women from both lower and upper socioeconomic groups were asked to keep a calendar in which they recorded all bodily states and dysfunctions. Only a small percentage even reported the dysmenorrhoea as a 'dysfunction', and among the lower income group only 18% even mentioned the menses or its accompaniments. Definitions of what constitutes an 'abnormal' pain, and which therefore requires medical attention and treatment, tend to be culturally defined, and to vary over time. As Zola notes, 'the degree of recognition and treatment of certain gynaecological problems may be traced to the prevailing definition of what constitutes "the necessary part of the business of being a woman"'. This in turn may be influenced by the social and economic context in which the women's lives are embedded. Other definitions of 'abnormal' pain depend on cultural definitions of body image, and the structure and function of the body. Commonly held beliefs that 'the heart' occupies the entire chest, for example, may lead to an interpretation of all pains in this area as 'heart trouble' or a 'heart attack'. Elsewhere[8] I have described the case of a man with psychosomatic chest pains who clung to the idea that he had 'trouble with the heart', despite numerous diagnostic tests which excluded cardiac disease, because he still had 'pain over my heart'.

Zborowski[9] has pointed out that a culture's *expectations* and acceptance of pain as a normal part of life will determine whether it is seen as a clinical problem which requires a clinical solution. Cultures or groups that emphasize military achievements, for example, both expect and accept battle wounds, while more peaceful cultures may expect them, but not accept them without complaint. Similarly, he notes how in Poland and in some other countries labour pains are both expected and accepted, while in the USA they are not accepted and analgesia is frequently demanded. These attitudes towards pain are acquired early in life, and are an essential part of any culture's child-rearing practices.

Although physical pain is a particularly vivid and emotionally laden symptom, it can only be understood in a cultural context by seeing it as part of the wider spectrum of *misfortune*; pain, like illness generally, is only a special type of suffering. As such, it can provoke the same types of questions in the victim as do other forms of misfortune: 'Why has it happened to me?' or 'What have I done to deserve this?' Where pain is seen as divine punishment for a behavioural lapse, the victims may be unwilling to seek relief for it; experiencing the pain without complaint becomes, in itself, a form of expiation. Alternatively they may demand more painful treatments from a physician, such as a surgical operation or an injection. If pain is seen as the result of moral transgressions, the response might also be self-imposed penitence, fasting or prayer – rather than consultation with a health professional. If interpersonal malevolence, such as 'sorcery', 'witchcraft' or 'hexing', is thought to have caused a pain, the strategy for pain relief may be an indirect one – by a ritual of exorcism, for example.

In many cultures, because pain is seen as only one type of suffering within the wider spectrum of misfortune, it is *linked* with the other forms of suffering in a number of ways. These include having a common aetiology (such as divine punishment or witchcraft) and therefore requiring a similar form of treatment (prayer, penitence or exorcism). This wider view of pain is common in non-Western societies, and members of these societies may find the secular Western treatment of pain – the prescribing of a pain-relieving drug – both incomplete and unsatisfying. Although Western medicine does acknowledge the existence of 'psychosomatic' or 'psychogenic' pain, its attitude to 'organic' pain does not take into account the social, moral and psychological elements that many people associate with pain. Nevertheless, the idiom of pain in modern English does still show linkages to other forms of suffering, including emotional distress, interpersonal conflicts and unexpected misfortune. These are often described using the metaphor of physical pain: 'I was sore at him', 'she hurt him deeply', 'a biting comment', 'a painful experience', 'a mere pin-prick', 'it was a blow to me', 'tortured soul' and 'heartsore'. In more traditional societies, the link between physical pain and social, moral and religious aspects of the culture is likely to be much more direct, and to influence closely how people perceive their own ill-health.

The types, and availability, of potential healers or helpers also determine whether a person will display pain behaviour, and in what settings. For example, such behaviour is more likely to bring sympathetic help from a doctor or nurse in a hospital than from a punitive army sergeant. The personality of the clinician, as well as whether he or she comes from a similar culture and social class to the sufferer, may influence the decision to display it or not. Such behaviour may be displayed to one clinician, but not to an unsympathetic colleague, leading to different evaluations of the patient's condition by the two clinicians.

A further factor determining whether private pain is made public is the perceived *intensity* of the pain sensation itself. There is some evidence that this perception (and 'pain tolerance') can be influenced by culture. In a review of the literature on culture and pain, Wolff and Langley[10] point out the paucity of adequately controlled experimental studies in this area. However, the studies that have been done confirm that 'cultural factors in terms of attitudinal variables, whether explicit or implicit, do indeed exert significant influences on pain perception'. Also, as Lewis[11] has noted, the intensity of a pain sensation does not follow automatically from the extent and nature of an injury. Beliefs about the meaning and significance of a pain, the context in which it occurs, and the emotions associated with that context, can all affect pain sensation: 'Fear of implications for the future may intensify awareness of pain in the surgical patient, or, by contrast, the hope and likely chance of escape from deadly risks of battle may diminish the injured soldier's sense of pain and his complaints, though the injury be similar in both cases.' A common example of this is soldiers who only notice that they have been wounded once the battle is over; the intensity of emotional involvement in the battle may divert attention, at least temporarily, from a painful wound. In certain states of religious trance or meditation the intensity of pain perception can also be reduced, although the physiological reasons for this are not well understood. Examples of this phenomenon are the *yogis* and *fakirs* of India, or the fire-walkers of Sri Lanka, who all undergo self-inflicted pain or discomfort, apparently without experiencing the full intensity of the pain.

Attitudes and expectations of a particular healer or treatment can also influence the intensity of pain, as in *placebo analgesia*; here, a pharmacologically inactive drug in which the patient 'believes' causes subjective pain relief in the sufferer. Levine *et al.*[12] have suggested that the release of endorphins within the brain is the physiological mechanism underlying placebo analgesia, because it can be counteracted by the use of nalorphine. Whatever the underlying mechanism, the perception of the intensity of a pain, as well as the meanings associated with it, may influence whether a privately experienced pain is shared with other people.

The presentation of public pain

Each culture or group has its own unique language of distress. Its members have their own specific way of signalling, both verbally and non-verbally, that they are in pain or discomfort. The *form* that this pain behaviour will take is largely culturally determined, as is the *response* to this behaviour. As Landy[13] puts it, this depends, among other factors, on 'whether their culture values or disvalues the display of emotional expression and response to injury'. Some cultural groups expect an extravagant display of emotionality in the presence of pain, others value stoicism, restraint and the playing down of their symptoms. In his study of reactions to pain by Italian Americans and Irish Americans, Zola[6] has pointed out that the Italian response was marked by 'expressiveness and expansiveness', which he sees as a defence mechanism ('dramatization') – a way of coping with anxiety 'by repeatedly over-expressing it and thereby dissipating it'. In contrast, the Irish tended to ignore and underplay their bodily complaints: for example, 'I ignore it like I do most things'. They tended to deny or play down the presence of pain; 'It was more a throbbing than a pain . . . not really pain, it feels more like sand in my eye'. Zola sees this denial as a defence mechanism against the 'oppressive sense of guilt' which he, and other researchers, see as a feature of rural Irish culture. These two different languages of distress may have negative effects on the types of medical treatment that these patients are given – especially by clinicians from different cultural backgrounds. The

Italian Americans for example, might be dismissed as 'over-emotional' or 'hypochondriacal' by a clinician who values stoicism and restraint, and the Irish Americans might have their suffering (private pain) ignored as they continually underplay it. Zola warns that this might perpetuate their suffering by creating a 'self-fulfilling prophecy'.

Pain behaviour may be *non-verbal*, and this too can be patterned by culture. In his study of bodily gestures, le Barre[14] has pointed out that while gestures do differ cross-culturally they can only be interpreted by taking into account the context in which they appear. For example, in the Argentine, shaking one of the hands smartly so that the fingers make an audible clacking sound can mean 'Wonderful', but can also signify pain when one says *'Ai yai'* following an injury. Therefore, non-verbal languages of distress include not only gestures, but also facial expressions, bodily posture and exclamations, all of which take their meaning from the context in which they appear. They may also include other changes in behaviour, such as withdrawal, fasting, prayer or recourse to self-medication.

Because pain behaviour, whether verbal or not, is often standardized within a culture, it is open to imitation by those who wish to get sympathy or attract attention: that is, by displaying public pain without any underlying private pain. Examples of this are the hypochondriac, the malingerer or the actor. The person with Munchausen syndrome, for example, may exactly mimic 'real' pain behaviour and therefore undergo repeated surgical operations or investigations before being discovered.[15] Pain behaviour may also mask an underlying psychological state, such as an extreme anxiety state or depression, as in *somatization* (see Chapter 10). In this case, the primary symptom complained of will not be 'anxiety' or 'depression', but rather their physical concomitants such as weakness, breathlessness, sweating or vague aches and pains. This type of somatization is common among low-income groups in the Western world, but is also a feature of many other cultures. For example, in Chinese culture in Taiwan the open display of emotional distress is not encouraged. Instead, these states are expressed in a mainly somatic or physical language of distress. In Taiwan, Chinese culture, as Kleinman says, 'defines the somatic complaint as *the* primary illness problem', even if psychological symptoms are also present; in one period, 70% of the patients who visited the Psychiatry Clinic at the National Taiwan University Hospital initially complained of physical symptoms.[16] In this and other cultures, a depressed person may complain of vague fleeting pains, or 'pains everywhere', for which no physical cause can be found. Just as culture can influence somatization, so can the personality and background of the clinician. A doctor orientated towards purely physical explanations of ill-health, for example, may acknowledge only somatic symptoms, in contrast to a colleague more interested in psychodynamic processes.

How pain is described is influenced by a number of factors, including language facility, familiarity with medical terms, individual experiences of pain, and lay beliefs about the structure and function of the body (such as the 'glove-and-stocking' distribution of hysterical pain or anaesthesia). The use of technical terms borrowed from medicine to describe a pain may also confuse the clinician: the patient who says 'I've had another migraine, doctor' may be using the term to describe a wide variety of head pains, not only migraine. The cues from clinicians that help shape a diffuse, especially psychosomatic, pain into a recognizable medical form, are questions like: 'Does it travel down your left arm?', 'Does it come on when you climb stairs?', or 'Does it feel like a tight band across your chest?' Medical history taking, examinations, and diagnostic tests may all unwittingly train patients to identify and describe the characteristic form of a particular type of pain, such as 'angina', 'colic' or 'migraine'.[8] Clinicians should therefore be aware of this process and the difficulties it poses for diagnosis.

Social aspects of pain

Public pain implies a *social* relationship, of whatever duration, between the sufferer and another person or persons. The nature of this relationship will determine whether the pain is revealed in the first place, how it is revealed, and the nature of the response to it. Lewis[11] notes how the *expectations* of the sufferer are important here, particularly the likely response to his pain, and the social costs and benefits of revealing it: 'Possibilities of care, of sympathy, the allocation of responsibility for sickness in others, affect how people show their illness'. People will receive maximum attention and sympathy if their pain behaviour matches the society's view of *how* people in pain should draw attention to their suffering – whether by an extravagant display of emotions, or by a quiet change in behaviour. As Zola[6] puts it: 'It is the "fit" of certain signs with a society's major values which accounts for the degree of attention they receive'. There is thus a

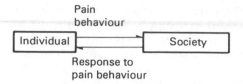

Figure 7.1 Pain behaviour relationship between the individual and society

dynamic between the individual and society (illustrated in Figure 7.1) whereby pain behaviour, and the reactions to it, influence each other over time.

The types of permissible pain behaviour within a society are learned in childhood and infancy. Engel[3] points out that pain plays an important role in the total psychological development of the individual: 'It is . . . intimately concerned with learning about the environment and its dangers . . . and about the body and its limitations'. It is integral to all early relationships: in infancy, pain leads to crying, which leads to a response from the mother or another person. In early childhood pain and punishment become linked: pain is inflicted for 'bad' behaviour by the adult world. Pain may therefore signal to the individual that he is bad and should therefore feel guilty; it may also become an important medium for the expiation of guilt. Pain is also part of relationships of aggression and power, and of sexual relationships. Engel has described the 'pain-prone patient', who is particularly liable to 'psychogenic pain', and whose personality is characterized by strong feelings of guilt. In his view this patient is more likely to complain of pains of one sort or another as a means of self-punishment and atonement; penitence, self-denial and self-deprecation may all be used as forms of self-inflicted punishments to ease the feelings of guilt. One could hypothesize that cultures characterized by a pervasive sense of guilt are also those that value 'painful' rituals of atonement and prayer, including fasting, abstinence, isolation, poverty and even self-flagellation.

Child-rearing practices help to shape attitudes towards and expectations of pain later in life: particularly, as Zborowski[9] notes, the cultural values and attitudes of parents, parent substitutes, siblings and peer groups. In his 1952 study (described below) a group of Jewish American and Italian American parents manifested 'over-protective and over-concerned attitudes towards the child's health, participation in sports, games, fights, etc.' The child was often reminded to avoid colds, injuries, fights and other threatening situations. Crying in complaint was quickly responded to with sympathy and concern. The parents therefore fostered an over-awareness of pain and other deviations from normal, as well as anxiety about their possible significance. By contrast, 'Old American' families were less over-protective; the child was told 'not to run to mother with every little thing', to expect pain in sports and games, and not to react in too emotional a way to them. All these culturally defined languages of distress will influence how private pain is signalled to others, and the types of reaction expected from them. Problems might arise, however, if the sufferer and society have different cultural origins, or come from different social classes, with different expectations of how a person in pain should behave, and how they should be treated.

In some cultural groups, individual sufferers are encouraged to turn their private pain into public pain within a ritual context of healing. This is seen in some of the public rituals of healing in Africa and Latin America, described in Chapter 4. It is also true of some religious groups in the West. Skultans,[17] for example, describes how women in a Welsh spiritualist church are encouraged to share their painful symptoms with one another, and to become 'possessed' by the pain of an ill member, and thus – by sharing it amongst themselves – to help to lessen her private pain.

Case history: Cultural components of pain in New York, USA

Zborowski,[9] in 1952, examined the cultural components of the experience of pain among three groups of patients in New York City: Italian Americans, Jewish Americans and mainly Protestant 'Old Americans'. Marked differences in pain behaviour, and in attitudes towards pain, were found between the groups. Both Italians and Jews tended to be very emotional in response to pain, and to exaggerate their pain experience, leading some of the doctors to conclude that they had a lower threshold of pain than other groups. However, this emotional display, although similar in the two groups, was based on different attitudes towards pain.

The Italians were mainly concerned with the immediacy of the pain experience, especially the pain sensation itself. When in pain they complained a great deal, drawing attention to their suffering by groaning, moaning, crying, etc., but once they were given analgesics, and the pain wore off, they quickly forgot their suffering and returned to normal behaviour. The anxieties of the Italian patients had centred on the effects of the experience on their immediate situation, such as occupation and economic situation. In contrast, Jewish patients were mainly concerned with the *meaning* and significance of the pain 'in relation to their health, welfare and, eventually, for the welfare of the families'. Their anxieties were concentrated on the implications for the future of the pain experience. Several of the Jewish patients were reluctant to accept analgesia, as they were anxious about its side-effects, and concerned that the drug treated only the pain and not the underlying disease. Even after the pain was relieved, many of these patients continued to display the same depressed and worried behaviour 'because they felt that though the pain was currently absent it may recur as long as the disease was not cured completely'. Some tended also to over-exaggerate their physical symptoms, not as an indication of the amount of pain experienced but as a means of ensuring that the pathological causes of the pain would be adequately taken care of. In contrast, the Italians seemed more trusting that the doctor would acknowledge their pain and take steps to relieve it; their emotional display was designed to mobilize efforts towards relieving the immediate pain sensation.

From these data, Zborowski concludes that:

1. 'Similar reactions to pain manifested by members of different ethnocultural groups do not necessarily reflect similar attitudes to pain'.
2. 'Reactive patterns similar in terms of their manifestations may have different functions and serve different purposes in various cultures'.

In contrast to these two groups, the Old Americans – those that had been 'Americanized' for several generations – tended to be less emotional in reporting pain, and to adopt a detached air in describing their pain, its character, duration and location. They saw no point in over-exaggerating their pain because 'it won't help anybody'. Withdrawal from society was a common reaction to severe pain. They often had a more idealized picture of how a person *should* react to pain and what the appropriate 'American' response should be. As one patient put it, 'I react like a good American'. In hospital, they tended to avoid being a 'nuisance' and to cooperate closely with the ward staff (who also often had 'Old American' attitudes). Like the Jewish Americans, their anxiety was future-orientated, although they tended to be more optimistic. They were more positive towards hospitalization, unlike the other two groups, who were 'disturbed by the impersonal character of the hospital and by the necessity of being treated there instead of at home'. As Zborowski notes, these differences in pain behaviour between Old Americans and others tend to disappear over time: 'the further is the individual from the immigrant generation the more American is his behaviour'. Therefore, as this study was carried out as long ago as 1952, many of its findings may no longer be relevant to a modern patient population.

The studies quoted in this chapter illustrate how both pain behaviour and attitudes towards pain may differ among social and cultural groups. Doctors and nurses should therefore be aware of these cultural influences in evaluating people in pain. However, each case should be assessed individually, and one should always avoid using stereotypes or generalizations in predicting how an individual from a particular social or cultural background will respond to being in pain.

Recommended reading

Engel, G. L. (1950) 'Psychogenic' pain and the pain-prone patient. *Am. J. Med.* **26**, 899–909

Wolff, B. B. and Langley, S. (1977) Cultural factors and the responses to pain. In: Landy, D. (ed.) *Culture, Disease, and Healing: Studies in Medical Anthropology.* New York: Macmillan, pp. 313–319

Zborowski, M. (1952) Cultural components in responses to pain. *J. Soc. Issues* **8**, 16–30

Chapter 8

Culture and pharmacology

In many cases, the effect of a medication on human physiology and emotional state does not depend solely on its pharmacological properties. A number of other factors, such as personality, social or cultural backgrounds, can either enhance or reduce this effect, and are responsible for the wide variability in people's response to medication. In this chapter I will examine some of these *non*-pharmacological influences, in relation to placebos, psychotropic and narcotic drugs, alcohol and tobacco.

'Total drug effect'

Claridge[1] has pointed out that the effect of any medication on an individual (its 'total drug effect') depends on a number of elements *in addition* to its pharmacological properties. These are:

1. The attributes of the drug itself (such as taste, shape, colour, name).
2. The attributes of the patient receiving the drug (such as experience, education, personality, sociocultural background).
3. The attributes of the person prescribing or dispensing the drug (such as personality, professional status or sense of authority).
4. The setting in which the drug is administered – the 'drug situation' (such as a doctor's office, laboratory or social occasion).

Because the total drug effect is dependent on the mix of these influences in a particular case, there can be wide variation in how different people respond to the same medication. However, in the case of very powerful drugs, such as certain poisons, the effect is entirely due to its pharmacological actions.

Placebo effect

The placebo effect can be understood as the total drug effect, but *without* the presence of a drug. Much research has been carried out in recent years into this phenomenon. This research, carried out mainly in medical settings, has also shed light on other phenomena, such as drug addiction and habituation, alcoholism, and the therapeutic effects of healing rituals in many cultures. In the medical literature placebos are often viewed merely as pharmacologically inert substances administered as part of a double-blind trial of a new drug. Other writers have pointed out that the placebo effect is much wider than this. Wolf,[2] for example, defines it as 'any effect attributable to a pill, potion or procedure, but not its pharmacodynamic or specific properties'. For Shapiro[3] it is 'the psychological, physiological or psychophysiological effect of any medication or procedure given with therapeutic intent, which is independent of or minimally related to the pharmacologic effects of the medication or to the specific effects of the procedure, and which operates through a psychological mechanism'. It is therefore the *belief* of those receiving (and/or administering) a placebo substance or procedure in the *efficacy* of that placebo which can have both psychological and physiological effects.

In one review of the literature, Benson and Epstein[4] point out that placebos may affect practically any organ system in the body. Placebos have been reported to provide relief in a variety of conditions, including angina pectoris, rheumatoid and degenerative arthritis, pain, hay fever, headache, cough, peptic ulcer and essential hypertension. Their psychological effects include the relief of anxiety, depression and even schizophrenia. Other studies indicate that placebos can even cause side-effects (such as drowsiness)[5] or psychological dependence on them[6] – and both these phenomena are examples of the *nocebo* effect, described in Chapter 11. Although the power of the placebo effect has been widely reported, its exact mechanism is still not clearly understood. Some attempt, though, has been made to explain placebo analgesia from a scientific perspective. In a study by Levine *et al.*,[7] for example, postoperative dental pain was relieved by placebos, but this effect disappeared when the patients were given naloxone. It was hypothesized that placebo analgesia was mediated by endogenous opiates, or endorphins, whose effect was counteracted by the naloxone. Other physiological effects of placebos are still being investigated.

For the placebo effect to occur a certain atmosphere or setting is required. Placebos, whether medications or procedures, are generally *culture-bound*; that is, they are administered within a specific social and cultural setting which validates both the placebo and the person administering it. Placebos that work in one cultural group may not, therefore, have any effect in another. According to Adler and Hammett,[8] the placebo effect is an essential component in all forms of healing, and from a wider perspective it is an important component of everyday life. They see all forms of therapy, cross-culturally, as having two characteristics:

1. Participation by all those taking part (patient, healer, spectators) in a shared cognitive system.
2. Access to a relationship with a culturally sanctioned parental figure (the healer).

The shared cognitive system refers to the cultural world-view of the group; how they perceive, interpret and understand reality, especially the occurrence of ill-health and other misfortunes.

In some societies this world-view is rationalistic, in others it is more mystical; in either case, the perspective on ill-health is part of their wider view of how the world operates, or how things 'hang together'. This world-view 'enables man to locate himself spatially and historically', and 'provides a conceptual–perceptual structure beyond the limits of which few men transgress even in imagination'. This cognitive system, shared with other members of one's culture or society, makes the chaos of life (and of ill-health) understandable, and gives a sense of security and *meaning* to people's lives.

The other component of the placebo effect is the emotional dependence of members of society on prominent people, such as healers; whatever their form, sacred or secular, the healers occupy a social niche of respect, reverence and influence comparable with the parental role. The therapeutic potency of this relationship is probably due to 'a reactivation of the feelings of basic trust adherent to the original mother–infant dyad'. In Adler and Hammett's view, both these aspects 'are the necessary and sufficient components of the placebo effect': what people take from a placebo may be what they need from life – a sense of meaning and security derived from membership of a group with a shared world-view, and a relationship with a caring, parental-type authority figure. Both these aspects are also part of Western healing rituals, such as the doctor–patient consultation.

All medications prescribed in this specialized setting are likely to have some placebo effect. In Joyce's view,[9] there is a placebo or symbolic element in *all* drugs prescribed by doctors, whether they are pharmacologically active or not. He estimates that nearly one in five of all prescriptions written by general practitioners in the UK are for their placebo or 'symbolic' functions, and that there are at least 500 000 people in Britain who each year are 'symbol-dependent' patients. In his view, any drug given for more than two years has a large symbolic component for the individual taking it. Any drug prescribed by a doctor can be seen as a 'multi-vocal' symbol, having a range of *meanings* for the individual patient. Some of these are discussed below, in the section on drug dependence.

The placebo effect of the drug itself has been studied by several researchers. For example, Schapira et al.[10] studied the effect of the *colour* of drugs used for treating anxiety in 48 patients at a psychiatric out-patient department. It was found that anxiety symptoms and phobic symptoms seemed to respond best to green tablets, while depressive symptoms responded best to yellow. The yellow tablets were least preferred by patients for alleviating their anxiety. The authors conclude that one 'cannot ignore any ancillary factor which might enhance the response of patients to drug treatment'. In another study, by Branthwaite and Cooper,[11] self-prescribed analgesic tablets used for headaches were found to vary in their effectiveness, depending on whether the analgesic was labelled as a well known, widely marketed proprietary analgesic. Patients found these 'branded' or labelled analgesics much more effective in relieving headaches than unbranded forms of the same drug. The brand name can be seen as having a symbolic aspect for those that take it, and to stand for a drug with a general reputation for efficiency over many years. Another example of the potency of branded drugs in the eyes of their users was shown in a study by Jefferys et al.[12] of self-medication on an English working-class housing estate. Aspirins were found to be widely used for a range of complaints, including insomnia, anxiety and 'nerves'. In my own study[13] of a group of long-term users of psychotropic drugs, 36% said they would take a proprietary analgesic (such as Aspro, Panadol or Veganin) for the relief of insomnia or anxiety if their psychotropic was withdrawn or unobtainable.

The attributes of the *patient* receiving the drug can also influence the placebo response. Among these are, as Claridge[14] puts it, the patient's 'attitude towards and knowledge of drugs, (and) what he has been told about the particular drug he is taking'. Also relevant is whether he is part of the same shared cognitive system as the prescriber, and certain traits of his personality. Various attempts have been made to define the 'placebo type' of personality, who is more likely to show this response. Among the attributes mentioned are over-anxiety, emotional dependency, immaturity, poor personal relationships and low self-esteem. As Adler and Hammett have noted, the placebo may supply some of what is lacking in their lives: a sense of meaning, security, belonging, and a caring relationship with a 'parental' prescriber. One should note that *all* ill people display some of these characteristics to a lesser or greater extent, especially in the presence of severe illness. This sense of anxiety, vulnerability and dependence may enhance the placebo effect in a ritual of healing.

The characteristics of the *prescriber* or healer are crucial to the placebo effect, especially if their healing role is validated by their society. This validation is likely to be displayed by the use of certain ritual symbols, such as a white coat, stethoscope or prescription pad. By manipulating these potent symbols in a healing context the prescriber is both expressing and reaffirming certain basic values of the society, and enhancing a feeling of security and continuity on which the placebo effect depends (see Chapter 9). Their age, appearance, clothing, manner and air of authority are also relevant here, as are their own beliefs and expectations of the drug or procedure. As Claridge points out, the authority of the prescriber can also be used to manipulate *how* people respond to a particular drug: 'Deliberately manipulating the individual subject's motives or expectations is one way . . . in which drug effects can be enhanced, diminished or reversed.'[15]

Rapport, mutual confidence and understanding between prescriber and patient also contribute to the placebo effect. For this effect to be maximized there must be a congruence between the doctor's approach to therapy and the patient's attitudes towards illness and expectations of the treatment. This atmosphere of prescribing is complemented by the social environment in which *ingestion* of the medication actually takes place. The patients' perception of other people's behaviour with whom they are interacting may affect their response to the drug. This type of response is more clearly seen in the public healing rituals of some small-scale non-Western societies, where the patient is surrounded by a crowd of friends and relatives who share expectations of the treatment's efficacy. However, even in a Western setting the experience and expectation of a patient's family and friends of a particular drug (or doctor) may influence the degree of the placebo response.

In summary, the placebo effect may be seen with either

pharmacologically inactive or active preparations, although its effects have been more vividly described with the former. It is also a feature of double-blind trials of new drugs, where about one-third of the sample usually respond to a placebo. It is fashionable for some doctors, trained to look only for physiological data, to dismiss this phenomenon as 'only a placebo effect' (and therefore not *real* medicine). Nevertheless it should be noted that the therapeutic effects of belief, expectations and a good healer–patient relationship have been utilized by healers in every human culture, in all parts of the world, and throughout human history.

Case history: Placebo effect in angina pectoris

The placebo effect depends on the beliefs and expectations of a physician, as well as those of the patients. This is illustrated in a study by Benson and McCallie[16] of the effectiveness of various types of therapy for angina pectoris. Many of these have been tried only to be abandoned later on. They include: heart muscle extract, various hormones, X-irradiation, anticoagulants, monoamine oxidase inhibitors, thyroidectomies, radioactive iodine, sympathectomies and many other treatments. When each of these has been introduced, their proponents (or 'enthusiasts') have reported remarkable successes in their initial trials of treatment. Most of these non-blind or single-blind trials fail to control the strong placebo effect evoked by the investigators' expectations of success. Later, when more controlled trials are done by 'sceptics' – more sceptical investigators, who operate under circumstances that minimize the placebo effect – the therapy is found to be no better than inert, control placebos. Quantitatively, there is a consistent pattern of a 70–90% success reported initially by the enthusiasts, which is reduced in the sceptics' trial to 30–40% 'baseline' placebo effectiveness. This 30%, as already mentioned, is the usual proportion of 'placebo types' in a group, or the degree of 'placebo effect' from any drug or procedure.

Benson and McCallie have analysed the results of five erstwhile treatments for angina pectoris, all of which 'are now believed to have no specific physiologic efficacy, yet at one time all were found to be effective and were used extensively'. These were: the xanthines, khellin, vitamin E, ligation of the internal mammary artery, and implantation of this artery. Vitamin E, for example, was introduced as a therapy for angina in 1946. Initial enthusiastic reports noted that 90% of 84 patients benefited from several months' treatment with it. Over the years, several more trials were carried out which gradually reduced its level of effectiveness. By the 1970s controlled trials were showing it to be no better than placebo pills. That is, 'the discrepancy between the results of advocates and sceptics may be attributed, in part, to the greater degree of placebo effect evoked by the enthusiasts'. Over 80% of patients initially reported subjective improvement in symptoms, from any of these five treatments. There were also objective improvements, such as increased exercise tolerance, reduced nitroglycerin usage, and improved electrocardiograph results. In some cases these lasted up to one year.

The authors point out that 'the placebo effect will most likely persist as long as the psychologic context in which it was evoked remains unchanged. Patient and physician belief in the efficacy of the therapy and a continuously strong physician–patient relation should maintain the effects for long periods.' This can even occur in the presence of angiographically verified coronary artery disease. They also point out that the history of angina treatments demonstrates that 'the advent of a "new" procedure may impair the effectiveness of an old one', and that the expectation of better results transfers the placebo effect to the new procedure. They quote Trousseau's remark that 'you should treat as many patients as possible with the new drugs while they still have the power to heal'.

Drug dependence and addiction

Psychological dependence on drugs has been defined by Lader[17] as: 'the need the patient experiences for the psychological effects of a drug. This need can be of two types. The patient may crave the drug-induced symptoms or changes in mood – a feeling of euphoria or a lessening of tension, for example. Or the patient may take the drug to stave off the symptoms of withdrawal.' Both personality and sociocultural factors are as important as the pharmacology of the drug used, in both psychological dependence *and* physical addiction. In some cases the pharmacology can be irrelevant, as in psychological dependence on a placebo, or on a drug taken for years that no longer has any physical effect. In understanding these phenomena, the social

and cultural contexts in which drugs are prescribed, administered or taken – all of which contribute to the total drug effect –
need to be taken into account.

Some of these factors have been examined in the case of
psychotropic drugs, such as tranquillizers and sleeping tablets.
These drugs form the single largest group of drugs prescribed
each year in the Western world, and this has increased steadily
in the past 20 years. In the UK, for example, from 1965 to 1970,
prescriptions for tranquillizers increased by 59% and for
non-barbiturate hypnotics by 145%.[18] In 1972, 45.3 million
prescriptions for psychotropics were issued by the NHS general
practitioners in England alone (17.7% of the total number of
prescriptions).[19] In the USA, benzodiazepine psychotropics are
the most commonly prescribed drugs,[20] and in 1973 it was
estimated that prescriptions for one of these, diazepam
(Valium), was increasing at a rate of 7 million annually.[21] Many
of these drugs are given by regular repeat prescriptions or
'refills', and are taken for many years. In Parish's study in
Birmingham,[22] 14.9% of the patient sample had taken psychotropics regularly for one year or more, and 4.9% for five years or
more. Yet Williams,[23] of the Institute of Psychiatry in London,
quotes studies showing that most hypnotics lose their 'sleep-
promoting properties' within 3–14 days of continuous use by
the patient, and that there was little convincing evidence that
benzodiazepines were effective in the treatment of anxiety after
four months' continuous treatment. It would therefore seem
that many people are taking psychotropics for reasons other
than their pharmacological effect. The symbolic meaning of the
drug for the individual taking it is an important component of
the phenomenon of psychological dependence.

Both the psychotropic drug and the prescription for it can be
viewed as 'multi-vocal' ritual symbols (see Chapter 9), the power
of which is conferred in the ritual of prescribing – and which
signify many different things for the patients and for those
around them. Ostensibly the drug is meant to have a particular
physical effect (its 'manifest function'), but it may have other
dimensions of meaning ('latent functions') for those ingesting it.
It may symbolize, for example, that the patient is 'ill'; that all
personal failures are due to this 'illness' (or to the drug's
side-effects); that he or she deserves sympathy and attention
from family and friends; that the doctor – a powerful, respected,
healing figure – is still interested in him or her; and that modern
science (which produced the drug) is powerful, reliable and
efficient. Smith,[24] in reviewing the literature on this subject, lists

27 of these 'latent functions', as well as seven more 'manifest' ones. Perhaps most importantly, the drug carries with it some of the healing attributes of the doctor who prescribed it.

Psychotropic drug use is embedded in a matrix of *social* values and expectations. The drug can be used to improve social relationships, by bringing one's behaviour (and emotions) into conformity with an idealized model of 'normal' behaviour. In my own study[13] of 50 long-term users of psychotropics, for example, the drugs were often taken for their believed effect on relationships with others. With the drug, the patient was 'normal', self-controlled, good to live with, nurturing, non-complaining, sociable and assertive. Without it the opposite would occur, with damaging effects on their relationships. For example, *without* the psychotropic drug: 'I'd be nervy, impatient with other people', 'I'd be nasty, jumpy, not nice to live with', 'I wouldn't want to see people', 'I couldn't help those I love'.

At a study at the Addiction Research Foundation in Toronto, by Cooperstock and Lennard,[25] the findings were similar. Tranquillizers were taken as an 'aid in the maintenance of a nurturing, caring role', especially by women in role conflicts between work and home. Men saw tranquillizers particularly 'as a means of controlling somatic symptoms in order to perform their occupational role'. In both these studies, psychotropic drugs were seen as a means (both pharmacological and symbolic) of meeting social expectations, whether at work or within the family. These expectations are part of a culture's view of what constitutes normal, acceptable behaviour, and how this is to be attained. Several authors have pointed out that in Western industrialized society there is widespread social support for what Pellegrino[26] terms 'chemical coping' – that is, the regular use of medications (including alcohol, tobacco and psychotropics) to improve one's emotional state and social relationships and help one conform to societal norms. Warburton[27] has called this phenomenon 'the chemical road to success'.

Social acceptance of psychotropic drug-taking as a normal part of life can lessen the stigma of psychological dependence on them. In my psychotropic drug study,[13] for example, 72% of the sample knew of another person taking the same drug, and 88% were known by others to be taking a psychotropic. Only 18% reported disapproval by others of their taking the drug, 10% reported approval, and 29% said that those who knew did not care either way. In this sample, at least, psychotropic drug ingestion took place openly, and in the absence of any major moral disapproval. This climate of acceptance makes possible 'fashions' in drug taking, and facilitates the *exchange* of drugs between patients. In Warburton's study in Reading,[27] 68% of young adults interviewed admitted receiving psychotropics from friends or relatives.

This 'normalization' of drugs in Western culture is illustrated by lay beliefs about what is, and what is not, 'a drug'. In Jones' study,[28] for example, while 80% of patients interviewed agreed that heroin was 'a drug', only 50% classified morphine, sleeping tablets and tranquillizers as such, while only one-third saw aspirin as a drug. While 84% of patients in my study saw psychotropics as drugs, they were at pains to point out that it was *not* a powerful or 'hard' drug, that is something they had little control over, and which interfered with consciousness: 'It's just a calmer, a help. I can cut it off when I want to', and 'It's soft, sweet. It's different. It's softer' (than other drugs).

The social values that support this normalization may partly be *learned* from doctors, who in turn may be influenced by colleagues, and by the advertising of the pharmaceutical industry. Parish[22] has suggested that, in prescribing these drugs for personal problems, doctors are communicating a model on how to deal with these problems, not by confronting them but by taking a drug. The issuing of repeat prescriptions or refills can also be interpreted by patients as tacit approval of psychological dependence. Patients' experiences of taking psychotropics, with medical sanction, can have cumulative effects. As Joyce points out, 'People who have had one favourable outcome from drug treatment will more probably experience such an outcome on subsequent occasions as well', and this can lay the foundations for future dependence. In Tyrer's view[29] this dependence on psychotropics is more likely if the drug is prescribed in a fixed dosage regimen (where it becomes a fixed point around which the day is organized) and for a long period of time.

In physical dependence, or *addiction*, social and cultural factors also play an important role. Claridge has pointed out that the distinction between psychological and physical dependence may be more theoretical than real: 'Medically recognized addiction is only the pathological end-part of a continuum of drug-taking that involves us all. Even the most upright of citizens have their chemical comforters, most of which are psychologically harmless when taken in small quantities'.[30] These chemical comforters include tea, coffee, tobacco, psychotropic drugs and, of course, alcohol. Cultures differ on what particular comforter is most commonly used, and under what circumstances, and there are usually tacit rules controlling their use. In the case of 'hard' drugs, such as heroin or morphine, the sociocultural matrix in which drug-taking occurs also has its tacit rules and sanctions. Addicts often form an outcast subculture, with their own particular view of the world.[31] These subcultures may play an important part in the spread of certain disease, such as infectious hepatitis. Recently, there has been increased research on the role of needle sharing among intravenous drug users in the spread of AIDS: in Edinburgh, for example, it has been estimated that about 60% of injecting drug users in the city are HIV positive.[32]

The extent to which individual addicts are integrated into this subculture may determine whether they are able to give up hard drugs or not. If for any reason the subculture is dismantled, addicts may overcome their physical addiction with unexpected ease. For example, Robins et al.[33] did a follow-up study (1973) of drug use by US servicemen returned from Vietnam. They studied 943 men who had returned to the USA from Vietnam in 1971, 8–12 months after their return. Of these, 495 had had urine tests positive for opiates at the time of departure from Vietnam; and three-quarters of these felt that they had been addicted to narcotics in Vietnam. In the 8–12 months after their return, one-third had had more experience with opiates, but only 7% of the group showed signs of physical dependence. Almost none of the urine-positive group expressed a desire for treatment, or addiction rehabilitation programmes. As Robins et al. point out, this result is surprising 'in the light of the common belief that dependence on narcotics is easily acquired and virtually impossible to rid oneself of, [yet] most of the men who used narcotics heavily in Vietnam stopped when they left Vietnam and had not begun again 8–12 months later'. Part of the explanation for this is probably that the milieu in Vietnam – psychologically, socially and economically – was favourable towards the persistence of an addict subculture without, as the authors put it, 'the deterrents of high prices, impure drugs, or the presence of disapproving family'.

Physical addiction, therefore, is not just a physical phenomenon; it also requires certain social or cultural factors for its persistence. A further example of this is a case quoted by Jackson,[34] from St. Louis in the mid-1960s. Here the lifestyle and activities of heroin addicts remained, unexpectedly, unchanged, when the supply of heroin in the city dried up. It was temporarily replaced by metamphetamine – the pharmacological effect of which is the polar opposite of that of heroin – but the addicts carried on behaving exactly as before: 'they went to the same shooting galleries to shoot up, scored from the same connections, and bought the magic white powder (metamphetamine instead of heroin) in the same little glassine envelopes they knew so well'. As Jackson concludes, 'the addicts maintained the heroin subculture on a metamphetamine metabolism; obviously the subculture had had powerful and spectacular magic working for it'.

Case history: Addict subculture in Lexington, Kentucky, USA

The power, and nature, of an addict subculture has been studied by Freeland and Rosenstiel,[35] at the Clinical Research Center in Lexington, Kentucky. They found that self-defined groups, such as narcotic addicts, 'tend to justify their own way of life by stereotyping the behaviour of others in a negative fashion'. The power of culturally based stereotypes to influence one's life and one's perceptions depends on how committed one is to that way of life. In the case of the narcotic addicts, this commitment was intense and all-embracing. Their cultural (or rather subcultural) belief system embodied a strong we–they dichotomy. 'They' were the 'squares', whose life was seen as being boring, passive, hypocritical, fear-ridden and subordinate. This negative picture was contrasted with their own idealized self-image as 'hustlers', that is 'an active, dominant, capable, self-motivated person who is highly aware of his surroundings and in control of them'. They saw themselves as living 'the fast life': a hustler first, and an addict second. Hustlers were seen as having a specialized type of knowledge about the world which 'maximizes one's abilities as a predator'. In the authors' view, the maintenance of this we–they dichotomy, and the stereotypes of the square and the hustler, will tend to minimize the impact of any therapeutic or rehabilitative programmes directed towards the addicts.

As a strategy to overcome this situation, they organized lengthy discussions on these stereotypes between the addict group and a group of 'squares'. The aim was to reduce the addicts' tendency to stereotype by reducing their ethnocentrism, that is by providing them with alternative ways of seeing the world, derived from other groups. The 'squares' included medical staff and students, as well as others in churches and schools. Both groups were encouraged to discuss the stereotypes of the others, and to examine how these stereotypes affected their interactions. The addicts were also shown films of other societies, and it was pointed out that stereotyping was a universal human feature though it could be dangerous and inhibit communication. The outcome of this process was to convince the addict group that they could modify their lifestyle 'without being doomed to a life of subservience, boredom, inactivity, and passivity', and this was a major step in their rehabilitation into everyday life. It was also helpful in enhancing rapport between addict patients and medical staff. This study, like the others mentioned above, stresses the importance of the *non*-pharmacological variables in producing and maintaining drug addiction; in any individual addict, this will includes a mix of sociocultural, economic, geographical and personality variables.

Alcohol use and abuse

Excessive alcohol usage is a feature of many groups and individuals world-wide, especially those of lower social status and income. Various studies of the problem have indicated that the incidence of alcoholism, and the regular consumption of alcohol on ritual and other occasions, differs markedly between social and cultural groups. In the USA, for example, Italian Americans and Jewish Americans have low rates of alcoholism, while Irish Americans[36] and some Native Americans[37] have very high rates. The reasons for these differences must be found in the ways that alcohol intake is embedded in the matrix of cultural values and expectations of these groups.

The effect of alcohol on the individual drinker depends, as with all total drug effects, on a number of factors: physical, psychological and sociocultural. The *physical* factors include the body build of the drinker, the presence or absence of liver damage, whether drinking took place on an empty stomach or not, and possibly an inherited intolerance of alcohol. They also include the pharmacological properties of the drink itself, especially its volume, type and concentration. These physical and pharmacological factors are not enough, however, to explain how and why people drink, and how it affects their behaviour. One should also consider the *sociocultural* characteristics of the drinkers, their family and friends, and the setting in which drinking takes place. In particular, the attitudes of the cultural group towards two different types of drinking – 'normal' and 'abnormal' – should be examined.

'Normal' drinking refers to the everyday use of alcohol at mealtimes, or on social and ritual occasions. In these cases, the moderate use of alcohol is an accepted part of daily life. However, the type and amount of alcohol, and when and by whom it is consumed, are strongly *controlled* by cultural rules and sanctions. In 'abnormal' drinking, these mores are transgressed and there is frequent and excessive intake of alcohol, with resultant *uncontrolled*, drunken behaviour. Cultural groups vary in how, and under what circumstances, abnormal drinking takes place, and in how they define the behavioural characteristics of drunkenness. The boundary between normal and abnormal drinking is not clear-cut, however. In an Irish wake, for example, drunkeness is sometimes acceptable, but it is considered abnormal in other contexts. O'Connor[38] has pointed out that 'if one looks at the patterns and attitudes of drinking in a society, one may come to some understanding of drinking pathologies or alcoholism'. That is, one should look at the culturally defined normal drinking behaviour of a group in order to understand the abnormal forms of drinking that may be found within it.

On this basis, O'Connor has classified cultures, in relation to drinking, into four main groups:

1. Abstinent cultures.
2. Ambivalent cultures.
3. Permissive cultures.
4. Over-permissive cultures.

This classification refers to attitudes towards drinking as a 'normal' part of everyday life, and towards drunkenness. In abstinent cultures the use of alcohol is strictly prohibited under any circumstances, and there are strong negative feelings towards alcohol use. Examples of this are the Muslim cultures of North Africa and the Middle East, and certain Protestant ascetic churches in the Western world (such as Baptists, Methodists, Mormons and Seventh Day Adventists). While 'normal' drinking is rare in these cultures, problem ('abnormal') drinking is slightly higher here than in more permissive cultures, especially as a result of personal problems. O'Connor quotes studies that show that in the Southern USA, which has a strong abstinence tradition, 'a relationship was found between parental disapproval of drinking and an increase in the percentage of problem drinkers'. Similarly, another study showed a high incidence of heavy drinking and intoxication among a group of Mormon students, because drinking by members of abstinent groups is not controlled by any drinking norms, therefore alcoholism is more likely among such groups.

Drinking norms are tacit rules about who can drink, in whose company, in which settings, and how much can be consumed. Alcoholism, therefore, is the over-use of alcohol, and behaviour *uncontrolled* by social norms.

Ambivalent cultures have two, mutually contradictory attitudes towards alcohol. O'Connor applies this label to the Irish. On the one hand, drinking is a normal part of Irish life: 'from the womb to the tomb the Irish were seen to use drink at christenings, weddings and funerals. All social and economic life was centred around the use of alcohol.' On the other hand, there has been strong disapproval of *all* drinking by various abstinent temperance movements in the past 150 years. This has led to the absence of a consistent, generalized and coherent attitude in Ireland towards alcohol intake. In this situation, 'the culture does not have a well integrated system of controls, the individual is left in a situation of ambivalence which may be conducive to alcoholism'.

In a *permissive* culture, by contrast, there are norms, customs, values and sanctions relating to drinking which are widely shared by the group. Everyone is allowed to drink, but only in a controlled way and on certain occasions. In this type of culture, the moderate intake of alcohol at mealtimes, and on certain social or festive occasions, is encouraged as being normal – though there are strong sanctions against drunkenness or other forms of uncontrolled drinking behaviour. In these groups, such as Italians, Spaniards, Portuguese and orthodox Jews, the rate of alcoholism is low. For example, as Knupfer and Room[36] point out, Italian Americans see wine as a type of food, to be consumed only as part of a meal, while among orthodox Jews wine is an integral part of many religious rituals. Both groups tend to despise drunken behaviour. Among both, intoxication is regarded as a personal and family disgrace, and the use of wine between meals is frowned upon. France, too, is a permissive culture towards drink, though in O'Connor's view it is *over-permissive*. Although less wine is taken in France than in Italy, the pattern of drinking in the two countries is different, and alcoholism is much higher in France. Not only are French attitudes towards normal drinking favourable, but cultural attitudes 'are also favourable to other forms of deviant behaviour while drinking'. Drinking is also associated with virility, and 'there is widespread social acceptance of intoxication as fashionable, humorous or at least tolerable'.

In general, therefore, both permissive and over-permissive cultures, where drinking *is* allowed (but only in a controlled form), have lower rates of alcoholism – that is, abnormal, uncontrolled drinking behaviour – than either abstinent or ambivalent cultures. These sociocultural patterns are passed on from generation to generation, and partly determine whether a particular member of the society is likely to seek solace in drink at times of crisis or unhappiness.

The differences in alcohol use and abuse among ethnic and cultural groups in the USA have been examined by Greeley and McCready,[39] using data gathered by the National Opinion Research Center. The study was based on almost one thousand families of Irish, Jewish, Italian and Swedish origin. They have developed a model to examine how children learn drinking behaviour, and to explain much of the ethnic diversity in drinking patterns that has been found. In their view, five variables, from both the individual's upbringing and their present situation, can influence drinking behaviour, both normal and uncontrolled:

1. *Family drinking.* Whether and how frequently both parents drink; a 'drinking problem' within the family; and parental approval of their children drinking.
2. *Family structure.* In particular the 'decision-making style' in the home, that is whether decisions regarding the children are made by one parent or jointly by both; and also the degree of explicit affection and mutual support within the family.
3. *Personality variables.* Particularly orientations towards achievement, efficacy and authority. It has been suggested that an authoritarian family structure produces men with a particular type of personality, especially a great need to be the only (and powerful) decision-maker, and that this attitude may predispose to problem drinking.
4. *Spouse's drinking behaviour.* Alcoholism is more likely if a spouse drinks heavily as well.
5. *Drinking environment* in which the person lives; that is the prevalence of drinking and the availability of drink in their sociocultural environment, including social, ritual or festive occasions.

These five groups of variables, taken together, account for many of the differences in drinking patterns, and rates of alcoholism, among ethnic and cultural groups; they may also help us to understand why an individual in a particular group is at risk of becoming a problem drinker.

O'Connor[38] has developed a similar model to show 'that for groups that use alcohol to a significant degree, the lowest incidence of alcoholism is associated with certain habits and attitudes'. These include:

1. Exposure of the children to alcohol early in life, within a strong family or religious group.
2. Use of this alcohol in a very diluted form (to give low blood-alcohol levels).
3. Alcohol viewed mainly as a 'food', and usually consumed with meals.
4. The parents presenting an example of moderate drinking.
5. Drinking not being given any moral importance, as either a virtue or a sin.
6. Drinking not being considered proof of adulthood or virility.
7. Abstinence being socially acceptable.
8. Drunkenness being socially unacceptable and not considered 'stylish, comical or tolerable'.
9. Wide agreement among members of the group on 'the ground rules of drinking' – that is, the norms governing drinking behaviour.

A further factor governing drinking behaviour is the *setting* in which it takes place (such as a pub, club, bar, restaurant or home) and the social function performed by these settings. Each of these contexts has its own implicit rules governing the drinking behaviour that takes place within them. Drinking patterns in public settings, such as bars or clubs, are often independent of the drinkers' sociocultural background (although there are more ethnic settings, such as 'Irish pubs'). For example, Thomas[40] studied public drinking in bars and taverns in an urban working-class community of 50 000 people in New England, with the pseudonym 'Clyde Cove'. He found that these 'laboring-men's bars' functioned mainly as social clubs after work, where working-class men could meet together in an atmosphere of relative equality and mutual acceptance. In this setting, alcohol was merely a social lubricant, and not the main reason why the men came together. As Thomas puts it: 'in the after-work hours of 4–6 p.m., nothing more is derived from bar life than a light form of *communitas* and a short period of time-out from the workaday world'. There were implicit rules governing their normal drinking behaviour, and drunkeness or 'problem' drinking was very infrequent, and was considered to be deviant behaviour within the bar. The bar customers were drawn from many ethnic groups, but ethnicity did not affect the content of bar life, and in many bars blacks and whites drank freely together.

In another study, in England, Hunt and Satterlee[41] describe the different social uses of alcohol in two pubs in a village in Cambridgeshire. The one pub, 'The Griffin', was frequented mainly by newcomers to the village, who were predominately upwardly mobile and middle class, and about one-third of them were women. Here alcohol was a way of creating – and sustaining – new relationships, especially by the ritual of 'round buying', which involved taking turns to buy drinks for as many as 20 people in the group. Much of their bonhomie spilled over into social events in each others' homes, either before or after the pub. By contrast, the clientele of 'The Three Barrels' were predominately male, mainly working class and middle-aged. Most of them had been born in the village, lived nearby, had known one another for many years, and were often related to one another. In this ambience, round buying was rare and unnecessary, since group cohesion was already maintained by a shared history, by shared kinship and shared neighbourhood. In each pub, therefore, alcohol had a different meaning, and played a different social role in maintaining the cohesion of the group of drinkers.

From an anthropological perspective, therefore, alcohol intake should always be viewed against its social and cultural background. This includes patterns of normal and abnormal drinking, the settings in which they occur, and the values associated with them. Other relevant factors are the *meanings* given to drinking by individuals or groups, such as a proof of virility, manhood, adulthood or rebelliousness. All these elements, in addition to personality traits and socioeconomic status, should be taken into account in understanding why and how a particular individual abuses alcohol.

Smoking behaviour

Tobacco smoking, like tea, coffee, alcohol and psychotropic drugs, is a commonly used chemical comforter. As with the other comforters, psychological dependence on smoking cannot be explained only by reference to the pharmacological properties of nicotine or tobacco. Sociocultural factors also play an important role in determining who smokes, under what circumstances, and for what reasons. As with alcohol use, it is important to understand the symbolic meanings of cigarette smoking – for individual smokers, and for those around them.

In the USA, cigarette smoking is believed to be the single largest cause of disease and death,[42] and the annual cost of morbidity from smoking-related diseases has been estimated at 27 billion dollars.[43] There are several studies that examine the demographic characteristics of these smokers, especially their age, sex, education, marital state and socioeconomic position, and from these data one can infer some of the influences on smoking behaviour. Reeder[44] of the University of California, Los Angeles, has reviewed most of the available literature on this subject. He points out that in the USA and Europe consumption of cigarettes has increased three-fold since 1930, despite anti-smoking propaganda. While the proportion of adult smokers in the USA has dropped, that of teenagers has risen. The proportion of smokers has been declining among men, but increasing among women. Men and women who were 21 in the late 1970s now smoke at equal rates, but many men in their 50s have given up the habit. Smoking rates are lowest among better educated groups, but this is less true for women. In general, there is a greater prevalence of smoking among women employed outside the home as compared with housewives, and female white collar workers are more likely to smoke than women in other occupations. Men in upper income categories were *less* likely to smoke, while women in the same bracket are *more* likely to be current smokers. Reeder relates these contradictory statistics to the changing sex roles of women, a greater proportion of whom (in the USA) have a college education and paid employment. There is a general trend towards equality 'in virtually all domains of social and economic life', and smoking rates reflect this equality. However, 'in the case of socioeconomic status the pattern is delayed, so that the smoking behaviour may be perceived as in some way an indicator of increased social power and/or independence – even before there is equality in economic status'.

Other studies reviewed by Reeder relate heavy smoking to a perception of powerlessness by the smokers, and a sense of 'anomie' and futility in their daily lives. Other correlations of high adult smoking rates were a drop in socioeconomic status (in men), and experiences of divorce or separation. Among teenagers, those less academically successful, or from one-parent families, were more likely to smoke. As with alcohol, teenagers were more likely to smoke if parents, siblings and friends already did so, the likely mechanisms in this case being imitation and role-modelling behaviour.

Considerable numbers of people still continue to smoke, despite all the health warnings from government and other agencies about its dangers. Some studies indicate that many smokers still do not believe that smoking could damage their health. For example, Marsh and Matheson[45] studied beliefs about smoking among 2700 British smokers and 1200 non-smokers, aged 16–66 years. Forty-five per cent of the smokers rejected outright the concept that they were more liable to heart disease because of their smoking, and 33% that smoking made them more prone to lung cancer. Overall, only 14% completely accepted the idea that smoking causes heart disease, and 11% that it causes lung cancer.

Doherty and Whitehead[46] suggest that cigarette smoking may also persist because it can be a way of communicating a wide range of social messages, especially among family and friends. Among other messages, smoking may signal to other people: 'Let's talk', 'Let's relax together', 'I need to be alone', 'I'm my own person', 'Be aware that I'm upset', or even 'I'm not going to tell you how I'm feeling'. Smoking, like alcohol, may therefore play a variety of social roles, and may help define a sense of social cohesion or of social withdrawal.

Cigarette smoking, however, does not persist only because of smokers' anomie, ignorance, or use of cigarettes as a social message. An overall picture of smoking must include the economic interests involved in tobacco production and use. In 1986 the *Bulletin of the Pan American Health Organization*[47] reviewed tobacco use world-wide, based on data from the World Health Organisation. They point out that tobacco is produced in about 120 countries, and that the contribution of developing countries to world tobacco production increased from 50% in 1963 to 63% in 1983. The major tobacco producing and consuming countries are China, the USA, the USSR, India and Brazil. About 37% of the world's cigarettes are produced by state-controlled industries in centrally planned countries, and a further 17% are manufactured by state monopolies whose aim is to maximize government revenue. The remainder of the market is dominated by seven international conglomerates. In many countries, the tobacco industry provides thousands of jobs, and it also provides income for the advertising industry, tax revenue for governments, and foreign currency for nations short on foreign exchange. Against this economic background, the *Bulletin* deplores 'the common government reluctance to act on tobacco, which is demonstrably a cause of avoidable disease and death on a scale unmatched by any other currently available product for human consumption'.

Sacramental drugs

In many cultures, drugs are used as sacramental substances, intrinsic to the rituals of religion, divination and healing, and to certain social interactions. Like the social foods described in Chapter 3, their ingestion may contribute to the continuity and cohesion of a particular group of people. World-wide, the most common ritual drug is obviously alcohol, and some of its social and religious uses have been described above. Other common substances important to the rituals of social encounters are the chemical comforters tobacco, tea and coffee.

In some cultural groups, hallucinogenic drugs are used to obtain states of transcendence and fervour, and in their trance state those who take them are 'possessed' by the power inherent in the drug. Such rituals may take many hours, or even days, to perform. Sometimes the drug is used only by a shaman or ritual healer, whose visions will reveal the source of individual or collective misfortune. Dobkin de Rios,[48] for example, describes the use of the hallucinogen *ayahuasca* by folk healers (*ayahuas-queros*) in an urban slum in Iquitos, Peru. As part of the ritual of healing, the healer imbibes the *ayahuasca* and the visionary content of his drug experience will help identify the cause of an individual's illness (such as witchcraft, evil eye, or *susto*), and how it should then be dealt with.

In Medieval Europe, certain hallucinogens were used as part of 'witches' brew' or as unguents rubbed into the skin. They included belladona (*Atropa belladona*), henbane (*Hyoscyamus niger*), mandrake (*Mandragora officinarum*) and the fly agaric mushroom (*Amanita muscaria*).

Among the more well known hallucinogenic drugs used in a ritual context today are: marihuana (*Cannabis sativa* and *Cannabis indica*) known as *hashish* or *kif* in the Middle East and North Africa, and as *ganja* among Rastafarians in the Caribbean;[49] psilocybin (*Psilocybe mexicana Heim*) among some Mexican Indian groups; peyote cactus (*Lophophora williamsii*) among Native Americans in the south-western USA, members of the Native American Church (which claims about 250 000 members);[50] *ayahuasca* or *yagé vine* (*Banisteriopsis caapsis* and *B. inebrians*), a hallucinatory drink used by South America Indians (especially in Brazil, Ecuador, Peru and Colombia);[51] and Jimson weed (*Datura stramonium*) used among the Algonquin Indians in the north-eastern USA, and other species of *Datura* used in parts of South America, Africa and Asia.[52]

In recent years, use of many of these hallucinogenic plants has spread beyond their groups of origin, and their original ritual context. In the industrialized world, many have been used as recreational drugs, in either their original or synthetic forms. In some susceptible individuals they are known to have caused addiction, habituation, acute psychosis, suicidal behaviour and various other disorders.

Recommended reading

Benson, H. and Epstein, M. D. (1975) The placebo effect: a neglected asset in the care of patients. *JAMA* **232**, 1225–1227

Claridge, G. (1970) *Drugs and Human Behaviour*. London: Allen Lane. A good summary of research into the placebo effect in Chapter 2.

Helman, C. G. (1981) 'Tonic', 'food' and 'fuel': social and symbolic aspects of the long-term use of psychotropic drugs. *Soc. Sci. Med.* **15B**, 521–533. A study of the symbolic meanings of psychotropic drugs for those who use them regularly.

O'Connor, J. (1975) Social and cultural factors influencing drinking behaviour. *Irish J. Med. Sci.* Suppl. (June), 65–71

Chapter 9

Ritual and the management of misfortune

Rituals are a feature of all human societies, large and small. They are an important part of the way that any social group celebrates, maintains and renews the world in which they live, and the way they deal with the dangers that threaten that world. Rituals occur in many settings, take on many forms, and perform many functions, both sacred and secular. In this chapter I will be describing the type of rituals that relate to health and illness, and the management of misfortune.

What is ritual?

Anthropologists have defined the various attributes of ritual in a number of ways, and they have pointed out that, for those that take part in it, ritual has important social, psychological and symbolic dimensions. A key characteristic of any rituals is that they are a form of repetitive behaviour that does not have a direct overt technical effect. For example, brushing one's teeth at the same time each night is a repetitive form of behaviour, but not a ritual. It is designed to have a specific physical effect: the removal of food and bacteria from the teeth. If, however, this action is accompanied by others which do not directly contribute towards the effect – such as always using a toothbrush of a particular colour, or saying certain words or prayers before, during or after brushing the teeth – then these extraneous actions can be thought of as having a private *ritual* significance for the person. In some cases *all* actions in a repetitive pattern of behaviour have no technological effect – as in private prayers or religious observance, or in some of the actions of the obsessive compulsive neurotic. In general, though, this form of private ritual behaviour is of less interest to anthropologists than the *public* rituals which take place in the presence of one or more other people.

Loudon[1] has defined these public rituals as 'those aspects of prescribed and repetitive formal behaviour, that is those aspects of certain customs, which have no direct technological consequences and which are symbolic'. That is, 'the behaviour or actions say something about the state of affairs, particularly about the social conditions of those taking part in the ritual'. In a social setting, rituals both express and renew certain basic values of that society, especially regarding the relationships of man to man, man to nature, and man to the supernatural world, relationships that are integral to the functioning of any human group. As Turner[2] puts it, 'ritual is a periodic restatement of the terms in which men of a particular culture must interact if there is to be any kind of coherent social life'. He sees two functions of ritual: an expressive function and a creative function. In its *expressive* aspect, it 'portrays in symbolic form certain key values and cultural orientations'. That is, it expresses these basic values in a dramatic form, and *communicates* them to both participants and spectators. Leach[3] and other anthropologists see this aspect of ritual as being the most important. For them ritual has some of the properties of a language, which can only be understood within a specific cultural context, and only by those who can 'decode' its meaning. As Leach[3] puts it, 'we must know a lot about the cultural context, the setting of the stage, before we can even begin to decode the message'. In its creative aspect ritual, according to Turner, 'actually creates, or re-creates, the categories through which men perceive reality – the axioms underlying the structure of society and the laws of the natural and moral orders'. It therefore restates, on a regular basis, certain values and principles of a society, and how its members should act *vis-à-vis* other men, gods, and the natural world, and it helps to re-create, in the minds of the participants, their collective view of the world.

The symbols of ritual

These two functions of ritual are achieved by the use of *symbols*. These include certain standardized objects, clothing, movements, gestures, words, sounds, songs, music and scents used in rituals, as well as the fixed order in which they appear. Turner[2] has examined the forms and meanings of ritual symbols, particularly those used in healing rituals. He points out that, especially in pre-literate societies, rituals have the important function of storing and transmitting information about the society; each ritual is an 'aggregation of symbols', and acts as a 'storehouse of traditional knowledge'. He sees each symbol as a 'storage unit' into which is packed the maximum amount of information. This is because ritual symbols are 'multi-vocal', that is they represent many things at the same time. Each symbol can be regarded as a multi-faceted mnemonic, with each facet 'corresponding to a specific cluster of values, norms, beliefs, sentiments, social roles and relationships within the cultural system of the community performing the ritual'. Therefore, to the outsider observing a ritual, there is more to the symbols than meets the eye. Each symbol has a whole range of associations for those taking part in the ritual; it tells them something about the values of their society, how it is organized, and how it views the natural and supernatural worlds. This restatement of basic values is particularly important at times of *danger* or uncertainty – when people feel that their world is threatened by misfortunes such as accident, famine, war, death, severe interpersonal conflicts or ill-health.

As mentioned above, ritual symbols can be 'decoded' only by looking at the context in which they appear. For example, a white coat worn in a hospital setting has a different range of associations from one worn by a supermarket attendant. Although both may be worn as a hygienic measure, the context in which they are worn adds many other associations to them. The white coat worn by a doctor in a healing context (hospital or doctor's office) may be regarded as a ritual *symbol*. While it does have a technical aspect – maintaining hygiene, and avoiding dirt and contamination – it also carries a number of associations with it. For those taking part in medical healing (doctors, nurses, patients) it *symbolizes* or represents a number of attributes associated with doctors in general. Some of these associations are shown in Table 9.1. The potency of this multi-vocal symbol is shown by its widespread use in television or newspaper advertisements for patent medicines, which feature an 'expert' whose white coat symbolizes 'science' and 'reliability'.

Similarly, these coats are often worn by medical secretaries and receptionists, though this is often not crucial for hygienic reasons. Here the coat symbolizes membership (however peripheral) of the healing profession, and carries with it some of the attributes of doctors. Because of the proliferation of white coats among hospital nurses, paramedical staff and technicians, however, other subsidiary symbols, such as a stethoscope, bleeper, or specially coloured name tag, are required to complete the 'message' to others involved in the healing context.

Table 9.1 Some associations of the physician's white coat as ritual symbol

A training in medicine
A licence to practise medicine
Membership of the medical profession
Being answerable to a professional organization
A repository of specialized and inaccessible knowledge
Power to:
  take a medical history
  obtain intimate details of patients' lives
  examine patients' bodies
  order a wide range of tests
  prescribe medication or other treatments
  make life or death decisions
  control those lower in professional hierarchy, e.g. junior doctors, nurses,
    medical students
Orientation towards caring, and the relief of suffering
A scientific orientation in concepts and techniques
Confidentiality
Reliability, efficiency
Emotional and sexual detachment
Cleanliness
Respectability and high social status
Familiarity with situations of illness, suffering or death

The sum of these symbols communicates information about the wearer of the coat, and also reinforces ideas of how 'a doctor' should dress and behave. These symbols refer less to the individual doctor than to the attributes of his or her *role* as representative of that special category of persons who constitute the official healing profession, a group that is empowered to use the forces of science or technology for the benefit of their patients. Thus the individual doctor employs the potent symbols of medical science, such as a white coat or a stethoscope, in rituals of healing in the same way that a non-Western healer employs certain religious symbols or artefacts (such as certain plants, talismans, divination stones, holy texts or statuettes) which also symbolize powerful healing forces (such as gods, spirits or ancestors). In this way, the use of these symbols brings the wider values of the society directly into the doctor–patient interaction.

Turner[4] has pointed out another attribute of ritual symbols: 'polarization of meaning'. This refers to the 'clustering' of the associations of a particular multi-vocal symbol around two opposite poles. At one pole the symbol is associated with 'social and moral facts', at the other with 'physiological facts'. This is seen in both healing rituals and 'rites of social transition'. For example, in some societies in girl's first menstruation, the menarche, is marked by a specific ritual. Some of the symbols used in this ritual are associated, in the minds of the participants, both with the *physiological* event (the menarche) and the *social* event of her new membership of the community of adult, fertile women. The ritual symbol acts as a 'bridge' linking the physiological and social stages of human life. These stages include birth, puberty, marriage and death. The symbols are a way of integrating physiological changes (especially at puberty), which might potentially be socially disruptive if left unchecked, with the laws and values that help keep the society together. As Turner puts it, 'powerful drives and emotions associated with human physiology, especially with the physiology of reproduction, are divested in the ritual process of their antisocial quality and attached to components of the normative order'.[4] In the Western world many of the rituals that used to mark life stages such as birth, puberty or death have disappeared; this means that these major life changes are not surrounded by ritual symbolism that gives meaning to the event far beyond its physiological significance. In contrast, in many non-Western societies, the symbols associated with physiological changes link these changes to wider social or cosmological events: pregnancy, for example, is not only a physical event, but is also the social transition of 'woman' to 'mother'; death is a physical event, but is sometimes seen as a simultaneous 'birth' into the society of ancestors. Some of these rituals will be described further in this chapter.

Case history: Colour symbolism of Zulu medicines

To illustrate the multi-vocal and bi-polar aspects of ritual symbols I have selected Harriet Ngubane's description[5] of the symbols used in healing rituals by the Zulu of Southern Africa. In this community, it is the *colour* of the medicines rather than their pharmacological properties that is considered their most important attribute. This colour symbolism is particularly important in medicines used for prophylactic purposes, or in dealing with illnesses thought to have a supernatural origin. The medicines are divided into three groups, black (*mnyama*), red (*bomvu*) and white (*mhlope*), and each colour is associated with a cluster of meanings, physiological, social and cosmological. Black represents night-time, darkness, dirt, pollution, faeces, death and danger. Defaecation, dirt and death can be seen as antisocial elements, all of which should be absent from normal social encounters. Also, night is the time when people cannot see, when they withdraw from their usual social activities; at night, sick people become sicker and sorcerers are said to work. Ancestral spirits visit their descendants in dreams, so that sleep is a point of contact with the dead; sleep, as Ngubane says, 'may be regarded as a miniature death that takes a person away from the conscious life of the day'. In contrast, white symbolizes the good things of life, good health and good fortune. It represents daylight, and the events that take place during it like eating or social interactions. During the day people participate in social activities and live their lives. They see clearly and there is no sense of danger. White represents the social values of life, eating, and seeing. The third colour, red, symbolizes the states of transition between black and white, much as sunset or sunrise between day and night. It represents an in-between position, slightly more dangerous than white, but less so than black. It also stands for other states of transition or transformation, such as growth, regeneration and rebirth. The association of blood with states of transition (such as birth or a fatal wound) are also relevant here. In treating an ill person, the Zulu healer aims to restore health, which is seen as a *balance* between the person and the environment. This is achieved by expelling from the body what is bad, by the use of black and red remedies, and then strengthening the body by the use of white medicines. The medicines are always used in a fixed order – black, red, white. This is meant to achieve a transformation from illness to health, 'from the darkness of night to the goodness of daylight', from death to life, from danger to safety, from antisocial to social behaviour. As Ngubane puts it: 'the daylight represents life and good health. To be (mystically) ill is likened to moving away from the daylight into the dimness of the sunset and on into the night . . . The practitioner endeavours to drive a patient out of the mystical darkness by black medicines, through the reddish twilight of the sunrise by red medicines, and back into daylight and life by white medicines.'

Types of ritual

While there are many types of private ritual, anthropologists have described three main types of public ritual:

1. Cosmic cycle or calendrical rituals.

2. Rituals of social transition (*rites de passage*).
3. Rituals of misfortune.

Calendrical rituals

Calendrical rituals celebrate changes in the cosmic cycle, such as the changing of seasons, the division of the year into segments such as months, weeks or days, as well as certain festivals and holy days. The identity and world-view of the group is linked symbolically to events in the cosmic cycle, or to certain specified points within that cycle. Examples of this are harvest festivals, mid-summer festivals, holy days such as Christmas or Easter, or commemorative days such as Thanksgiving or Remembrance Sunday. These social occasions are usually based on the cycle of the seasons, or the position of the moon, sun or planetary bodies. In many of these rituals, the symbols used link the social and cosmological dimensions, and help reinforce and re-create the social organization and values of the society.

Rituals of social transition

The rituals of social transition are present in one form or another in every society. They relate changes in the human life-cycle to changes in social position within the society, by linking the physiological to the social aspects of an individual's life. Examples of this are rituals associated with pregnancy, birth, puberty, menarche, weddings, funerals and severe ill-health. In each of these stages, the ritual signals the *transition* of the individual from one status to another, such as that from 'wife' to 'mother' in pregnancy. As Standing[6] points out, the ritual taboos and prescriptions surrounding pregnancy in many societies help prepare the woman, in terms of her behaviour, for her future role as 'a mother', as well as dramatizing this change in status to the society at large. In Western society, puberty rituals, such as Confirmations or Barmitzvahs, still exist, and signal the transition between child and young adult; birth rituals, such as baptism, christening or circumcision, signal 'social birth' (new membership of society), shortly after biological birth.

Leach[7] sees the origin of these transition rituals in the human tendency to divide things or actions into categories, each with its own boundary and name (see Chapter 1). As he puts it: 'when we use symbols (either verbal or non-verbal) to distinguish one class of things or actions from another we are creating artificial boundaries in a field which is "naturally" continuous'. These 'boundaries' in the continuous field of perception are characterized by a sense of ambiguity and danger. When things lie in the 'no man's land' between definitions or categories, when they are 'neither fish nor fowl', they provoke a sense of uneasiness, especially in those who prefer things to be more clearly defined. This process, according to Leach, applies also to the progress of the individual through various social identities during the course of their life – such as 'child', 'adult', 'mother' and 'widow'. In the period of transition *between* these identities the individual is considered to be in an interval of 'social timelessness', in a vulnerable, 'abnormal' position, dangerous both to themselves and to others. For this reason, special 'rituals of social transition' are invoked which mark the event, and protect both individual and society by various ritual taboos and observances. For example, many Western wedding customs still specify that in order to avoid 'bad luck' the bride should not be seen by her groom the night before the wedding, and she is kept protectively veiled until well into the wedding ceremony, after which she is no longer considered vulnerable. In many non-Western societies, the vulnerable 'period of transition' may last for months or even years.

In Leach's view,[7] most ritual occasions in any society are concerned with this 'movement across social boundaries from one social status to another'. In these circumstances, ritual has two functions: 'proclaiming the change in status' and 'magically bringing it about', though the two are closely related. To the participants, the belief is that without the ritual the change would somehow not take place.

States of social transition

Van Gennep[8] has described three stages in these *rites de passage*. They are: *separation, transition* and *incorporation*. In the first stage, the person is removed from his or her normal social life, and set apart by various customs and taboos for a variable period of time. After this stage of *transition*, other rituals celebrate the third stage of *incorporation*, whereby the person is returned to normal society, and into their new social role. Often this last stage is marked by ritual bathing or other rites of symbolic purification. Based on Van Gennep's and Leach's work, the three stages of these rituals of social transition are illustrated in Figure 9.1.

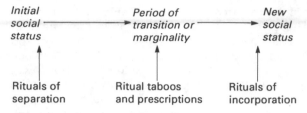

Figure 9.1 Rituals of social transition

Rituals of pregnancy and childbirth

In all societies, pregnancy and childbirth are more than just biological events. As described in Chapter 6, they are also *social* events – the transition of the woman (especially with a first birth) from the social status of 'woman' to that of 'mother'. During pregnancy, the woman is in a state of transition between these two social statuses. In this state of limbo, she is often considered to be in an ambiguous and socially abnormal situation – vulnerable to outside dangers, and sometimes dangerous to other people. In many traditional societies, pregnant women withdraw from social activities, and live somewhat apart from other people, subject to certain taboos about diet, dress and behaviour. These taboos are designed to protect the pregnancy, but they are also ways of marking the transition between social statuses. In some cases, these taboos may extend well into the postpartum period. Among the Zulu people of Southern Africa, for example, a women is considered to be still vulnerable to outside dangers until all her postpartum bleeding ceases.[9] Furthermore, this blood is considered to be dangerous to her husband's virility, as well as to plants in the field, and even to livestock.

Many of the practices and beliefs associated with modern Western obstetrics can also be seen as having an important ritual component,[10] and the ritual symbols used here are those of medical science and technology. Some of the culturally specific 'messages' transmitted by these symbols have been described in more detail in Chapter 6. Overall, pregnancy and childbirth in the Western world are as ritualized, in their own way, as they are elsewhere. As Kitzinger[11] has put it: 'baptism, circumcision, naming ceremonies, segregation of the new mother and baby, churching of women, taboos on sexual intercourse following birth, even the postnatal checkup, are all often complicated steps in a kind of dance which continues until mother and child

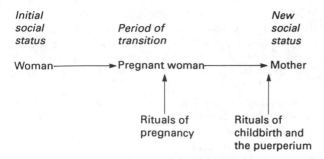

Figure 9.2 Rituals of pregnancy and childbirth

are safely established in their correct social places and are considered no longer at risk'.

The three main stages of social transition in pregnancy and childbirth are illustrated in Figure 9.2.

Rituals of death and mourning

Hertz[12] has examined one form of rituals of social transition: those associated with death and mourning. He has examined the funerary customs of many societies, and sees common themes among them. In most human societies people have, in effect, two types of death: one biological and the other social. Between these two there is a variable period of time, which may be days, months or even years. While biological death is the end of the human organism, 'social death' is the end of the person's social identity. This takes place at a series of ceremonies, including the funeral, whereby the society bids farewell to one of its members, and reasserts its continuity without him. Hertz points out that in most non-Western societies, death is seen, not as a single event in time but as a *process* whereby the deceased is slowly transferred from the land of the living into the land of the dead. Simultaneously, there is a transition between social identities, from living person to dead ancestor. During the period between biological death and final social death, the deceased's soul is often considered to be in a state of limbo, still a partial member of society, and potentially dangerous to other people as it roams free and unburied. In this transitional phase the soul still has some social rights, especially over its bereaved relatives. They have to perform certain ceremonies, act or dress in a special way, and generally withdraw from ordinary life. Like the soul they, too, are in a socially ambiguous state between identities, dangerous both to themselves and to others. In many cultures a widowed woman is prohibited from remarrying for a specified period after her husband's death. In Hertz's view she is considered to be in a transitional state, still married to the soul of her husband until his final moment of social death.

In the Malay archipelago, the corpse is given a first, temporary burial while it decomposes, before being reburied months or even years later at a final ceremony. During the period between the two funerals 'the deceased continues to belong more or less exclusively to the world he has just left. To the living falls the duty of providing for him; twice a day till the final ceremony . . . [they] bring him his usual meal.' During this period 'the deceased is looked upon as having not yet completely ended his earthly existence'. The final funeral ends this existence, and its ritual is one of *incorporation*, whereby the deceased is initiated or 'reborn' into the society of dead ancestors, and the mourners reincorporated into normal society and liberated from the special taboos and restrictions of their transitional state. The final ceremony also removes the danger from the soul, which is no longer in limbo.

Eisenbruch[13] has described some of the culturally patterned ways of taking leave of the deceased, among different social and cultural groups in the USA – including urban blacks, Chinese, Italians, Greeks, Haitians, Latinos, and south-east Asian refugees – and shown the wide variations in their bereavement beliefs and customs. In the UK, Skultans[14] has also described some of the range of bereavement practices among different cultural groups. The Irish *wake*, for example, involves watching of the corpse by relatives for several days and nights, and sometimes involves feasting and drinking. Among Greek Cypriots there is 'socially patterned weeping and wailing', followed by a defined period of mourning and wearing black. Among orthodox Jews, the *shib'ah* has a precise structure of mourning, lasting seven days from the funeral, during which time the bereaved remain at home and are visited by consolers. Mourning dress is worn until the 30th day, and recreation and amusement are forbidden for one year. In this case the transitional period lasts from the funeral (shortly after biological death) until the tombstone is dedicated a year later, and mourning officially ends. The dedication of the tombstone can be seen as the last of a series of 'funerals', during which the deceased gradually leaves the world of the living. In this group, as in others, 'social death' takes place slowly, in a series of culturally defined stages.

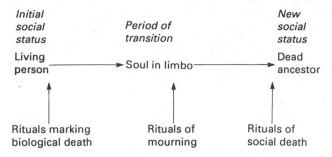

Figure 9.3 Stages of social death

As these examples illustrate, there is a wide variation in bereavement practices in different social and cultural groups. Therefore, as Eisenbruch[15] has pointed out, although there are certain constancies in how human beings grieve, one cannot assume that the states of grieving in different cultures occur at the same rate, or even in exactly the same sequence.

The three main stages in the process of social death are illustrated in Figure 9.3.

Rituals of hospitalization

Many *healing rituals* are also rituals of social transition, whereby an 'ill person' is transformed into a 'healthy person'. This often involves the patient's withdrawal from everyday life, while certain treatments are followed and taboos observed. If the patient recovers, he is ritually re-incorporated into normal society, but in the phase of transition the sufferer is considered especially vulnerable, as well as dangerous to other people. To some extent the hospital can be seen as a setting for these rites of social transition. A patient admitted to hospital leaves his normal life behind, and enters a state of limbo characterized by a sense of vulnerability and danger. As with other institutions, such as the army or prison, they undergo a standardized ritual of entry, by which they are divested of many of the props of their social identity. Their clothing is removed, and replaced by a uniform of bathrobe and slippers. In the ward they are allocated a number, and transformed into a 'case' for diagnosis and treatment. When they have recovered they regain their own clothes and rejoin their community in the new social identity of a 'healthy' or 'cured' person. While hospital treatment is designed to provide intensive medical care and observation, and

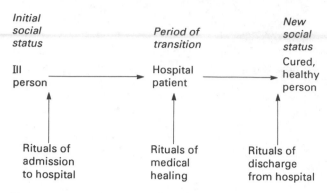

Figure 9.4 Hospitalization as a ritual of social transition

to remove patients with infectious diseases from the community, it also follows Van Gennep's three stages of separation, transition and incorporation, as illustrated in Figure 9.4. Clinicians should be aware of these social dimensions of hospitalization, especially patients' feelings of unease or anxiety about their ambiguous or abnormal social status.

Rituals of misfortune

These usually come into play at times of unexpected crisis or misfortune, such as accidents or severe ill-health. Loudon[1] sees two functions of this type of ritual: a manifest function (the solution of specific problems) and a latent function ('the re-establishment of disturbed relationships between human beings). In non-industrial societies, they also function to restore disturbed relationships with the social and supernatural worlds. As Foster and Anderson[16] point out, in these societies 'illnesses are often interpreted as reflecting stress or tears in the social fabric. The purpose of curing therefore goes well beyond the limited goal of restoring the sick person to health; it constitutes social therapy for the entire group, reassuring all onlookers that the interpersonal stresses that have led to illness are being healed.' Illness is therefore seen as a *social* event. The illness of one member, especially if blamed on witchcraft or sorcery resulting from interpersonal conflicts, threatens the cohesion and continuity of the group. The group has an interest in finding and resolving the cause of the illness, and restoring both the victim, and themselves, to health. As a result, such healing rituals usually take place in *public*, in marked contrast to the privacy and confidentiality that characterize doctor–patient consultations in the Western world. The aim of these public rituals is to visibly restore the harmonious relationships between man and man, man and the deities, and man and the natural world.

Rituals of misfortune usually have two consecutive phases: the phase of *diagnosis* or divination of the cause of the misfortune, and the *treatment* of the effects of the misfortune and removal of the cause. In the case of ill-health the first phase includes giving the condition a label or identity within the cultural frame of reference. This implies a concept of how misfortune is caused, its probable natural history and its prognosis, which is shared by healer, patient and spectators. There are many techniques used by different cultures to diagnose ill-health, ranging from divinatory séances to the use of sophisticated diagnostic technology. For example, Beattie[17] describes a divinatory séance among the Nyoro people in Uganda, where the diviner goes into a trance, speaking in a small falsetto voice and using a special vocabulary 'so people knew that the spirit had come into his head, and they began to ask him questions'. These questions related to the diagnosis of a variety of misfortunes, such as marital conflicts, theft and ill-health. It was the 'spirit' who diagnosed their cause and prescribed treatment speaking publicly through the mouth of the diviner. In contrast, the private diagnosis of Western medicine refers mainly to disorders of the patient's body or emotions; in general, both his mystico-religious beliefs and his social relationships are not considered major factors in his diagnosis and treatment. In both cases, there is an overlap between these rituals and rites of social transition; many involve the transition of the sufferer from the social identity of 'ill person' towards that of 'cured' person, via the three stages described by Van Gennep.

Technical aspects of ritual

In looking at all forms of healing ritual it is important to distinguish the ritual aspect from the practical or *technical* aspect that often coexists with it. In practice the division between the two is not absolute: a purely sacred ritual can have the practical, technical effect of permanently altering people's behaviour or emotional state, for example. The technical aspect is often interwoven with the ritual, and includes such practical techniques as the use of medicines, surgical operations, inhalations, massages, cupping, injections and bonesetting, as well as techniques of psychotherapy and midwifery. Even in the most 'primitive' society, where the purely ritual aspect of healing is strongest, there is likely to be a component of shrewd observations and experience on the part of the healer as to why and how people get ill, some knowledge of human nature, and a mastery of certain theatrical and practical techniques. In Western society, diagnosis and treatment also take place in 'ritual time' and 'ritual space'; that is, at certain times and in certain settings carefully marked off from the rest of everyday life (such as a hospital clinic, or a doctor's office). In this setting, even the most technical treatments are influenced by the ritual atmosphere, and this is clearly illustrated in the case of the placebo effect. Also, as Balint[18] has pointed out, the most important 'drug' that can be administered in this setting is the personality of the doctor.

Functions of ritual

Rituals fulfil many functions, both for the individual and for society. Depending on the perspective from which one views them, these functions can be classified into three overlapping groups: *psychological, social* and *protective.*

Psychological functions

In situations of unexpected misfortune or ill-health, rituals provide a standardized way of explaining and controlling the unknown. The sudden onset of illness causes feelings of uncertainty and anxiety in the victim, and his or her family. They ask: 'What has happened?' 'Why has it happened?' 'Is it dangerous?' Part of the function of a healing ritual (as well as treating the condition) is to provide explanations for the illness in terms of the cultural outlook of the patient. That is, to convert the chaos of symptoms and signs into a recognizable, culturally validated condition, whether it is 'pneumonia' or *susto,* with a name and a known cause, treatment and prognosis. In this way the uncertainty and anxiety of patient and family are reduced, by converting the unknown into the known. As Balint[19] puts it, in the consultation 'the patient is still frightened and lost, desperately in need of help. His chief problem, which he cannot solve without help, is: What is his illness, the thing that has caused his pains and frightens him?' Only after the condition is given a name does the patient ask for treatment to relieve his distress. As Phineas Parkhurst Quimby, a famous folk healer born in New England in 1802, said: 'I tell the patient his troubles, and what he thinks is his disease, and my explanation is the cure. If I succeed in correcting his errors I change the fluids in the system, and establish the patient in health. The truth is the cure.'[20]

Ritual also lessens anxiety at times of physiological change, such as pregnancy. These rituals, many of them public, help to control the sense of anxiety or unease associated with this vulnerable 'transitional' state. Standing[6] has noted how it is impossible to eradicate *all* risk in pregnancy, but following prescribed rituals and taboos at least provides some kind of assurance that everything possible is being done to minimize that risk. Some diagnostic rituals can also be used to explain misfortune or failure *post hoc*, and thus lessen feelings of guilt or responsibility. For example, in some communities a woman who has given birth to a deformed child might be told that she had been bewitched by an unknown person during pregnancy, and that therefore the deformity was not her fault.

At times of extreme crisis, such as bereavement, rituals also provide a standardized mode of behaviour which helps to relieve the sense of uncertainty or loss. Everyone knows what to do, and how to act under those circumstances, and this restores a sense of order and continuity to their lives. It also enables the bereaved to slowly adjust to the fact of death, and to see it as the end of one cycle, but the beginning of another. This gradual acceptance occurs in well defined ritual stages, which vary between cultures.[13,14] The normal phases of grieving (at least in most Western communities) – from 'numbness' to 'reorganiza-tion' – described by Parkes[21] can therefore be placed in a ritual context, and at each stage the mourners can be given much-needed social support and understanding. For example, in previous generations in the UK, the status of mourner was signalled by wearing a black dress or black arm-band. This marked the mourner out from other people, and ensured a special, protective attitude towards him or her. Skultans[14] has speculated that the increased risk of death among the recently bereaved (see Chapter 11) may be partly due to the disappear-ance of this type of protective ritual. She points out that in modern, middle-class Britain, while 'some rituals are main-tained at the actual time of death and funeral in that the family gathers and mourning dress is worn . . . the absence of ritual is most marked during the subsequent period of mourning. Most noticeably, the bereaved are given no guidance on how to behave in their precarious position; they are not, as in non-industrialized societies, set apart from the rest of the society for a prescribed period of time, nor are they given ritual protection in this severe crisis'. There is little outward change in behaviour and dress, and often grieving is seen as a 'pathological' state, to be treated by antidepressants. Mourning rituals that encourage emotional display of grief, and define precisely when the mourning period ends, probably limit the possibility of excessive or pathological mourning.

Rituals also provide a way of expressing and relieving unpleasant emotions; that is, they have a *cathartic* effect. This is especially true of the public rituals of small-scale societies. As Beattie puts it, 'they provide a way of expressing, and so of relieving, some of the interpersonal stresses and strains which are inseparable from life in a small-scale society'. This 'safety valve' function benefits both the individual and society, especially in many small-scale non-Western societies. Here, diagnosis and treatment take place in the presence of *all* the family, friends and neighbours of the patient, and their part in the aetiology of the illness is openly discussed, as well as what they can do to help the patient. In Western clinical practice, as Turner[22] remarks, 'relief might be given to many sufferers from neurotic illness if all those involved in their social networks could meet together and publicly confess their ill will towards the patient and endure in turn the recital of his grudges against them'.

Finally, the rituals of healing can also function to reduce anxiety and uncertainty in the healer himself. Bosk[23] has suggested that many of the 'occupational rituals' of American physicians – such as case conferences, grand rounds, and mortality and morbidity conferences – help the physicians to cope with anxiety and uncertainty, and to make the necessary treatment decisions, while Katz's study[24] of surgical rituals in the USA has come to the same conclusion.

Social functions

These overlap with the psychological functions. Particularly in small-scale societies, the cohesion of the group is threatened by interpersonal conflicts. By ascribing ill-health to these conflicts, the group can use this misfortune to bring conflicts into the open, and publicly resolve them; this is a feature of societies where ill-health is ascribed to interpersonal malevolence, such as witchcraft or sorcery. Illness also creates a temporary caring community around the victim, and old antagonisms are forgotten, at least for the moment. Because ill-health reminds the community of its own vulnerability to death and decay, both rituals of misfortune and those of social transition (such as mourning rites) help reassert the continuity and survival of the group after the illness or death of one of its members.

Another social function of rituals is to create, or re-create, the basic axioms on which the society is based. By the use of multi-vocal symbols the rituals dramatize these basic values, and remind people of them. According to Turner,[2] the way a society lives can be seen as an attempted imitation of models portrayed and animated by ritual. As such, rituals can modify behaviour towards a more sociable form, and resolve the tensions between self-interest and the interests of the group. In the colour symbolism of Zulu healing, for example, the colours are always used in the sequence black, red, white; that is, from 'antisocial' symbols, through a 'red' transitional phase, towards more positive 'social' symbols. From defaecation, death and dirt towards life, eating and cleanliness. In other societies, rituals of social transition help control or tame potentially antisocial sexual impulses at puberty, by restrictive taboos during the period of 'becoming an adult'.

Protective functions

Rituals dealing with ill-health can protect the participants in two ways, either psychologically or physically. The role of rituals in protecting against the anxiety and uncertainty associated with illness, death and other misfortune has already been described. In other ways, ritual observances can protect the ill or weak person from physical dangers such as infection. Some of the rituals surrounding pregnancy, birth or the postpartum period, for example, may protect the woman and her child from sources of infection, or injury, especially if they involve withdrawal from normal social life. Secluding an ill person, as part of a ritual of social transition, may also limit the spread of infectious diseases to the community. However, a healing ritual held in public may have exactly the opposite effect. Other protective functions arise from cleansing and purification rites which, although carried out for ritual purposes, may also remove dirt and bacteria and promote physical cleanliness.

This section has listed some of the main functions of ritual – psychological, social and protective – especially in rituals of illness and misfortune. If Douglas[25] is correct, and the industrialized world is moving away from ritual and 'there is a lack of commitment to common symbols', then the individual's management of misfortune, disease, death and the stages in the human life-cycle might all become more difficult.

In the following case histories, two types of ritual of misfortune are contrasted: a public healing ceremony in a non-Western community, and the more private diagnostic ritual in a Western society.

Case history: Curative rites among the Ndembu of Zambia

Turner[22] describes curative rites among the Ndembu people of Zambia. The Ndembu ascribe all persistent or severe ill-health to *social* causes, such as the secret malevolence of sorcerers or witches, or punishment by the spirits of ancestors. These spirits cause sickness in an individual if his family and kin are 'not living well together', and are involved in grudges or quarrelling. Because death, disease and other misfortunes are usually 'ascribed to exacerbated tensions in social relations', diagnosis (divination) takes place publicly, and becomes 'a form of social analysis', while therapies are directed to 'sealing up the breaches in social relationships simultaneously with ridding the patient . . . of his pathological symptoms'. The Ndembu ritual specialist, the *chimbuki*, conducts a divinatory séance attended by the victim, his kin and neighbours. The diviner is already familiar with the social position of the patient, who his relatives are, the conflicts that surround him, and other information gained from the gossip and opinions of the patient's neighbours and relatives. By questioning these people, and by shrewd observation, he builds up a picture of the patient's 'social field' and its various tensions. Actual divination takes place by peering into medicated water in an old meal mortar, in which he claims to see the 'shadow-soul' of the afflicting ancestral spirit. He may also detect witches or sorcerers who have caused the illness, among the spectators. The diviner calls all the relatives of the patient before a sacred shrine to the ancestors, and induces them to confess any grudges . . . and hard feelings they may nourish against the patient. The patient, too, must publicly acknowledge his own grudges against his fellow villagers if he is to be free of his affliction. By this process, all the hidden social tensions of the group are publicly aired, and gradually resolved. Treatment involves rituals of exorcism, to withdraw evil influences from the patient's body. It also includes the use of certain herbal and other medicines, manipulation and cupping, and certain substances applied to the skin. These remedies are accompanied by dances and songs, the aim of which is the purification of both the victim and the group. Turner doubts whether the medicines he saw used in these rituals have much pharmacological effect, but he points out the psychotherapeutic benefits, to both the victim and the community, of the public expression and resolution of interpersonal conflicts, and the degree of attention paid to the victim during the ceremony.

Case history: Consultation with a general practitioner in the UK

The consultation between the average British general practitioner (GP) or family physician and his or her patients is markedly different from the Ndembu example, but it too is a form of healing ritual. Consultations take place at defined times and places (the office or surgery), and are governed by implicit and explicit rules of behaviour, deference, dress and subject matter to be discussed. Events take place in a fixed order: entering the surgery, giving one's name to a receptionist, sitting in a waiting room, being called in turn to see the doctor, entering the doctor's room, exchanging formal greetings, and then beginning the consultation. From this point onwards, Byrne[26] has described six stages in the procedure:

1. The establishment of rapport between GP and patient.
2. Discovering why the patient has come.
3. The doctor's verbal and/or physical examination.
4. Both parties' 'consideration of the patient's condition'.
5. The doctor detailing treatment or further tests.
6. The termination of the consultation, usually by the doctor.

The patient's symptoms and signs are recorded, during the consultation, in the 'medical card', and the present condition is seen against the background of previous illnesses recorded there. Particular attention is paid to questions like, 'When did the pain begin?', When did you first notice the swelling?', as part of the verbal diagnosis. As Foster and Anderson[27] point out, this 'historical' approach is characteristic of Western diagnosis; in other cultures, the healer is expected to 'know' all about the patient's condition, without asking so many probing questions. As well as gathering clinical information by history-taking, physical examination or tests, GPs, like the Ndembu *chimbuki*, use 'informal' knowledge gathered over the years in the community. As a result, assessment of a patient is not only based on the consultation, but on the GP's knowledge of the patient's environment, family, work, past medical history, pattern of behaviour, and the culture of the neighbourhood.

The consultation is characterized by privacy and confidentiality, and usually involves only one patient and one doctor at a time. Its form is the ritual exchange of information between the two: symptoms and complaints flow in one direction, diagnoses and advice in the other. The patient receives practical advice ('Spend a day in bed') or a prescription for medication. The prescription form itself resembles a contract, with the name of the doctor, the name of the patient, and the prescribed medication linking the two written on it. It is assumed that the authority of the doctor extends beyond the consultation, because the drug must be taken as prescribed once the patient gets home. As with other healing rituals, the consultation takes place at specified times, and in a setting set aside for this purpose. The GP's room, although designed for a 'technical' purpose, includes many objects that will not be used in a particular consultation, and can therefore take on the significance of ritual symbols. These may include: a framed diploma on the wall; a stethoscope; an otoscope and ophthalmoscope; a sphygmomanometer; tongue depressors; scalpels, forceps, needles and syringes; a glass cabinet full of instruments; bottles of antiseptic and other medicines; one or more telephones; a bookshelf filled with impressive textbooks or journals; a large desk; sheaves of special forms, or notepaper; an ink pad and rubber stamps; and a pile of the previous patients' 'medical cards'.

In this formalized setting of ritual time and place, the patient's diffuse symptoms and signs are given a diagnostic label and organized into the named diseases of the medical model. As well as prescribed medication, the most powerful 'drug' administered in this setting is faith in the healing powers of the doctor.[18]

Recommended reading

Hertz, R. (1960) *Death and the Right Hand*. London: Cohen and West, pp. 27–86. A discussion of funeral rituals in different societies.
Katz, P. (1981) Ritual in the operating room. *Ethnology* **20,** 335–350. A study of surgical rituals in the USA.

Leach, E. (1968) Ritual. In: *International Encyclopaedia of the Social Sciences*. New York: Free Press/Macmillan, pp. 520–526. A summary of the various anthropological theories of ritual.
Turner, V.W. (1974) *The Ritual Process*. Harmondsworth: Penguin

Chapter 10

Cross-cultural psychiatry

Cross-cultural psychiatry is the study, and comparison, of mental illness in different cultures. It is one of the major branches of medical anthropology, and has been a valuable source of insight into the nature of health and ill-health in different parts of the world. Historically, research into the subject has been carried out by two different types of investigator. Firstly, Western-trained psychiatrists who have encountered unfamiliar, and sometimes bizarre, syndromes of psychological disturbance in parts of the non-Western world, and who have tried to understand these syndromes in terms of their own Western categories of mental illness – such as 'schizophrenia' or 'manic depressive psychosis'. Secondly, social anthropologists whose main interests have been the definitions of 'normality' and 'abnormality' in different cultures, the role of culture in shaping 'personality structure', and cultural influences on the aetiology, presentation and treatment of mental illness. Although these two approaches have led to different perspectives on the subject, they share a concern with two types of clinical problem:

1. The diagnosis and treatment of mental illness, where doctor and patient come from different cultural backgrounds.
2. The effect on mental health of migration, urbanization, and other forms of social change.

The focus of cross-cultural psychiatry is mainly on mental 'illness' – rather than on mental 'disease'. That is, it is concerned less with the organic aspects of psychological disorders than with the psychological, behavioural and sociocultural dimensions associated with them. Even when the condition clearly has an organic basis – as in neurosyphilis, delirium tremens or dementia – anthropologists are more interested in how *cultural* factors affect the patient's perceptions and behaviour, the content of the hallucinations or delusions, and the attitudes of others towards the patient.

In general, the relationship of culture to mental illness can be summarized as follows:

1. It defines 'normality' and 'abnormality' in a particular society.
2. It may be part of the aetiology of certain illnesses.
3. It influences the clinical presentation, and distribution, of mental illness.
4. It determines the ways that mental illness is recognized, labelled, explained and treated by other members of that society.

'Normality' *versus* 'abnormality'

Definitions of 'normality', like definitions of 'health', vary widely throughout the world; and in many cultures these two concepts overlap. Mention has already been made in Chapter 4 of some of the medical definitions of health that are based on the measurement of certain physiological and other variables that lie in the 'normal range' of the human organism. At its most reductionist, this approach concentrates mainly on the physical signs of brain dysfunction, before diagnosing mental illness. In this chapter, some of the other ways of looking at the problem will be examined, especially the *social* definitions of normality and abnormality. These definitions are based on shared beliefs within a cultural group as to what constitutes the ideal, 'proper' way for individuals to conduct their lives in relation to others. These beliefs provide a series of guidelines on how to be culturally normal and, as will be described below, how also to be temporarily abnormal. Normality is usually a multi-dimensional concept. Not only is the individual's behaviour relevant, but also dress, posture, hairstyle, smell, gestures, facial expression, tone of voice and use of language are all taken into account, as is their *appropriateness* to certain contexts and social relationships.

The social definition of normality is not uniform or static, however. Most cultures have a wide range of social norms which are considered appropriate for different age groups, genders, occupations, social ranks and cultural minorities within the society. Attitudes towards foreigners or outsiders often include stereotyped views of their 'normal' behaviour, which may be seen as bizarre, comical or even threatening. Societies with strict codes of normal behaviour often make provision for certain specified occasions where these codes are deliberately flouted or *inverted*, and abnormal behaviour becomes the temporary norm. Anthropologists have described many of these 'rites of reversal' or 'symbolic inversions', which Babcock[1] defines as: 'any act of expressive behaviour which inverts, contradicts, abrogates, or in some fashion presents an alternative to commonly held cultural codes, values and norms be they linguistic, literary or artistic, religious, or social and political'.

These special occasions – such as certain festivals, carnivals (particularly in Latin America and the Caribbean), bacchanalia, or *mardi gras* – sometimes involve an inversion of normal behaviour and roles. For example, in their study of the carnival in St. Vincent, West Indies, and *belsnickling* (a form of Christmas mumming) on La Have Islands, Nova Scotia, Abrahams and Bauman[2] point out that both involve 'a high degree of symbolic inversion, transvestism, men dressed as animals or super-natural beings, sexual license, and other behaviors that are the opposite of what is supposed to characterize everyday life'. In a Western setting, such temporarily abnormal social behaviour is found on April Fool's Day, fancy dress balls, university 'Rags', New Year's Eve parties and Halloween. Similar alterations or inversions of normal role behaviour are found in some of the spirit possession cults of African women, described by Lewis,[3] where women who seek power and aspire to roles otherwise monopolized by men 'act out thrusting male parts with impunity and with the full approval of the audience'. All these forms of public abnormal behaviour by large numbers of people are, however, also strictly *controlled* by norms, since their context and timing are structured in advance.

On a more individual level, displays of behaviour that are abnormal by the standards of everyday life must also be seen against the background of the culture in which they appear. Like the crowd behaviour at a rite of reversal, they are also controlled (to a variable extent) by implicit cultural norms, which determine how and when they may appear. In many cultures, especially non-Western ones, individuals involved in interpersonal conflicts, or who are experiencing feelings of unhappiness, guilt, anger or helplessness, are able to express these feelings in a standardized language of distress (see Chapter 5). This may be purely verbal, or involve extreme changes in dress, behaviour or posture. To the Western-trained observer, some of these languages of distress may closely resemble the diagnostic entities of the Western psychiatric model. For example, they may involve statements such as, 'I've been bewitched', 'I've been possessed by a spirit (or by God)', or 'I can hear the voices of my ancestors speaking to me'. In a Western setting, people making this type of statement are likely to be diagnosed as psychotic, probably schizophrenic.

However, one should remember that in many parts of the world people freely admit to being 'possessed' by supernatural forces, to having spirits speak and act through them, and to having had dreams or hallucinations that conveyed an important message to them. In most cases this is not considered to be pathognomonic of mental illness. One example of this is the widespread belief, especially in parts of Africa, of spirit possession as a cause of mental or physical ill-health. Women especially are the victims of possession by malign, pathogenic spirits that reveal their identity by the specific symptoms or behaviour changes that they cause. In these societies, as Lewis[3] notes, possession is a normative experience, and whether or not people are actually in a trance, they are only possessed when they consider they are, and when other members of their society endorse this claim. That is not to say that spirit possession is normal, in the sense that most people expect to be possessed during their life. Rather, it is a culturally specific way of presenting, and explaining, a range of physical and psychological disorders in certain circumstances. In these societies, writes Lewis, 'belief in spirits and in possession by them is normal and accepted. The reality of possession by spirits, or for that matter of witchcraft, constitutes an integral part of the total system of religious ideas and assumptions. Where people thus believe generally that affliction can be caused by possession by a malevolent spirit (or by witchcraft), disbelief in the power of spirits (or of witches) would be a striking abnormality, a bizarre and eccentric rejection of normal values. The cultural and mental alienation of such dissenters would in fact be roughly equivalent to that of those who in our secular society today believe themselves to be possessed or bewitched.'[3]

Possession, then, is an abnormal form of behaviour, but one which is in conformity with cultural values, and the expression of which is closely controlled by cultural norms. These norms provide guidelines as to who is allowed to be possessed, under what circumstances, and in what way, as well as how this possession is to be signalled to other people.

Another form of controlled abnormal behaviour is *glossolalia*, or 'speaking in unknown tongues'. To those who believe in it, it is thought to result from a supernatural power entering into the individual, with 'control of the organs of speech by the Holy Spirit, who prays through the speaker in a heavenly language'.[4] It is a dissociative, trance-like state in which the participants 'tend to have their eyes closed, they may make twitching movements and fall; they flush, sweat and may tear at their clothes'. It is a feature of religious practices in parts of India, the Caribbean, Africa, Southern Europe, North America and among many Pentecostal churches in the UK (including those of West Indian immigrants). There are believed to be about two million practitioners of glossolalia in the USA, in various denominations, including some Lutheran, Episcopalian and Presbyterian churches. Glossolalia usually takes place in a specified context (the church) and at specified times during the service. It can be seen as a form of 'controlled abnormality' which, to a Western-trained psychiatrist, might seem evidence of a mental illness. However, there is no evidence that this is the case; on the contrary, there is some evidence from various cultures that 'in any particular denomination, those members of it who speak in tongues are better adjusted than those who do not'.[4] In one study, a comparison between a group of schizophrenic patients from the Caribbean and West Indian Pentecostals suggested that the Pentecostals believed that the patients 'were unable to control their dissociative behaviour sufficiently to conform with the highly stylized rituals of glossolalia in church'.[4] Although both groups might appear to practice similar glossolalia, it was the culturally *uncontrolled* form that was regarded as mental illness by members of that community.

In every society there is a spectrum between what is regarded as normal and abnormal social behaviour. However, as the example of glossolalia illustrates, there is also a spectrum of abnormal behaviour, from controlled to uncontrolled forms of abnormality. As with the abnormal drinking behaviour (drunkenness) described in Chapter 8, it is behaviour at the *uncontrolled* end of the spectrum that cultures regard as a major social problem and that they label as either 'mad' or 'bad'. As Foster and Anderson[5] put it, 'there is no culture in which men and women remain oblivious to erratic, disturbed, threatening or bizarre behaviour in their midst, whatever the culturally defined context of that behaviour'. According to Kiev,[6] the symptoms that would suggest mental disorder include uncontrollable anxiety, depression and agitation, delirium and other gross breaks of contact with reality, and violence (both to the community and to self). In one study by Edgerton,[7] lay beliefs about what behaviour constitutes madness or psychosis was examined in four East African tribes: two in Kenya, one in Uganda, and one in Tanzania (Tanganyika). It was found that all four societies shared a broad area of agreement as to what behaviours suggested a diagnosis of 'madness'. These included such actions as violent conduct, wandering around naked, 'talking nonsense' or 'sleeps and hides in the bush'. In each case the respondents qualified their description of psychotic behaviour by saying that it occurred 'without reason'. That is, violence, wandering around naked and so on occurred without an apparent purpose, and in the absence of any identifiable external cause (such as witchcraft, drunkenness or simply malicious intent). Edgerton notes how this catalogue of abnormal behaviours is not markedly at variance with Western definitions of psychosis, particularly schizophrenia. In these cultures, behaviour was labelled as madness if it was not controlled by cultural norms, and had no discernible cause or purpose.

Abnormal behaviours at the controlled end of the spectrum frequently overlap with religious and cosmological practices. Examples of this are glossolalia, the use of hallucinogens and marihuana in religious rituals (see Chapter 8), some forms of spirit possession, and the healing rites of the *shaman*. The latter is a form of sacred folk healer who is found in many cultures, and has been more fully described elsewhere in this book. The shaman is a 'master of spirits' who becomes voluntarily possessed by them in controlled circumstances and who, in a divinatory séance, both diagnoses and treats the misfortune (and illness) of the community. To a Western psychiatrist, the behaviour of the shaman during a trance may closely resemble that of the schizophrenic. However, as Lewis[3] points out, shamans in their ritual performances act in conformity with cultural beliefs and practices and, in the selection of shamans, frankly psychotic or schizophrenic individuals are screened out as being too idiosyncratic and unreliable for the rigour of the shamanic role.

At various points along the spectrum of abnormal social behaviours, the different *culture-bound* mental illnesses can be located. These conditions, which are described more fully below, are under the control of social norms to a variable extent. For example, their timing and setting may be unpredictable, but the clinical presentation of their symptoms and behaviour changes is patterned by culture. Also, unlike the severe uncontrolled psychosis in the East African example, a culturally explicable cause for them can be found, such as *susto* following an unexpected accident or fright, or *evil eye* resulting from an extravagant lifestyle that attracted envy. These conditions do not occur in the formalized setting of temple or ritual, but cultural factors influence their presentation, recognition and treatment.

Comparison of psychological disorders

Given the marked variation in cultural definitions of 'normal' and 'abnormal' throughout the world, can one make meaningful comparisons between mental illness in different groups and societies? Landy[8] has summarized two of the questions faced by medical anthropologists and cross-cultural psychiatrists who have examined this problem:

1. 'Can we speak of some aspects of behaviour as normal or abnormal in a panhuman sense?' (that is, specific to the human species).
2. 'Are the psychoses of Western psychiatric experience and nosology universal and transcultural, or are they strongly shaped by cultural pressures and conditioning?'

The answers to both these questions are important, because they determine whether one can adequately diagnose and treat mental illness cross-culturally. They would also shed light on why some forms of mental illness seem to be more common in some parts of the world than in others.

In examining notions of abnormality in the section above, most of the attention has been on abnormal *social behaviour*, rather than on organic disorders or on emotional state. For most medical anthropologists the social and cultural dimensions of mental illness are the main area of study. This is because cultural factors influence the clinical presentation, and recognition, of many of these disorders – even those with an organic basis. In addition, in many parts of the Third World (and elsewhere) mental illness is perceived as 'abnormal action' rather than 'mistaken belief'.[9] Diagnosing mental illness by psychological state (such as the presence of a delusion) may be difficult where the content of the delusion is shared by other members of the society. For example, in some cultures a person who accuses a neighbour of having bewitched him may initially be perceived as acting in an acceptable, rational way (for that society). He will only be viewed as mad or psychotic if his accusations are then followed by 'mal-adaptive personal violence rather than the employment of the accepted communal technique for dealing with sorcery'.[9] In this case, the diagnosis of mental illness by a Western-trained doctor would depend not only on his own clinical observations – based on assessment of the affected person's behaviour, biological changes (such as anorexia, insomnia and loss of libido) and response to certain psychological tests – but also on how the affected person's *behaviour* is perceived by his *own* community. The problem therefore – in comparing mental illness in different societies – is whether to compare Western clinical evaluations of patients in different cultures, or the perceptions by various cultures of those that they regard as mentally ill. Those who have examined this problem have tended to take one of three approaches.

The biological approach

This sees the diagnostic categories of the Western psychiatric model as being universally applicable to mankind, despite local variations due to cultural factors, since they have a *biological* basis. In Kiev's view,[10] the *form* of psychiatric disorders remains essentially constant throughout the world, irrespective of the cultural context in which they appear. For example, 'the schizophrenic and manic-depressive psychotic disorders are fixed in form by the biological nature of man', while the secondary features of mental illness, such as the *content* of delusions and hallucinations are, by contrast, influenced by cultural factors. On this basis, Kiev[11] is able to classify the various 'culture-bound disorders' within the diagnostic categories of the Western model. For example, *koro, susto* and bewitchment are forms of 'anxiety', the Japanese *shinkeishitsu* is an 'obsessional-compulsive neurosis', *evil eye* and *voodoo death* examples of 'phobic states', and *spirit possession, amok* in Malaya, and *Hsieh ping* in China are all examples of 'dissociative states'. In Kiev's opinion, these conditions 'are not new diagnostic entitles; they are in fact similar to those already known in the West'. This approach, which is similar to the view of 'diseases' as universal entities (see Chapter 5), has been criticized for the primacy it gives to the Western diagnostic and labelling system. In addition, Western categories of mental illness are also 'culture-bound', as well as being the product of specific social and historical circumstances, and are therefore not necessarily 'panhuman' in their applicability. For example, Kleinman[12] has criticized the WHO International Pilot Study of Schizophrenia, which compares schizophrenia in a number of Western and non-Western societies. He points out that the study enforces a definition of schizophrenic symptomatology, and that this definition may distort the findings by 'patterning the behaviour observed by the investigators and systematically filtering out local cultural influences in order to preserve a homogeneous cross-cultural sample'. Applying the Western model of, say, schizophrenia to other parts of the world may therefore be an example of what Kleinman[13] terms a *category fallacy* – that is, 'the reification of a nosological category developed for a particular cultural group that is then applied to members of another culture for whom it lacks coherence and its validity has not been established'. The danger of category fallacies is therefore implicit in much of the biological approach, and in its attempt to fit 'exotic' illnesses into a universal diagnostic framework.[14]

A further critique of the biological approach is that the same mental illness may play *different* social roles in different societies. For a fuller understanding of an episode of that mental illness in another culture, one must always know something of the *context* – social, cultural, political and economic – in which it has taken place. For example, in some small-scale societies a psychotic episode may be viewed as evidence of an underlying social conflict, which must be resolved by a public ritual, while the same psychosis is unlikely to play so central a role in the life of a Western urban community.

The social labelling approach

This perspective, developed by sociologists, sees mental illness as a 'myth', essentially a *social* rather than a biological fact, and one which can appear with or without biological components. Society decides what symptoms or behaviour patterns are to be defined as 'deviant', or as that special type of deviance 'mental illness'. This mental illness does not appear until it is so labelled, and had no prior existence. Once the diagnostic label is applied, it is difficult to discard. According to Waxler,[15] mental illness is only defined relative to the society in which it is found, and cannot be said to have a 'universal' existence. She notes how, in Western societies, social withdrawal, lack of energy and feelings of sadness are commonly labelled 'depression', while in Sri Lanka the same phenomena receive less attention and very little treatment. The definition of mental illness is thus culture-specific. The process of labelling involves a first stage where an individual's minor deviant behaviour is labelled as mental illness. There are, however, certain 'culture-specific contingencies' under which potential deviants are immune from this labelling, and these include the individual's power relative to the labeller (based on his or her age, sex, race, economic position, etc.). Once an individual is labelled as mentally ill, he is subject to a number of cultural cues which tells him *how* to play his role, that is, 'the mentally ill person learns how to be sick in a way his particular society understands'. Once labelled, the individual is dependent on the society at large for de-labelling him and releasing him from the sick role. In some cases he may never be able to free himself from this role. The value of the social labelling perspective is that it sheds light on the *social* construction and maintenance of the symptomatology of mental illness. Because this mental illness exists only by virtue of the society that defines it, mental illness is a relative concept and cannot easily be compared between different societies. This perspective has been criticized for its neglect of the biological aspect of mental illness, especially in those conditions where this is a definite feature (such as brain tumours, delirium tremens or dementias). It also ignores the more extreme psychoses, which do seem to be universal in distribution.

The combined approach

This utilizes elements of both the biological and the social labelling perspectives and is the one most medical anthropologists would agree with. In this view, there *are* certain universals in abnormal behaviour, particularly extreme disturbances in conduct, thought or affect. While there is wide variation in their form and distribution, the Western categories of major psychoses, such as schizophrenia and manic depressive psychosis, *are* found throughout the world, though of course they may be given different labels in different cultures. An example of this – the similarity to Western definitions of psychosis of folk categories of 'mad' behaviour in four East African tribes – has already been described above. The major psychoses, therefore, as well as disorders arising from organic brain disease, seem to be recognized in all societies, although their clinical presentations are usually influenced by the local culture. For example, a psychotic in a tribal society may say that his behaviour is being controlled by powerful witches or sorcerers, while a Western psychotic may feel controlled by spacemen, Martians or flying saucers. Those who suffer these extreme psychological disorders are usually perceived by their own cultures as exhibiting uncontrolled abnormal forms of social behaviour. To a variable extent their clinical pictures can be compared between societies. Foster and Anderson[5] have suggested that this comparison should be between their *symptom patterns* rather than between diagnostic categories (such as schizophrenia); on this basis, the problem of trying to fit other cultures' mental illnesses into Western diagnostic categories can be overcome.

The comparison of symptom patterns can also be carried out for the culture-bound disorders, to be described below, many of which could be classified as neuroses or functional psychoses in the Western psychiatric model. These conditions, especially those with a preponderance of neurotic or somatic symptoms, are probably more difficult to compare than are the major psychoses. Many of them seem to be unique clusters of symptoms and behaviour changes, which make sense only within a particular context, and within a particular culture, and have no equivalent in other societies. The specific symptom patterns of *susto*, for example, are unlikely to be found in the UK, at least not among the native-born population. Not only does culture closely pattern their clinical presentations, but the *meanings* of these conditions for the victim, family and community are difficult for a Western observer to evaluate or to quantify. Nevertheless, anthropologists like Rubel[16] believe that these folk illnesses have a fairly constant clinical presentation within a culture, and can therefore be quantified and investigated using standard epidemiological techniques (see Chapter 12).

Cultural influences on psychiatric diagnosis

Before psychological disorders can be compared they have to be diagnosed. In recent years a number of studies have indicated some of the difficulties in standardizing psychiatric diagnoses, particularly among psychiatrists working in different countries. Variations in the clinical criteria used to diagnose schizophrenia, for example, have been found between British and American psychiatrists, and among psychiatrists working within these countries. Some of the diagnostic categories in French psychiatry – such as 'chronic delusional states' (*délires chroniques*) and 'transitory delusional states' (*bouffées delirantes*) – are significantly different from the diagnostic categories of Anglo-American psychiatry.[17] A further example is the diagnostic category 'sluggish schizophrenia' in Soviet psychiatry, which is virtually limited to the USSR.[18] All of these discrepancies in diagnostic behaviour among psychiatrists are important, because they affect both the treatment and the prognosis of mental illness, as well as the reliability of comparing morbidity statistics for these conditions between different countries.

Part of the reason for these differences lies in the nature of psychiatric diagnosis, and the categories into which it places psychological disorders. Unlike the diagnosis of medical 'diseases', there is often little evidence of typical biological malfunctioning. Where biological evidence does exist, it is often difficult to relate this to specific clinical symptoms. Most psychiatric diagnosis is based on the doctor's subjective evaluation of the patient's appearance, speech and behaviour, as well as performance in certain standardized psychometric tests. The aim is to fit the symptoms and signs into a known category of mental illness, by their similarity to the 'typical', textbook description of the condition. However, according to Kendell,[19] the way that psychiatrists learn how to do this may actually make diagnostic differences among them more likely. He points out how the majority of patients encountered by trainee psychiatrists do *not* possess the typical cluster of symptoms of a particular condition. They may have some of the symptoms but not others, or have symptoms typical of another condition. As a result, trainee psychiatrists learn how to assign diagnoses largely by the example of their clinical teachers: 'He sees what sorts of patients his teachers regard as schizophrenics, and copies them'. So although young psychiatrists see many typical cases of various disorders during their studies, their diagnostic behaviour tends to be modelled on that of their teachers, rather than using the stricter criteria of their textbooks. As a result, 'diagnostic concepts are not securely anchored. They are at the mercy of the personal views and idiosyncrasies of influential teachers, of therapeutic fashions and innovations, of changing assumptions about aetiology, and many other less tangible influences to boot.'[19]

Among these influences, Kendell[20] cites the personality and experience of the psychiatrist, the length of the diagnostic interview, and styles of information-gathering and decision-making. To this list one can add social class, ethnic or cultural background (especially its definitions of normality and abnormality), prejudices, religious or political affiliations, and the context in which diagnosis takes place.

An example of how these influences work in practice was provided by Temerlin's[21] classic experiment in 1968. Three groups of psychiatrists and clinical psychologists were each shown a videotaped interview with an actor who had been trained to give a convincing account of normal behaviour. Before the viewing, one of the audiences was allowed to overhear a high-prestige figure comment that the patient was 'a very interesting man because he looked neurotic but actually was quite psychotic'. The second group were allowed to overhear the remark, 'I think this is a very rare person, a perfectly healthy man', while the third group was given no suggestions at all. All three audiences were asked to diagnose the 'patient's' condition. In the first group of 95 people, 60 diagnosed a neurosis or personality disorder, 27 diagnosed psychosis (usually schizophrenia), and only eight stated that he was mentally normal. In the second group, all 20 people diagnosed the 'patient' as normal, while only 12 of the 21 members of the third group also diagnosed normality: the other nine diagnosed neurosis or personality disorders.

Another factor enhancing the subjective element in psychiatric diagnosis is the diffuse and changeable nature of the diagnostic categories themselves. Kendell[22] points out that many of these categories tend to overlap, and ill people may fit into different categories at different times, as their illnesses evolve. Each category or syndrome is made up of the typical clinical features, but as he notes: 'Many of these clinical features, like depression and anxiety, are graded traits present to varying extents in different people and at different times. Furthermore, few of them are pathognomonic of individual illnesses. In general, it is the overall pattern of symptomatology and its evolution over time that distinguishes one category of illness from another, rather than the presence of key individual symptoms.'

However, psychiatrists differ on whether to adopt this historical approach, or whether to focus mainly on the individual's current mental state – as indicated by the degree of 'insight' displayed, or behaviour at the clinical interview. There is also a difference of opinion as to what explanatory model should be used to shape this diffuse clinical picture into a recognizable diagnostic entity. Eisenberg[23] points out that Western psychiatry is not an internally consistent body of knowledge, and includes within it many different ways of viewing mental illness. For example, its perspective on the psychoses includes 'multiple and manifestly contradictory models', such as the medical (biological) model, the psychodynamic model, the behavioural model, and the social labelling model. Each of these approaches emphasizes a different aspect of the clinical picture, and proposes a different line of treatment. The choice of explanatory model, and of diagnostic label, may sometimes be as much a matter of temperament as of training.

Political and moral considerations also play a part in the

choice of diagnosis. In some cases psychiatrists may be called upon to decide whether a particular form of socially deviant behaviour is mad or bad. In the Western world this is common as part of the judiciary system, but has also been applied to such conditions as homosexuality, alcoholism, truancy or obesity. Szasz[24] has argued also that confining lawbreakers to psychiatric hospitals, ostensibly for treatment – that is, labelling them as mad rather than bad – is just another form of punishment, but without the benefits of a proper defence and a proper trial. Psychiatrists making these decisions are likely to be under the influence of social and political forces, the opinions of their colleagues, and their own moral viewpoints. In some societies, many forms of political dissent are labelled as mental illness. The state and its supporters are assumed to have a monopoly of truth, and disagreement with them is considered pathognomonic of psychosis. Wing[25] has described a number of these cases in different countries where state psychiatrists have labelled dissent as madness, especially in the Soviet Union – for example, according to Merskey and Shafran,[18] political dissidents in the USSR have often been diagnosed as suffering from 'sluggish schizophrenia'. In their study of mental illness among immigrants to the UK, Littlewood and Lipsedge[9] also suggest that psychiatry can sometimes be used as a form of social control, misinterpreting the religious and other behaviour of some West Indian patients, as well as their response to discrimination, as evidence of schizophrenia. By contrast with the high rate of schizophrenia among West Indians, depression is rarely diagnosed, and the authors suggest that 'whatever the empirical justification, the frequent diagnosis in black patients of schizophrenia (bizarre, irrational, outside) and the infrequent diagnosis of depression (acceptable, understandable, inside) validates our stereotypes'.[26] In dealing with immigrants and the poor, they warn against psychiatry's role in 'disguising disadvantage as disease'. Eisenberg[23] mentions a further example of how deviant behaviour can be given a moral or medical diagnosis: the same constellation of symptoms and signs (including weakness, sweating, palpitations, chest pain on effort) can, in the absence of physical findings, be diagnosed either as neurocirculatory aesthenia or Da Costa's syndrome (and thus as a medical problem), or as the symptoms of cowardice if they appear in a soldier on the battlefield. More recently, Blackburn[27] has suggested that the psychiatric definition of the psychopathic personality is also 'little more than a moral judgement masquerading as a clinical diagnosis'.

Looked at in perspective, there are a number of factors which can affect the standardization of psychiatric diagnostic concepts between different cultures. These include the lack of hard physiological data, the vagueness of diagnostic categories, the range of explanatory models available, the subjective aspect in diagnosis, and the influence of social, cultural and political forces on the process of diagnosis. Some of the differences in diagnosis between psychiatrists in different countries, and within one country, are illustrated in the following case histories.

Case history: Differences in psychiatric diagnosis in the UK and the USA – 1

Cooper et al.[28] examined some of the reasons for the marked variations in the frequency of various diagnoses made by British and American hospital psychiatrists. Hospitals in the two countries differ in their admission rates (as noted on the hospital records) for the condition 'manic-depressive psychosis'. In the UK, for some age groups, admission for this condition is more than ten times more frequent than in American state mental hospitals. The authors posed the problem: 'Are the differences in official statistics due to differences between the doctors and the recording systems, or do both play a part?' That is, was the actual prevalence of manic-depressive psychosis different in the two cities (London and New York), or were the differences in admission rates caused by the diagnostic terms and concepts used by the two groups of hospital psychiatrists? At a mental hospital in each city, 145 consecutive admissions were studied, in the age range of 35–59 years. These were assessed by the project psychiatrists, and diagnosed according to objective, standardized criteria. These diagnoses were then compared with those given by the hospital psychiatrists. Hospital staff in both cities were found to diagnose schizophrenia more frequently and 'affective disorders' (including manic depressive psychosis and depressive neurosis) less frequently than did the project psychiatrists. Both these trends were more marked in the New York sample. While differences in the incidence of the various disorders *were* found by the project staff between the cities, these differences were less significant than the hospital diagnoses suggest. The hospital psychiatrists appeared to exaggerate these differences by diagnozing schizophrenia more readily in New York, and affective illness more readily in

London. The study does not reveal, however, how the cultural differences between the two groups of psychiatrists affected their diagnostic behaviour.

Case history: Differences in psychiatric diagnosis in the UK and the USA – 2

Katz et al.[29] examined the process of psychiatric diagnosis in more detail, among both British and American psychiatrists. The study aimed to discover whether disagreements among these diagnoses were 'a function of differences in their actual perception of the patient or. . . simply a matter of their assigning different designations to patients on whose symptoms and behaviour they are in agreement'. Groups of British and American psychiatrists were shown films of interviews with patients, and asked to note down all pathological symptoms and to make a diagnosis. Marked disagreements in diagnosis between the two groups were found, as well as different patterns of symptomatology perceived. The British saw less pathology generally, and less evidence of the key diagnostic symptoms 'retardation' and 'apathy', and little or no 'paranoid projection' or 'perceptual distortion'. On the other hand, they saw more of the symptom 'anxious intropunitiveness' than did the Americans. Perceiving fewer of these key symptoms led the British psychiatrists to diagnose schizophrenia less frequently. For example, one patient was diagnosed as schizophrenic by one-third of the Americans, but by none of the British. The authors conclude that 'ethnic background apparently influences choice of diagnosis and perception of symptomatology'.

Case history: Differences in diagnosis by psychiatrists in the UK

Copeland et al.[30] studied differences in diagnostic behaviour among 200 British psychiatrists, all of whom had had at least four years in full-time practice, and possessed similar qualifications. They were shown videotapes of interviews with three patients, and asked to rate their abnormal traits on a standardized scale, and to assign the patients to diagnostic categories. There was fairly good agreement on diagnoses among the sample, except that psychiatrists trained in Glasgow had a significant tendency to make a diagnosis of 'affective illness' in one of the tapes, where the choice of diagnosis was between affective illness and schizophrenia. In addition, psychiatrists trained at the Maudsley Hospital, London, gave lower ratings of abnormal behaviour on the patients than the rest, while older psychiatrists – and those with psychotherapeutic training – rated a higher level of abnormalities than did younger psychiatrists. The authors point out that rating behaviour as abnormal is 'likely to be affected by the rater's attitude towards illness and health and what is normal and abnormal'. The survey illustrates therefore that differences in these attitudes are associated with differences in postgraduate psychiatric training, as well as with age.

Cultural patterning of psychological disorders

Each culture provides its members with ways of becoming ill, of shaping their suffering into a recognizable illness entity, of explaining its cause, and of getting some treatment for it. Some of the issues raised by this process, in the case of physical illness, have already been discussed in Chapter 5 – and they apply equally to cases of psychological disorder. Lay explanations of these conditions fall into the same aetiological categories: personal behaviour, and influences in the natural, social and supernatural worlds. Mental illness can therefore be explained by, for example, spirit possession, witchcraft, the breaking of religious taboos, divine retribution, and the capture of one's soul by a malevolent spirit. Foster and Anderson[5] point out how these types of 'personalistic' explanations for mental illness are much more common in the non-Western world; in contrast, the Western perspective on mental illness emphasizes psychological factors, life experiences, and the effects of 'stress' as major aetiological factors.

As with physical illness, cultures determine the language of distress in which psychological distress is *communicated* to other people. This language includes the many culturally specific definitions of abnormality, such as major changes in behaviour, speech, dress or personal hygiene. When it includes the verbal expression of emotional distress, including the description of hallucinations and delusions, it usually draws heavily on the symbols, imagery and motifs of the patient's cultural milieu. For example, in Littlewood and Lipsedge's[31] study, 40% of their patients with severe psychoses who had been born in the Caribbean and in Africa, structured their illness in terms of a religious experience – compared with only 20% of the white patients born in the UK. Similarly, Scheper-Hughes[32] points out that in rural Kerry, in western Ireland, psychiatric patients showed a greater tendency to delusions of a religious nature, including the motifs of the Virgin and the Saviour, than would occur among American schizophrenics, who would be more likely to have 'secular or electromagnetic persecution delusions'. While possession by a malign spirit may be reported in parts of Africa, possession by Martians or extraterrestials is more likely among Western psychotics. Each culture provides a repertoire of symbols and imagery in which mental illness can be articulated – even at the 'uncontrolled abnormality' end of the spectrum. As with the ritual symbols described in the previous chapter, the symbols in which mental illness is expressed show 'polarization of meaning'. On the one hand they stand for personal psychological or emotional concerns; on the other they stand for the social and cultural values of the wider society. Where the mentally ill person comes from a cultural or ethnic minority, they often have to utilize the symbols of the dominant majority culture to articulate their psychological distress and obtain help.[33] That is, they have to internalize (or appear to internalize) the value system of the dominant culture, and to utilize the vocabulary that goes with these values. This process is illustrated in the following case history.

Case history: 'Beatrice Jackson'

Littlewood[34] describes the case of 'Beatrice Jackson', the 34-year-old daughter of a black Jamaican Baptist minister, who had lived in London for 15 years. She was a widow who lived alone with her son, working at a dress factory far from home. She was often lonely and depressed, guilty about her estrangement for various reasons from her father in the Caribbean. She was very religious and frequently attended church. After her father died she became increasingly guilty, constantly ruminating over her past life. She developed pain in her womb, and persuaded a gynaecologist to do a hysterectomy, so 'clearing all that away'. The pains now shifted to her back, and she continued to ask for further operations to remove the trouble. Her psychotic breakdown was precipitated by her son's criticism of the white police during a riot, which she bitterly contested. The following day she was admitted to a mental hospital, talking incoherently and threatening to kill herself, and shouting that her son was not hers because he was black, and that black people were ugly although *she* was not as she was not black. In hospital she became more attached to the white medical and nursing staff, helping them as far as she could and taking their part against the patients in any dispute. By contrast, she kept on getting into arguments with the West Indian staff, refusing to carry out requests for them which she readily agreed to if asked by a white nurse.

Closer analysis of the case revealed that Beatrice saw the world literally in black and white terms. She had internalized the dominant symbolism of both colonial Jamaica and of the England she had encountered, where 'black' represents badness, 'sin, sexual indulgence and dirt'. In religion, black represents hatred, evil, devils, darkness and mourning (and evil people are 'blackhearted'). By contrast, 'white' is associated with 'religion, purity and renunciation'; it also stands for purity and joy, and both brides and angels are dressed in white. In the Caribbean, popular magazines often advertise 'skin lightening creams and hair straighteners', and a lighter coloured skin is a highly valued social asset. Beatrice had internalized this dichotomy, and had hoped to become 'white inside' by strict adherence to religious values, but could not match this by social acceptance from the white world outside. She felt that part of her remained 'black' (and therefore evil, unacceptable) and located the trouble in her sexual organs, blaming these for the carnal feeling which 'is in conflict with that part of her which seems to have managed to become white'. Her son's repudiation of the police, the representatives of white society, seemed to threaten her category system of white = good, black = bad and she could no longer reconcile her inner symbolic system, the outer social reality, and her emotional relationships. Thus 'her system collapsed'. In hospital she attempted to restate her value system, identifying once again with the white staff, and blaming her psychotic episode on the machinations of the (black) Devil. According to Littlewood, at each stage of her life problems, Beatrice attempted to adapt to, and make sense of, the outer reality of her life in terms of the black/white symbolic system that she had internalized. Eventually, though, it became increasingly difficult to reconcile external reality with her system of explanations, and a psychotic episode was precipitated.

Somatization

A problem frequently encountered in making psychiatric diagnoses cross-culturally is that of *somatization* (see Chapters 5 and 7), the cultural patterning of psychological disorders into a language of distress of mainly physical symptoms and signs. This has been reported from many cultures, especially from the Far East,[35] and from lower socioeconomic groups in the Western world. It is particularly a feature of the clinical presentation of depression. These depressed patients often complain of a variety of diffuse and often changeable physical symptoms: such as 'tired all the time', headaches, palpitations, weight loss, dizziness, vague aches and pains, and so on. They frequently deny feeling depressed, or having any personal problems. Kleinman[36] points out how different cultures pattern unpleasant effects, such as depression, in different ways. In some groups or cultures somatization represents a culturally specific way of coping with these effects, and functions to 'reduce or entirely block introspection as well as direct expression'. Unpleasant effects are expressed in a non-psychological idiom: 'I've got a pain' instead of 'I feel depressed'. In the USA, as Kleinman points out, such somatization is more common among poorer social classes who are blue-collar workers with a high school education or less and who have more 'traditional' lifestyles, while *psychologization* (viewing depression as a psychological problem) is more common among upper middle-class professionals and executives with a college or graduate school education. However, even though it is the notional opposite of somatization, psychologization (the use of psychological terms or concepts to describe subjective mental states) is also often couched in a somatic or non-psychological idiom. For example, in my own study[37] in Massachusetts, patients with psychosomatic disorders often described their emotions and feelings as if they were tangible 'things' that somehow entered them and caused damage to their bodies: 'I tend to hold lots of things inside. . . anger, tension, hostility, any kind of fear – I think of them as being crammed into my colon', 'I put negative feelings inside myself. . . Doctors often say anger gets stored in the colon'. In everyday English, too, psychological distress is often expressed in a somatic idiom. Examples of this include: 'broken hearted', 'a pain in the neck', 'full of joy', 'can't stomach something', 'a painful experience' and 'hungry for attention'.

Kleinman[36] has also described somatization in Taiwan, where it is extremely common. According to him, in both Hokkien and Chinese, the two languages spoken on the island, there is an impoverishment of words referring to psychological states, and often words meaning 'troubled' or 'anxious' express these emotions in terms of bodily organs. Self-scrutiny is not encouraged, and as an American psychiatrist working there he found it 'extremely difficult to elicit personal ideas and feelings' from his Taiwanese patients. The use of somatization as a language of distress, expressing a psychological disorder, is illustrated in another Chinese example, this time from Hong Kong.

Case history: Depression in Hong Kong

Lau et al.[38] studied 213 cases of depression (142 women, 71 men), presenting to a private general practice in Hong Kong, in a period of six months. The chief complaints that had prompted them to consult their doctor were: epigastric discomfort (18.7%), dizziness (12.2%), headache (9.8%), insomnia (8.4%), general malaise (7.5%), feverishness (4.7%), cough (4.7%), menstrual disturbances (3.3%) and low back pain (3.3%). Somatic symptoms were complained of initially by 96% of the sample. Practically no depressed patient mentioned emotional distress initially as the chief complaint. Many of the sample had pain as the sole or coexisting complaint – 85% in all had pains or aches of some description. Headaches, for example, were present in 85.4% of the sample. The authors warn of the dangers of missing the diagnosis of depression, because of the façade of somatic symptoms.

Hussain and Gomersall[39] also point out that depression among Asian immigrants to the UK may manifest primarily as somatic symptoms. The symptoms that occur most commonly among depressed Asian patients are generalized weakness, 'bowel consciousness', exaggerated fear of a heart attack, and concern about the health of genital organs, loss of semen in urine or nocturnal emissions.

Culture-bound psychological disorders

The culture-bound disorders are a group of folk illnesses, each of which is unique to a particular culture or geographical area. Each is a specific cluster of symptoms, signs or behavioural changes recognized by members of those cultural groups, and responded to in a standardized way (see Chapter 5). They usually have a range of symbolic meanings – moral, social or psychological – for both the victims and those around them. They often link an individual case of illness with wider concerns, including the relationship with the community, with supernatural forces, and with the natural environment. In many cases they play an important role in expressing – and resolving – both antisocial emotions and social conflicts in a culturally patterned way. The conditions in this group range from purely behavioural or emotional disorders to those with a large somatic component. Among the dozens that have been described[40] are: *amok*, a spree of sudden violent attacks on people, animals and inanimate objects, which afflicts men in Malaysia; *hsieh-ping*, a trance state among Chinese, where patients believe themselves possessed by dead relatives or friends whom they have offended; *koro*, a delusion among Chinese men that the penis will retract into the abdomen and ultimately cause death; *mal ojo* or *evil eye* among Latin Americans (and other groups) where illness is blamed on the 'strong glance' of an envious person; *latah*, a syndrome of hyper-suggestibility and imitative behaviour, found in South East Asia; *voodoo death*, in the Caribbean and elsewhere, where death follows a curse from a powerful sorcerer; *shinkeishitsu*, a form of anxiety and obsessional neurosis among young Japanese; *windigo*, a compulsive desire to eat human flesh, among the Algonkian-speaking Indians of central and north-eastern Canada; and *susto* (or 'fright'), a belief in 'loss of soul', in most of Latin America.

Culture-bound syndromes are by no means all as exotic as this list suggests. Elsewhere in this book it has been suggested that a number of common behaviours, idioms of distress, perceptions of bodily states, and also certain diagnostic categories can all – in certain contexts – be regarded as Western culture-bound disorders. These include obesity, anorexia nervosa, premenstrual syndrome, and the type A behaviour pattern. In a review of this subject, Littlewood and Lipsedge[41] have added to this list a number of other conditions common in contemporary Britain, including: *parasuicide* (an overdose with medically prescribed drugs), *agoraphobia* ('the housewives' disease'), *shoplifting* (by well-off, middle-aged women), *exhibitionism* (or 'flashing'), and *domestic sieges* (where a divorced man, denied access to his children, holds the family hostage in their home). In each of these, the authors see certain recurrent patterns of public behaviour, each of which encapsulates some of today's core cultural themes and values. Like the conditions mentioned earlier, they can therefore be regarded as culture-bound. Housewives' agoraphobia, for example, can be seen as both a ritual display of – and a protest against – the cultural pressures and injunctions on women, especially those which state that 'a woman's place is in the home'. By 'over-conforming' to this stereotype, the woman is able to dramatize her situation, mobilize a caring family around herself, and at the same time also restrict her husband's movements, by forcing him to stay at home and look after her.

In addition to these specific syndromes, both non-Western and Western, a more diffuse cultural patterning determines the language of distress in which certain types of psychological disorder are expressed in each society. In these cases, the mode of *presentation* is culture-bound, though not the exact pattern of symptomatology. Examples of this, quoted above, are the somatic presentation of depression among Chinese in Taiwan and Hong Kong, Asian immigrants in the UK, and working-class Americans.

An example of a well known, and widely spread culture-bound psychological disorder found in Latin America is *susto*, described in this case history.

Case history: *Susto* in Latin America

Rubel[16] has described the characteristics of *susto* (or 'magical fright'), which is also known as *pasmo, jani, espanto* and *pédida de la sombra*. It is found throughout Latin America, in both rural and urban areas, among both men and women, and among both Indians and non-Indians. It is also found among Hispanic Americans, especially those in California, Colorado, New Mexico and Texas. It is based on the belief that an individual is composed of a physical body and of one or more immaterial souls or spirits which, under some circumstances, may become detached from the body and wander freely. This may occur during sleep or dreaming, or as the consequence of an unsettling experience. Among Indians it is believed to be caused by the soul being 'captured' because wittingly or not the patient disturbed the spirit guardians of the earth, rivers, ponds, forests or animals. The soul is believed to be held captive 'until the affront has been expiated'. Among non-Indians this 'soul loss' is usually blamed on a sudden fright or unnerving experience. Its clinical picture consists of the patient:

1. Becoming restless during sleep.
2. During waking hours, complaining of depression, listless-ness, loss of appetite and lack of interest in dress and personal hygiene.

The healing rites, carried out usually by a folk healer or *curandero*, consist of an initial diagnostic session where the cause of the specific episode is identified and agreed, and then a healing session whereby the soul is 'coaxed and entreated to rejoin the patient's body'. The patient is massaged, rubbed and sweated to remove the illness from the body and to encourage the soul to return. Rubel relates the incidence of the condition to a number of epidemiological factors (see Chapter 12), including stressful social situations, especially where the individuals cannot meet the social expectations of their own family and cultural milieu.

As the examples above illustrate, culture-bound disorders can only be fully understood by looking at the *context* in which they appear. In some cases, this context may include many of the political, economic and social issues of the wider society. For example, De La Cancela *et al.*[42] have described *ataques de nervios* ('attacks of nerves') among Puerto Ricans and other Latinos in the USA. These are described as a specific and 'culturally meaningful way to express powerful emotion'. The attacks usually have an acute onset, with a variety of physical symptoms including: shaking, a feeling of heat or presssure in the chest, difficulty in moving limbs, numbness or paraesthesiae of hands or face, a feeling of the mind 'going blank', and sometimes a loss of consciousness, or abusive behaviour. These acute episodes usually follow the gradual build-up of *nervios* ('nerves'), from the general problems of one's life, especially with family relationships, housing or money. An attack is then usually precipitated by some specific stressful event. The authors point out that, for most Latinos, it is not seen as an illness needing medical attention, but rather as an expression of upset, anger, frustration or sadness at the stressful event – as well as a temporary escape from it, and a way of getting sympathy and help from other people. However, they suggest that one cannot only understand this disorder at the micro-level; one also needs to examine the social, political and economic status of Latinos in the USA, and 'the sense of hopelessness, helplessness, and lack of control' many of them experience. Stressful experiences in the countries of origin (especially in Central America), coupled with the effects of migration – such as the disruption of family life, unemployment, discrimination, over-crowded housing and shifts in gender roles – are all part of this wider context. Added to this is the sense of social and political helplessness, the constant 'demands to submerge cultural identity and assimilate to the United States culture', and the lack of respect accorded to their cultures of origin. The authors suggest, therefore, that as well as treating individuals with this condition, and their families, attention must also be paid to wider socioeconomic realities: 'in the long run *ataques* may be more effectively dealt with in the sociopolitical arena'. Therefore health providers 'need to engage in social action and advocacy focusing on the social problems and material conditions that give rise to *ataques de nervios'*.

Cultural healing of psychological disorders

In the Western industrial world most of the focus of psychiatry and psychology, with the exception of family therapy (see below), is on the individual patients. They are the main 'problem' for the therapists, and their emotional state, behaviour, insights and delusions are the main area of concern. Most of their diagnosis and treatment takes place in specialized settings, such as a doctor's office, far removed from their family and friends. Usually both privacy and confidentiality are features of these consultations, which often involve only one therapist and one patient at a time. Provided that both patient and therapist come from similar cultural milieus, they are likely to share many assumptions about the likely origin, nature and treatment of psychological disorders. As mentioned earlier in the discussion of the placebo effect (Chapter 8), the shared world-view and cognitive system are important elements in any healing ritual. In the case of some forms of psychoanalysis, the patient may have to *learn* this world-view and acquire an understanding of the concepts, symbols and vocabulary that comprise it.[43] This can be seen as a form of 'acculturation', whereby the patient acquires a new system for the explanation of misfortune (in this case his own), in terms of the Jungian, Freudian, Kleinian or Laingian models. This world-view, gradually shared by patient and therapist, is often inaccessible to the patient's family or community, who in any case are excluded from the therapist–patient consultations.

In parts of the non-Western world, particularly in rural or small-scale societies, the picture is very different. As noted in Chapter 5, illness – whether somatic or psychological – as well as its treatment is considered to be a more *social* event, which intimately involves the patient's family, friends and community. In many cases, ill-health is interpreted as indicating conflicts or tensions in the social fabric. Kleinman[44] uses the terms *cultural healing* when healing rituals attempt to repair these social tears, and 'reassert threatened values and arbitrate social tensions'. Healing takes place at many levels: not only is the patient restored to health but so is the community in which he or she lives. The aim of treatment, therefore, is to resolve the conflicts causing his illness, restore group cohesion, and integrate the patient back into normal society. Unlike the Western world, psychological disorders are often seen as *useful* to the community. For example, Waxler[15] notes how in small-scale societies mental illness is useful, even necessary: it incurs obligations between people (such as the obligations of family, friends and neighbours to attend and pay for a public healing ritual), and this has an *integrating* function – strengthening the ties within and between groups. In these societies, few other specialized institutions (such as a centralized legal, political and bureaucratic organization) exist to promote this integration, and deviance – such as mental illness – can play this role. This occurs within a shared cognitive system where everyone shares similar views of the aetiology of misfortune and ill-health. If mental illness in one individual is ascribed to sorcery or witchcraft from someone in another group (family, clan or tribe), the offender's group have incurred obligations to the victim's group, which must be repaid in a public ceremony. This process recreates the ties between groups, and also reasserts the boundaries between them. In this process, the mentally ill person is reintegrated into society. According to Waxler, this process and the key role of the family in caring for the patient means that in traditional, non-Western societies mental illness seems to be more easily cured and much more short-lived. She contrasts this with the West, where psychiatric treatment does not have this integrating function (which is fulfilled by the political, bureaucratic system and so on), and mental illness serves to *alienate* the sick individual even further from society. It establishes boundaries around the patient and does not create or re-establish social ties between kin and other groups (except perhaps within the nuclear family) or make clear the boundaries between groups. The Western psychotic is assumed to have a chronic, relapsing disease process which may always re-occur – and when recovered is 'a schizophrenic in remission', rather than 'a person who had schizophrenia'. She therefore relates this lack of an integrating function with the long illness careers of Western psychotics.

Kleinman[44] notes how 'cultural healing' may heal social stresses 'independently of the effects they have on the sick person who provides the occasion for their use'. In some societies the resolution of social conflicts may not be as beneficial to the mentally ill patient as Waxler suggests; it may involve imprisoning, killing or driving him from the community. For example, in the past those 'possessed' by evil spirits in New Hebrides and Fiji were routinely buried alive. However, in most non-industrialized societies, the mentally ill are usually well cared for within their families or communities.

Mental illness in these societies is usually dealt with by folk healers, such as the *tang-ki* in Taiwan, the Ndembu *chimbuki*, the Latin American *curandero* or the Zulu *isangoma*. Some of the practices and psychotherapeutic functions of these ritual healers have already been described. Perhaps the most famous is the *shaman*, who appears in many cultures, from Alaska to Africa. Like the mentally ill person who is possessed by spirits, the shaman also allows himself to become temporarily possessed by certain spirits. Lewis[45] points out that, in contrast with the patient, his possession is 'controlled' during the healing séance and this occurs when and where he chooses. In this condition of 'controlled abnormality' the fact that he is able to master or neutralize the spirits is of great reassurance to the community. He is also able to identify, and exorcise, malign spirits possessing the ill person, and in the process alleviate anxiety, fears, guilts and conflicts. Murphy[46] has described some of the psychotherapeutic aspects of shamanism, as part of his ritual of cultural healing. These include: working within the shared beliefs of the group, and thus reinforcing them; involving the individual as well as the community in the ritual, during which time the patient remains surrounded by familiar friends and relatives; becoming 'possessed' to illustrate his mastery over the other spirits causing ill-health; identifying, during his séance, the cause of mental illness (such as breach of a taboo) and prescribing the appropriate expiatory acts, which are believed to effect the cure and to demonstrate that the patient has indeed recovered. That is, 'through suggestion and the patient's personal involvement in the cure, these visible acts further promote in the patient a psychological realization that he is returning to a state of health'. According to Lewis, by the wide role that he plays in the religious life of his community, 'the shaman is not less than a psychiatrist, he is more'.

Few conclusive studies have been done of the therapeutic benefits of cultural healing for psychological disorders. In one detailed study of healing in a spiritualist temple in rural Mexico, Finkler[47] found that folk healing was ineffective for the psychoses, but useful as psychotherapy for 'neurotic disorders, psychophysiological problems and somatized syndromes'. It enabled patients to abandon their sick roles, return to normal behaviour, and eliminate the feeling of 'being sick'. In another study of therapeutic outcomes from treatment by a Taiwanese shaman, or *tang-ki*, Kleinman[48] found that cultural healing was effective for many episodes of neurosis and somatization, and its value was more in healing the illness, rather than curing the disease. Above all, cultural healing in non-Western societies fits the illness episode into a wider cultural context – explaining it in familiar terms, mobilizing social support about the victim, reaffirming basic values and group cohesion, and thus reducing anxiety in both the ill person and the family.

Anthropology and family therapy

Anthropology is essentially the study of groups, rather than of individuals – although sometimes individuals are studied within the context of certain groups. In all human societies, the primary social group is always the *family*. The composition of the family group varies greatly between cultures, as does the role that it plays in the lives of its members. Outside the urban areas of the industrialized world, where the nuclear family (two parents and their children) is often the norm, the extended multi-generational family is one of the commonest kinship patterns found world-wide. In poorer parts of the world, this larger family unit, though linked to the wider society, often acts as a miniature and self-contained community, or self-help group, whose members share many of their resources, and many of the tasks and responsibilities of everyday life. In whatever form it takes, and in whatever culture it appears, the family is always a *social*, as well as a biological unit, and it always includes members who are not biologically related to it. As well as marriage partners and their families of origin, it may also include honorary relatives or 'fictive kin', such as close friends or neighbours, or even health professionals.

In recent years there has been an increasing overlap in interest between medical anthropologists, family therapists and some psychiatrists. All three are interested in widening the definition of 'patient' beyond the individual, to include their family – and, where relevant, their community as well. For many clinicians, like some of the folk healers described in Chapter 4, the family –

and not the individual – has become the main focus for both diagnosis and treatment.

A useful way of looking at the family is to see it as a small-scale society, or even as a small tribe, with its own distinctive organization and culture. In many ways, what one may term this *family culture* is very similar to that of the wider society, but it also has certain unique and distinctive features of its own. As described at the beginning of this book, a culture includes a set of implicit and explicit guidelines telling one how to view the world, how to experience it emotionally, and how to behave in it – especially in relation to other people, to the natural world, and to supernatural entities or gods. Families, like larger cultural groups, also have their own particular view of the world, their own codes of behaviour, their own gender roles, their own concepts of time and space, their own private slang and language, their own history, and their own myths and rituals. They also have ways of communicating psychological distress to one another and to the outside world.

This family culture can be either protective or pathogenic of health, depending on the context. For example, certain types of family structure may contribute to the development of alcohol abuse among their children later in life (see Chapter 8), while others may protect against this.

The family can also be seen as a 'system', in which the pattern of interrelationships can have important influences on both health and disease.[49] This 'systems theory' or cybernetic model suggests that family dynamics are often aimed at maintaining a state of equilibrium between these various relationships – even at the cost of psychologically 'scapegoating' one of its members. For example, Minuchin *et al.*[50] have shown how certain types of family structure are more likely to cause psychosomatic disorders – such as anorexia nervosa – in some of its members. These 'psychosomatic families' maintain their cohesion, continuity and sense of equilibrium, not only by producing this disorder in one of its members, but also by helping to maintain it. The recovery of the 'identified patient' (in this case, the anorectic young girl) may well cause the break-up of such a pathological family. In this case, as in others, focusing only on the individual, and not the family, makes a fuller understanding of the problem difficult to achieve.

Byng-Hall[51] has described the concept of a *family script*, which is transmitted from generation to generation. These 'scripts' are ways of behaving, of viewing the world, and of reacting emotionally to it. As with culture in general, most of these scripts are outside conscious awareness. Their role is to provide a sense of stability and continuity, and a set of guidelines for performing the daily drama of a family's life. They often function to avoid potentially dangerous conflicts within the family. Each generation of the family knows their allocated role within this continuing drama, and sometimes this role may determine when and how they become ill, or even die. The script may also influence the clustering of certain symptoms within a particular family, and how these symptoms are passed on from parents to children.[52] Family scripts can be maintained by the family's own myths and folklore, which are passed on from generation to generation; in some cases, these myths may have originated centuries before the birth of its present members.[51] Many years later, these family myths may still be exerting a negative effect on both the mental and physical health of its members.

The relation of culture to family dynamics is complex, and to some extent controversial. In 1982, McGoldrick et al.[53] provided a comprehensive selection of mini-ethnographies of the family cultures of different American ethnic groups – such as 'the Irish family', 'the Italian family', and 'the British American family' – and the problems that family therapists face when dealing with each of them. Although it is certainly possible to make some generalizations about, say, Italian families, and the cultural themes they have in common, the danger of stereotyping *all* Italian families – mentioned in Chapter 1 – still applies. Furthermore, listing the supposed cultural traits of families from different ethnic groups often ignores major differences *between* families (based on region, economic position, social class, education, etc.) even if they come from the same ethnic group. Maranhao,[54] in his critique of McGoldrick's book, has also argued that 'family oriented ethnic groups' are sometimes described in it as if their differences from the Anglo-Saxon family type (with its emphasis on individual, rather than family, goals), were pathological by definition. Overall, in his view, knowledge of the cultural background of a family is useful, but not essential for therapy to take place – 'the interviewer does not have to know anthropology, but just be a sensitive family therapist'.

DiNicola[55] has suggested two alternative ways of describing the relationship between a family's mental health and its culture of origin. *Cultural costume* is 'the particular set of recipes the individuals or families of a community have to give meaning and shape to their experiences and to communicate these experiences through shared ceremonies, rituals and symbols'. It is therefore the repertoire of cultural beliefs and behaviours of which each family culture is a particular (and sometimes unique) expression. The cultural costume becomes *cultural camouflage* 'when culture is invoked as a smokescreen to obscure individual states of mind or patterns of interaction in the family'. That is, the family claims that pathological behaviour patterns within it are only normal expressions of its cultural background. DiNicola quotes, as examples of this: 'My husband drinks very hard, he's Irish', or 'My son had a breakdown because he stopped going to the Orthodox church and lost the Greek way'.

Lau,[56] like Maranhao, points out how West European or North American family therapists may misdiagnose family patterns from other cultures as pathological or deviant. This is especially likely where the family structure is less familiar to them, as in one-parent families (among some West Indians), or in multi-generational extended families (among Asians, Chinese and Greek Cypriots) who are living in the same household. She points out that, unlike in the post-industrial West, in many cultures 'breaks are not expected between the generations and continuity in the group depends on the presence of three generations'. Notions of individual autonomy and differentiation therefore have a different meaning, in these groups, from the Western nuclear family model. In dealing with the families from ethnic minorities, Barot[57] has further suggested that a focus on their culture may be insufficient, because one also requires a wider analysis of the institutional and structural factors – such as unemployment, racial discrimination, poor housing, inadequate social and health care facilities, and the effects of migration – which may also adversely affect their lives. Furthermore, these external factors may act to weaken the traditional culture and cohesion of those families, so that culture is no longer a viable explanations for many of the pathological breakdowns in family life.

As this section illustrates, therefore, one of the most fruitful areas of cooperation between psychology, psychiatry and medical anthropology is in the field of family therapy, and research in this area is likely to increase in the future.

Migration and mental illness

Studies done in various countries have indicated that immigrants often have a higher rate of mental illness than either the native-born population or the population in their countries of origin. This is indicated by higher rates of admission to mental hospitals and higher indices of alcoholism, drug addiction and attempted suicide. Some of these studies on immigrants to the UK, such as Asians, West Indians, Africans, Irish, Poles and Russians, are described in the next chapter. Some immigrant groups appear to be more vulnerable to some illnesses than to others; for example, Irish immigrants to the UK have significantly higher rates of alcoholism, while West Indians have the highest rate of schizophrenia of all the immigrant groups. In his study of mental illness among immigrants to Australia, carried out in Victoria, Krupinski[58] found that depressive states were particularly common among British and East European migrants, and the latter group also had the highest rate of schizophrenia. Overall, immigrants showed a much higher rate of psychological instability than exists in the Australian-born population.

Cox[59] has summarized the three hypotheses that seek to explain this high rate of mental illness associated with migration:

1. Certain mental disorders incite their victims to migrate (the *selection* hypothesis).
2. The process of migration creates mental stress, which may precipitate mental illness in susceptible individuals (the *stress* hypothesis).
3. There is a non-essential association between migration and certain other variables, such as age, class and culture conflict.

In the first group, restless and unstable people are believed to migrate more often, in an attempt to solve their personal problems. In another study in Australia, for example, Schaechter[60] found that 45.5% of non-British female immigrants admitted to a psychiatric hospital within three years of migration had had an established mental illness before migration. If 'suspected cases' of mental illness before arrival were added, the figure rose to 68.2%. Other studies, from different parts of the world, have shown that a certain percentage of immigrants *do* have a history of previous mental disorders in their countries of origin. The other, *stress* hypothesis, described in Chapter 11, emphasizes the role of changes in the migrants' 'life space', where the basic assumptions on which their world is founded can no longer be taken for granted. Littlewood and Lipsedge,[61] in their comprehensive study of mental illness among immigrants to the UK, point out that these disorders result from the complex interplay of many factors, including both 'selection' and 'stress'. These include material and environmental deprivation such as overcrowding, shared dwellings, lack of amenities, high unemployment, low family incomes, as well as racial discrimination, and conflict between immigrants and their local-born children. Language difficulties also play an important part, especially among female immigrants who arrive later in the country than do their menfolk, and who are often confined within the home and family. For example, in a study in Newcastle, Wright[62] found that 58% of Pakistani women spoke little or no English, and 15% of the men and 66% of the women had had little or no schooling and were entirely illiterate. These socioeconomic factors, coupled with the stress of culture change and the influence of selection, explain much of the increased rates of mental illness among first-generation immigrants. A further factor, mentioned earlier, is that diagnostic and admission rates in psychiatry may reflect moral or political prejudices, and misinterpret the immigrant's cultural beliefs, and reactions to his plight, as evidence of madness or badness.

Within the immigrant population, certain groups seem to have different rates, and forms, of mental illness, and the reasons for this are complex. According to Littlewood and Lipsedge, 'there appear to be no simple explanations for the different rates of mental illness applicable to all minority groups'. Some factors seem more significant in some groups than in others, and the best way to compare groups would be to add up all these negative factors (selection, stress, multiple deprivations, language difficulties, loss of status – both social and professional – clash between old and new cultural values, and so on) to find a 'score', indicating the risk factors for that community. For example, they note how West African students seem particularly vulnerable because of dissatisfaction with British food, weather, discrimination, economic and legal difficulties, experience of the 'typical British personality', sexual isolation, more mature age, middle-class aspirations, and fear of withdrawal of their grants if they fail their examinations. Those with the lowest rates of mental illness – the Chinese, Italians and Indians – have in common a great determination to migrate, migration for economic reasons, an intention to return home, little attempt at assimilation, and a high degree of 'entrepreneurial' activity. Immigrants who were forced to leave their countries as refugees, and who cannot return, are by contrast likely to have a higher rate of mental illness. Krupinski[58] has examined some of these variables among immigrant groups in Australia: he relates their high rates of mental illness to the fact that many are single young men migrating from the UK and Western Europe, among whom are a proportion of already unstable persons (including some chronic alcoholics arriving from the UK). The stresses of migration seem to affect migrants from Southern and Eastern Europe especially, particularly those in the latter group who had traumatic experiences in the War, or who had suffered loss in occupational status in Australia. Of East European migrants with university degrees, 70% now belonged to a lower socioeconomic class, compared with only 20% of British graduates. Krupinski also found that schizophrenia occurred most frequently among immigrant men 1–2 years after arrival, while in women the peak was found after 7–15 years. The late onset among women was ascribed to the onset of menopause, and the ending of the maternal role with the departure of grown-up children. In addition, a high proportion of non-British immigrant women could not speak English even after many years in the country, especially those from Southern Europe. As with the Pakistani women in Newcastle, their social and linguistic isolation was believed to contribute to their high rate of mental breakdown.

Looked at in perspective, migration seems to carry with it the increased risk of mental illness, for a variety of complex reasons. However, as some authors[63] have pointed out, studies of the mental health of immigrants are difficult to interpret unless one controls for such factors as age, social class, occupational status and ethnic group on one hand, and culturally biased diagnostic methods on the other. Without such controls, one cannot demonstrate clearly that there is a significant association between migration and the rates of mental illness among migrants. Although most of the studies of this problem have concentrated on the immigrants, and their response to their condition, the cultural attributes of the host community are just as important. Such factors as xenophobia, discrimination, racial prejudice[64] – both personal and institutionalized – are all likely to contribute towards the immigrant's mental and physical ill-health, as are the economic and political conditions prevailing in the host community.

Within the immigrant communities themselves, certain cultural traits are also likely to contribute to increased mental illness. These may include a rigid division among the sexes, the social isolation of women, multiple religious taboos and prescriptions, residential patterns which encourage several generations of a family to live in the same house, and pressure on children to succeed financially or academically. Some of these examples of 'culturogenic stress' will be reviewed in the next chapter.

Cross-cultural psychiatric diagnosis

This chapter has illustated some of the complexities in making cross-cultural psychiatric diagnoses – and especially the problems of defining normality and abnormality in the members of other cultures. A further problem is that clinicians may *over*-emphasize culture as an explanation for patients' behaviour, and thus ignore any underlying psychopathology.[65] In making cross-cultural diagnoses, therefore, the clinician should always be aware of:

1. The extent to which cultural factors affect some of the diagnostic categories and techniques of Western psychiatry.
2. The role of the patients' culture in helping them understand and communicate their psychological distress.
3. How the patients' beliefs and behaviour are viewed by other members of their cultural group, and whether their abnormality is viewed as beneficial to the group or not.
4. Whether the specific cluster of symptoms, signs and behavioural changes shown by the patients are interpreted by them, and by their community, as evidence of a 'culture-bound psychological disorder'.
5. Whether the patients' condition is indicative not of mental illness, but rather of the social, political and economic pressures on them.[64]

Recom·nended reading

Dow, J. (1986) Universal aspects of symbolic healing: a theoretical synthesis. *Am. Anthropol.* 88, 56–69. A comparison of common themes between Western psychotherapy, religious healing, and shamanism.

Foster, G. M. and Anderson, B. G. (1978) *Medical Anthropology.* New York: Wiley. *See* Chapter 5 on Ethnopsychiatry, for a good survey of the subject.

Littlewood, R. and Lipsedge, M. (1989) *Aliens and Alienists.* 2nd ed. London: Unwin Hyman. A study of mental illness among ethnic minorities in the UK, and the influences on how these illnesses are diagnosed.

Kleinman, A. and Good, B. (1985) *Culture and Depression.* Berkeley: University of California Press

Simons, R.C. and Hughes, C.C. (1985) *The Culture-Bound Syndromes.* Dordrecht: D. Reidel. A comprehensive survey of culture-bound syndromes in many parts of the world.

Chapter 11

Cultural aspects of stress

The nature of 'stress'

The concept of 'stress' was first described by Hans Selye in 1936,[1] and since then over 110 000 papers have been published on the subject.[2] In Selye's view, stress represents the generalized response of the organism to environmental demands. It is an inherent physiological mechanism which prepares the organism for action, and which comes into play when demands are placed on it. Not all stress is harmful to the organism: at a moderate level (*eustress*) it has a protective and adaptive function. At a higher level (*dystress*), though, the stress response can cause pathological changes, and even death. The actual environmental influence – whether physical, psychological or sociocultural – that produces stress, is termed a *stressor*. Selye has described the sequence of events whereby an organism responds to a stressor as the general adaptation syndrome (GAS). This usually has three stages:

1. The alarm reaction, whereby the organism becomes aware of a specific noxious stimulus.
2. The stage of resistance or adaptation, in which the organism recovers to a functional level superior to that before it was stressed.
3. The stage of exhaustion, where the recovery processes, under the continuing assault of stressors, are no longer able to cope and to restore homeostasis.

In this final stage, the physiological changes that have taken place in the organism now become pathological to it, and disease or death results. From a physiological point of view, the GAS is mediated via the adrenal medulla and the hypothalamic–pituitary–adrenocortical axis, and involves a wide range of physical changes.[3]

Selye's original model, although widely accepted as basic for all stress research, has been criticized on several counts, particularly for its over-emphasis on the physiological dimensions of the stress response. Psychologists such as Weinman[4] have pointed out the importance of the *psychological* responses or coping strategies of the individual confronted by a stressor. These range from an initial 'alarm and shock state' with feelings of anxiety or of being threatened, to attempts to cope with the subjectively unpleasant situation, to a range of more extreme psychological reactions such as depression, withdrawal, suicide or resort to chemical comforters. These responses are all influenced by the individual's personality, experience, education, social environment and cultural background; as such, they are of more interest to the social scientist than the purely physiological stress responses.

A further salient critique of Selye's model, and of much of the subsequent literature on stress, comes from the anthropologist Allan Young.[5] He argues that 'stressors' are often described as if they were abstract 'things', separated from a particular social and political context, and a particular time and place. Furthermore, the focus on these decontextualized stressors and their physiological effects may lead one to ignore the larger economic and other forces acting on the individual, which may also have an adverse effect on health.

Relation of stressors to stress response

By definition, a stressor according to Selye is an environmental influence or agent that produces a stress response in the organism. The range of possible stressors is therefore extremely wide, and one should include on the list such events as: severe illness or trauma, natural disasters, bereavements, divorce, marital conflicts, unemployment, retirement, interpersonal tensions at work, religious or other persecution, financial difficulties, changes in occupation, migration, wartime combat, and excessive exposure to heat, cold, damp or noise. However, the relationship between stressors and their response is more complex than this list suggests. For example, the same event might cause stress in one individual but not in another. Also, as Parkes[6] points out, stress can arise from usually positive experiences, such as promotions, engagements, the birth of a child, or winning a great deal of money, all of which involve a change in lifestyle. Individuals vary in how they cope with and adapt to these life changes, and to more adverse circumstances such as bereavement. In both cases, as the World Health Organisation[7] points out, stress – and the diseases that result from it – represents 'an unsuccessful attempt on the part of the body to deal with adverse factors in the environment'. Thus 'disease is the body's failure to become adapted to these adverse factors rather than the effect of the factors themselves'. There are many reasons for this failure of adaptation, including the physical, psychological and sociocultural characteristics of the individual. For example, elderly frail people are more likely to experience cold weather as stressful than younger, more robust people. Also, some situations (such as retirement) may cause a stress response in one person but not in another. Weinman notes that 'specific situations or objects are threatening to the individual because they are perceived as such rather than because of some inherent characteristic'.[4] Some of the social or cultural factors that predispose to or protect against the stress response will be described later in the chapter.

According to Selye,[2] the relationship between particular stressors and the response they elicit is marked by *non-specificity*. That is, one cannot predict what specific stress-related disease (such as peptic ulceration, psychiatric disorders, hypertension or coronary thrombosis) will result from a specific stressor (such as marital conflict, frustration at work, combat fatigue or burns). A stressor such as marital conflict may result in peptic ulceration in one individual and bronchial asthma in another. In psychosomatic research, this is known as the problem of 'organ choice', and many theories have been put forward to explain why one organ is 'chosen' and not another.[8] In practical terms, therefore, one can only link a stressor and its effect circumstantially, and to some extent only *post hoc*, although more experimental evidence is accumulating on the nature and incidence of this link. Stress can also be viewed either as a causal factor in disease or as a contributory one – by reducing the individual's 'resistance' to disease processes such as viral infection[9] or rheumatoid arthritis.[10] In other cases, an individual with a pre-existing organic disease might have a relapse in response to stress, as described by Trimble and Wilson-Barnet[11] in the case of epileptic seizures. Also, the physical disease itself may be a stressful experience which can delay recovery or cause other forms of ill-health – especially if it involves loss of income or of job security.

Stress and life changes

Many of the stressors mentioned above – such as bereavement, migration, or the birth of a child – involve prolonged, major *changes* in the patterns of people's lives. In recent years, more attention has been paid to the possible negative effects of these changes on both mental and physical health. From this point of view, stress represents an inadequate adaptation to change, an unsuccessful attempt on the part of the individual to cope with, and adapt to, the changed circumstances of their lives, whether this is promotion at work or the loneliness of widowhood. Parkes[6] provides a useful way of viewing these changes or 'psychosocial transitions': he points out that the change is likely to take place in that part of the world which impinges upon the self – the 'life space'. This consists of 'those parts of the environment with which the self interacts and in relation to which behaviour is organized; other persons, material possessions, the familiar world of home and place of work, and the individual's body and mind in so far as he can view these as separate from his self'. They also involve changes in the basic assumptions that people have made about their worlds; no longer can these assumptions be taken for granted. In Parkes' view, those psychosocial transitions most likely to cause stress are those which are lasting in their effects, take place over a relatively short period of time, and affect many of the assumptions that people make about their worlds. In that sense, the sudden, unexpected loss of a spouse or job is likely to be more stressful than other, slower transitions such as those involved in growth and maturation. Changes such as bereavement, redundancy or migration will involve many aspects of an individual's life space, such as social relationships, occupational status, financial security and living arrangements, and are more likely to provoke a stress response.

The effects of these changes on both mental and physical health have been studied by several investigators. In their study of bereavement, for example, Parkes *et al.*[12] examined the death rates of 4486 widowers of 55 years of age or older for nine years following the death of their wives. Of these, 213 died in the first six months of bereavement, 40% above the expected death rate for married men of the same ages. Death rate from degenerative heart disease was 67% above that expected. The mortality rate dropped to that of married men after the first year. The authors ascribe the increased death rate to 'the emotional effects of bereavement with the concomitant changes in psycho-endocrine function'. Other studies have reached similar conclusions: in a significant number of cases, ill-health is preceded by a high level of psychosocial transitions or 'life events', especially if these events are perceived as 'negative'.

The precise causal link between these life changes and the occurrence of ill-health remains unclear, although various hypotheses have been advanced. Murphy and Brown,[13] in examining the question 'whether stressful situations bring about episodes of illness associated with pathological structural changes occurring in a tissue, system or area of the body', point out that in most cases illness will not follow from an experience of stress, but where it does the link is likely to be a psychiatric disturbance. They cite evidence that individuals with psychiatric disorders have a significantly higher rate of organic illness, and hypothesize that 'stressful circumstances lead to organic illness by first producing a psychiatric disturbance'. In their study of 111 women in London, 81 had developed a new organic disease (from which they had previously not suffered) in the previous six months. Of this latter group, 30% (24) had had at least one severe 'life event' before the onset of ill-health, compared with 17% of a matched comparison group, although this association applied only to women between 18 and 50 years, where 38% had had at least one severe event, compared with 15% of a control group. In this age group, 30% had experienced the onset of psychiatric disturbance in an average period of seven weeks before the start of their illness, compared with an expected 2% in the control group. The authors conclude that 'it is the onset of psychiatric disturbance rather than a severe event that is the immediate cause of organic disorder for those (women) under 50'. The events most likely to cause psychiatric disorders are those involving long-term threat to the life space, such as an unplanned pregnancy, or terminal illness in a relative. However, the exact physiological mechanism – whereby life events, psychiatric disorder and organic illness are interlinked – remains unclear. Engel[14] has also pointed out how illness and sometimes death is preceded by a period of psychological disturbance, during which the person feels 'unable to cope', and which he terms the 'giving-up-given-up complex'. He suggests that this state 'plays some significant role in modifying the capacity of the organism to cope with concurrent pathogenic factors'. It is characterized by: a feeling of psychological impotence or helplessness ('giving-up'); a lowered self-image as one who is no longer competent, in control, or functioning in their usual manner; a loss of gratification from human relationships and social roles; a disruption of the sense of continuity between past, present and future; and a reactivation of earlier memories of helplessness, or giving-up. In this state, the person is less likely to deal with pathological processes, although the complex itself does not 'cause' disease directly but rather contributes towards its emergence. Once again, the precise physiological mechanism by which this occurs remains unclear. However, the three perspectives mentioned above – psychosocial transitions, life events and the giving-up-given-up complex – all provide useful ways of viewing the effects on health and illness of such dramatic changes in life space as migration, urbanization, conquest, rapid social or technological change, and voodoo death (to be described below).

Factors influencing the stress response

In Selye's model, stress represents a pathological response to environmental demands. However, this response is mediated by a number of other factors, including:

1. The characteristics of the individuals.
2. Their physical environment.
3. The social support available to them.
4. Their economic status.
5. Their cultural background.

The *individual's* characteristics that influence response to stress are partly physical (such as age, weight, build, genetic make-up and previous health), and partly psychological. Weinman[4] points out how differences in personality affect response to stress, from phlegmatic types to those whose response is primarily somatic – 'the gastric responders' or 'cardiovascular responders', for example. Infantile and childhood experiences also play a part, as does individuals' perception of whether they have control over their lives or not. In the work situation, for example, Karasek *et al.*[15] have related a low sense of personal control to high levels of stress response. To a variable degree, individuals' outlook on life, including their hopes, fears and ambitions, are conditioned by their sociocultural background, as well as their early upbringing.

Physical sources of stress include extreme heat, cold and damp, and sources of tissue damage such as pathogenic organisms, burns or trauma. In all these cases, the nature and extent of the environmental stressor will influence the severity of the stress response.

Social and *cultural* factors tend to overlap in practice, but will be considered separately. Several authors have noted the importance of *social support*, at all stages of life, in protecting against stress. Weinman[4] notes how 'insufficient early support can give rise to physical and behavioural abnormalities, including a reduced ability to withstand stress' later in life. Brown and Harris[16] have demonstrated that women who lost their mothers before the age of 11 are more vulnerable to depression in adulthood, and a close and confiding relationship with another person helps protect against stress and psychiatric disorder. Kiritz and Moos[17] also point out the relationships of social environment to stress. In their view, social support and a sense of group cohesion protect against stress, while a sense of personal responsibility for others increases the physiological stress response. Stress is also increased by work pressure (the pressure to complete a large number of transactions per unit time), by uncertainty (about the possibility of physical or psychological harm), and by change in psychosocial environments (such as job relocation or redundancy).

Economic factors are also relevant to the stress response: poverty and unemployment are potent stressors in any community, as is loss of income and financial insecurity resulting from either physical or mental ill-health.

Cultural factors play a complex role in the response to stress. In general, this role might be protective or pathogenic. Culture also helps to shape the *form* of the stress response into a recognizable language of distress. That is, different cultural groups exposed to similar stressors may display different types of stress response, as may men and women within the same cultural group. In their study of French, American, Filipino and Haitian college students, Guthrie et al.[18] found clustering of the different symptoms of stress in the four groups. The Americans, for example, reported more gastrointestinal symptoms, while the French reported more changes in mood or thought content. The Filipinos, especially the women, tended to emphasize cardiovascular symptoms, such as a rapid heartbeat and shortness of breath. Symptoms such as dizziness, headaches, nightmares and muscle twitches were more often complained of by women in all four groups, and the authors suggest that 'in certain societies it may be less socially acceptable for males to admit and experience this constellation of symptoms'. The cultural values of a group may also protect against stress: for example, by strengthening social and family cohesion and mutual support, which enable the individual to better cope with the viscissitudes of life. A culture's world-view can also have this effect, by placing individual suffering in the wider context of misfortune in general. This is characteristic of religious world-views, especially those with a fatalistic view of misfortune as being an expression of 'God's will'. Membership of a group with such a shared conceptual system also helps give meaning and coherence to daily life, and reduces the stress of uncertainty. Cultures that value meditation and contemplation, rather than competitiveness and material achievement, are probably less stressful overall to their members. A further factor is that in many societies the rearing of children (and the stress that goes with it) is shared among several adults of an extended family, as well as the parents themselves, and this may also have a protective function. In looking at non-Western or pre-industrial societies, however, one should avoid what Foster and Anderson[19] term 'the myth of the stress-free "primitive" existence'. Contrary to the WHO's contention[7] that stress as 'a traditional method of adaptation has become inadequate in the psychological, social and economic circumstances of modern society', the evidence is that traditional societies, too, have their share of damaging stressors.

'Culturogenic' stress

While culture can protect against stress, it can also make it more likely. That is, certain cultural beliefs, values and practices are likely to *increase* the number of stressors that the individual is exposed to. For example, each culture defines what constitutes 'success' (as opposed to 'failure'), 'prestige' (as opposed to 'loss of face'), 'good behaviour' (as opposed to 'bad'), and 'good news' (as opposed to 'bad tidings'), and there is considerable variation between these in different societies. In part of New Guinea, for example, failure to have enough pigs or yams to exchange with other tribal members on certain occasions may lead to a stressful loss of face; in the Western world, failure to 'keep up with the Joneses' in terms of consumer objects may also result in subjective stress. In each society, individuals try to reach the defined goals, levels of prestige and standards of behaviour that the cultural group expects of its members. Failure to reach these goals (even if these goals seem absurd to members of another society) may result in frustration, anxiety, depression, and even the giving-up-given-up complex described above. Some beliefs can be directly stressful, such as the belief that one has been cursed or hexed by a powerful person, against whom there is little defence. In some cases, as in voodoo death, this may result in the victim's death after a short period of time. Other cultural values that may induce stress are an emphasis on war-like activities, or intense competition for marriage partners, money, goods or prestige. The unequal distribution of wealth in a society, based on its 'economic culture', is usually stressful to its poorer members, whose lives are a daily struggle for existence, but economic privileges, too, sometimes involve high levels of stress, caused by competitiveness and fear of the poor.

In its effect upon the health of the individual, therefore, there are both negative and positive sides to belief; as Hahn and Kleinman[20] put it, 'belief kills; belief heals'. Those beliefs and behaviours which contribute to stress, and which are acquired by growing up within a particular society, can therefore be regarded as a form of culturally induced or *culturogenic* stress.

This type of stress is also an example of the *nocebo* phenomenon (from the Latin root, *noceo*, I hurt), which is the negative effect on health of beliefs and expectations – and therefore the exact reverse of the 'placebo' phenomenon (see Chapter 8).

Some examples

The most extreme form of culturogenic stress and the nocebo effect described by anthropologists is known as 'voodoo death', 'hex death' or 'magical death', but which Landy[21] prefers to term *sociocultural* death. This phenomenon has been reported from various parts of the world, including Latin America, Africa, the Caribbean and Australia, and is usually found in traditional, pre-industrial societies. In magical death a person who believes he or she has been marked out for death by sorcery sickens and dies within a short period, apparently of natural causes. Once victims and those around them believe that a fatal curse has been placed upon them all concerned regard them as doomed. As Landy puts it, a 'process is set in motion, usually by a supposed religious or social transgression that results in the transgressor being marked out for death by a sorcerer acting on behalf of society through a ritual of accusation and condemnation; then death occurs within a brief span, usually 24 to 48 hours'. The anthropologist Claude Lévi-Strauss[22] has described this process in more detail, beginning with the individual's awareness that he is doomed, according to the traditions of his culture. His family and friends share this belief, and gradually the community withdraws from him. Often they remind the unfortunate victim that he is doomed, and virtually dead. Then:

'Shortly thereafter, sacred rites are held to dispatch him to the realm of shadows. First brutally torn from all of his family and social ties and excluded from all functions and activities through which he experienced self-awareness, then banished by the same forces from the world of the living, the victim yields to the combined terror, the sudden total withdrawal of the multiple reference systems provided by the support of the group, and, finally, to the group's decisive reversal in proclaiming him – once a living man, with rights and obligations – dead and an object of fear, ritual, and taboo.'

This situation is a classic example of Engel's giving-up-given-up complex, which he sees as a life setting conducive both to illness and to sudden death. He has analysed the reports of 170 cases of sudden death[23] and finds certain common themes in most of them: they involve events that are impossible for the victim to ignore, the individual experiences or is threatened with overwhelming emotional excitation, and the person believes he no longer has control over the situation. Ten of the cases involved sudden death during loss of status or self-esteem; for example, two men who were confidently expecting promotion to important positions dropped dead when their expectations were unexpectedly dashed. Various hypotheses have been advanced to explain the mechanism of culturogenic sudden death. Cannon[24] believed it was due to overactivity of the sympathetic nervous system – the 'fight or flight' response – in a situation where the victim is (culturally) immobilized and can do neither. According to Engel,[25] it is due to vasovagal syncope and cardiac arrythmias in a patient with pre-existing cardiovascular disease; this occurs in cases of emotional arousal and psychological uncertainty, where both the sympathetic ('fight–flight') and parasympathetic ('conservation–withdrawal') systems are simultaneously activated. In Lex's[26] view this simultaneous activation takes place in the settings characteristic of magical death, and in this state the nervous system is 'tuned' or over-sensitized, and the individual is more vulnerable to suggestions that he will die by magical means; he is also vulnerable to acute parasympathetic hyper-reactivity, or vagal death.

Magical death is an extreme and dramatic form of the culturogenic stress response. It represents the reverse of Hertz's[27] model of bereavement (see Chapter 9), for here 'social death' precedes 'biological death' by a variable period of time. In a Western setting, long-term admission to a psychiatric institution or geriatric ward can also be seen as a form of sociocultural death; it involves a major change in life space and a new set of stressors for the inmates of these institutions, and has been well described in the work of Goffman.[28]

A modern form of social death is increasingly seen among the victims of AIDS. Cassens[29] describes the many stressful social consequences that may occur for homosexual men who have been diagnosed as having this condition. As well as the physical illness itself, they have to cope with guilt, anxiety, the fear of certain death, and the prejudices of other people (see Chapter 5). There is also a loss of privacy about their sexuality, possible loss of employment and rejection by family and friends, and constant exposure to lurid stories in the media – with their 'tones of sin and retribution' – which can only enhance their sense of social isolation and rejection.

Another, though less extreme, example of culturogenic stress is the damaging effect on health and behaviour of certain *diagnostic labels:* for example, telling a patient: 'You've got cancer', 'You've got a weak heart', or 'You've got hypertension'. In Waxler's view,[30] certain diagnostic labels can affect patients' symptoms, behaviour, social relationships, prognosis and self-perception, as well as the attitudes of others towards them. This may even occur in the absence of physical disease. In this case, the nocebo phenomenon results from lay beliefs about the origin, significance, severity and prognosis of a weak heart or hypertension, and about the behaviour appropriate to sufferers from that condition. Patients may see themselves as ill or disabled, while family and friends may begin treating them in a particular way – encouraging them to change diet or behaviour, or to take special precautions. Like the patients, their attitudes are shaped by cultural beliefs about the significance of certain diseases. In the case of children, this might have life-long effects: parents of a child labelled 'asthmatic' may – based on their own childhood memories of what asthma entailed – prohibit the child from a wide range of social or sporting activities. Diagnostic labels can thus become a form of self-fulfilling prophecy. Some individuals who are labelled as ill may become enmeshed within certain institutions that sustain the label rather than encourage its disappearance. Waxler notes how organizations such as Alcoholics Anonymous, for example, may inadvertently prolong an individual's label of illness because 'a large percentage of AA members' social lives centers on the organization and other members, thus isolating them from normal relationships and further strengthening their role as "alcoholics"'. She quotes another study of a group of

American farmers who had *no* evidence of cardiac disease, but who labelled themselves as having heart disease, following a misunderstanding of their doctor's diagnosis. As a result they took more 'heart-related precautions', and generally acted like cardiac invalids. As Waxler points out, the label itself – what the farmer or his family *believe* to be the case – has an important effect upon his behaviour, even when he has no symptoms and no disease. Another example of how labelling can affect everyday behaviour is described by Haynes *et al*.[31] who screened workers for hypertension in a large factory. In those (asymptomatic) patients who were told they had 'hypertension', absenteeism from work rose by 80%, greatly exceeding the 9% rise in absenteeism in the general employee population during the same period. Certain diagnostic labels, therefore, if they provoke anxiety and foreboding (such as 'cancer'), are likely to act as additional stressors, especially if the person is already physically ill.

A final example of how the cultural values of a society may contribute towards stress and disease in its members is seen in the case of coronary heart disease (CHD). This condition is believed to have a multifactorial aetiology, and a number of risk factors which predispose to its development have been described. These include the dietary intake of saturated fats, lack of exercise, cigarette smoking, raised serum cholesterol and hypertension. However, the work of Friedman and Rosenman[32] suggests that psychosocial patterns, especially behaviour patterns and personality type, also play a role in its aetiology, especially in susceptible individuals. They have described the characteristics of what they term the *type A behaviour pattern* (TABP) - in particular the chronic struggle to achieve an unlimited number of goals in as short a time as possible. These individuals displaying TABP show marked aggressiveness, ambition and competitive drive; they are work-orientated and 'workaholic' people, preoccupied with deadlines, and chronically impatient.[33] Their personal lives are emotionally parched and incomplete, and both family and leisure are less important to them than work and ambition. Long-term follow-up studies have shown that individuals with this behaviour pattern are about twice as likely to develop CHD as other adults of similar age group without these traits (known as the type B behaviour pattern).[33] Friedman and Rosenman believe that modern, Western industrial society encourages the development of type A traits, and rewards them. Those who exhibit them often become successful executives, professionals, politicians, managers, technocrats and salesmen. However, these rewards often involve constant anxiety about failure, demotion or loss of control. Appels[34] sees this type of personality as someone who cannot manage or handle the pressures of the industrialized, fast-moving and achievement-orientated society and who, by this very failure, shows the characteristics of this society in an excessive way. In his study of 22 societies he found that the mortality rate from CHD was positively correlated with a cultural emphasis in the societies on the 'need for achievement'. In the USA, Waldron[35] has examined the relationship of type A behaviour and gender within that country, where the risk of CHD is twice as great in men as in women. She suggests that while men's excess vulnerability may be partly due to hormonal factors, cultural factors also play a part. In particular, type A behaviour can contribute to success in traditional male roles and professions, but not in the traditional female role in society. Accordingly, parents and other socializing institutions may promote type A characteristics in boys, but not in girls – and later in life this may protect a higher proportion of women from risk of CHD.

It is possible therefore to view the type A behaviour pattern as a Western culture-bound syndrome (see Chapter 10), embodying many of the cultural values of an industrial, capitalist society, where competition, ambition, materialism and the time-urgency of rush hours and deadlines are all part of daily life. Furthermore, this model of stressful behaviour also embodies some of the *contradictions* within the cultural values of Western society, and the type A individual is the living embodiment of those contradictions. On one hand, for example, he conforms to the social values of his society – to what Weber[36] terms its 'philosophy of avarice' – and is rewarded for doing so, but on the other hand his hostile, competitive behaviour is also *anti*social, damaging to himself, his family, his friends, and to those he works with. It can be argued that this paradox of values – that some forms of antisocial behaviour are being constantly rewarded by society – is symbolically resolved (at least for a while) when he is 'punished' by suffering a heart attack, and emerges from the hospital as a chastened, fragile and less aggressive 'type B'.[37]

In the next chapter I will be discussing how some immigrants to the United States, such as the Japanese, seem to be partly protected by their cultural background against the risk of both type A behaviour and CHD, provided they retain many of their traditional cultural values.

Stress and migration

Migration from one culture to another is a stressful experience, involving major disruptions in the individual's life space. As Eitinger[38] notes, the new immigrant has to deal with isolation, helplessness and a feeling of insecurity in his surroundings, coupled with a flood of incomprehensible stimuli. Not only have they left family, friends and a familiar locality, but many of their assumptions about their world are no longer valid. They are often faced with language difficulties, with hostility or indifference from the host population, and with new cultural practices that may be at variance with their religious beliefs. Often, too, migration is not only between cultures, but from a small village community to a big metropolis; from the life of a peasant on his own little plot of land to that of an unskilled labourer in the big city. While some of the migrant's cultural values, such as an emphasis on family cohesion, may be protective against stress, the experience of migration is usually a profound psychosocial transition – analogous in some ways to bereavement or disablement. Eisenbruch[39] has coined the term *cultural bereavement* for those groups of people who have suffered a permanent and traumatic loss of their familiar land and culture. This applies especially to unwilling migrants such as refugees and exiles, suddenly uprooted during war or persecution. The stressful changes that such a group may undergo in its collective grief are analagous to those suffered by individual mourners, and may include pathological and atypical grief reactions.

Some of the stress responses, both physical and psychological, of immigrants to the UK and the USA have been examined in a number of studies.

Case history: Effect of migration on blood pressure

Cassell[40] has reviewed the research work done on the effect of migration on blood pressure. In one study, the blood pressure of black migrants from the Southern USA to Chicago was compared with that of Chicago-born blacks. It was found that the longer the period of city life, the higher was their blood pressure. In another study, the blood pressures of inhabitants of the Cape Verde Islands (off West Africa) were compared with those of Cape Verdeans who had migrated to the Eastern USA. The immigrants showed higher pressures at each age, and a sharper difference between young and old than did the islanders. Other studies showed higher rates of hypertension among Irish immigrants to the USA (32%) when compared with their brothers living in Ireland (21%). In Cassell's view, the findings of these studies are unlikely to be due to genetic differences between those who immigrate and those who stay behind, but possibly to genetic differences in the susceptibility to environmental influences among individual migrants. These influences include such physical factors as caloric intake, physical activity, salt intake and the absence of certain parasites and diseases in the host country which, in the country of origin, usually cause wasting, anaemia, and a fall in blood pressure. However, psychosocial factors also play a part, particularly the disappearance of a 'coherent value system', and its replacement by different values and different situations, where the migrant's traditional way of coping with life is no longer effective.

Case history: Mental illness among immigrants in Manchester, UK

Carpenter and Brockington[41] examined the incidence of mental illness among Asian, West Indian and African immigrants living in Manchester. It was found that the migrant populations had about twice the first admission rate to mental hospitals that British-born subjects had, especially those migrants aged 35–44, and also Asian women. Schizophrenia was particularly common among the immigrants, especially with delusions of persecution, a phenomenon noted in many other studies of migrants. The authors hypothesize that 'social and lingual isolation . . . insecurity and the attitudes of the milieu are the explanations for the development of persecutory delusions'.

Case history: psychiatric admission to hospitals of foreign-born people in Bradford, UK

Hitch and Rack[42] studied the rates of first admission to psychiatric hospitals in Bradford, and found that foreign-born people had substantially higher mental illness rates than British-born people. The rates of psychiatric breakdown of a sample of Polish and Russian refugees in Bradford were measured 25 years after they had settled in the UK. While both had higher rates of mental illness (especially schizophrenia and paranoia) than the British-born population, the Poles had a higher rate than the Russians. The most vulnerable group were the Polish women. The authors suggest that the difference between the immigrant groups is due partly to minimal cohesion among the Poles, but a strong sense of national, ethnic identity among the Russians (many of whom are Ukrainians). This ethnic social support not only affords a protection against environmental stress, it also bestows identity, though the Russians appear to have maintained this identity more than the Poles. Many years after migration, though, both immigrant groups are especially vulnerable to first-time mental illness. The authors suggest that 'the combination of wartime experiences and culture shock may have been met with adequate coping mechanisms, but nevertheless rendered the personality vulnerable to later stress'. In middle age, when children have moved away, and spouses or relatives have died, an immigrant who still speaks broken English and has no English friends will become particularly vulnerable to environmental stressors, with the consequent danger of mental or physical illness.

Case history: Attempted suicide among immigrants in Birmingham, UK

Burke, in his three studies, has examined the rate of attempted suicide among Irish,[43] Asian[44] and West Indian[45] immigrants in Birmingham. His findings indicate that immigrants have a higher rate of attempted suicide than the populations in their countries of origin, and this applies particularly to immigrant women. In Birmingham, those born in Northern Ireland or the Irish Republic have about a 30% higher rate than the native population (as measured in Edinburgh), and higher rates than in both Belfast and Dublin. Other indices of stress, such as the rates of alcoholism, drug addiction or mental illness, were also raised in this immigrant group. Asian immigrants (from India, Pakistan and Bangladesh) had a lower rate of attempted suicide than the native-born population, but their rate was higher than that of their countries of origin, especially among women. Burke points out that language difficulties for women may play a major part in this, because Asian men have usually migrated several years earlier, and have had a greater opportunity to learn the language and familiarize themselves with English culture. Immigrant women are often expected to remain at home and there is also some 'culture conflict' for younger Asian women and girls between the values of home and those of school or workplace. Among West Indians, too, attempted suicide was less common than among the native-born population, but West Indian women had a higher rate than women in the Caribbean; that is, the 'stresses that follow immigration and contribute to attempted suicide are more likely to affect women than men'. Part of the stress on young West Indians arises from the insecurity of low-paid jobs, fear of not being able to cope financially and emotionally, housing difficulties, and the absence of the extended family in an urban setting. All of these 'may effectively reduce the tolerance of immigrants in withstanding these stresses'.

While these studies are useful in illustrating the high level of stress responses among immigrants, they do not provide enough data on *how* the cultural practices and world-view of immigrants – and of the host community itself – interact in the migrant situation. For example, what cultural traits in immigrant communities protect them from stress, or predispose towards it? Do some cultural groups migrate less 'stressfully' than others? Is the status of the temporary migrant (such as *gastarbeiters*) less or more stressful than that of the permanent migrant, exile or refugee? What are the effects on immigrants' mental and physical health of discrimination and racial prejudice – both individual and institutional? Are some host cultures more stressful to immigrants than others?

A further factor, mentioned in Chapter 10, is that the medical and other authorities in the host community determine whether deviant behaviour among immigrants is regarded as mad or bad, and this can significantly affect the morbidity statistics among immigrant populations.

Lay models of 'stress'

In the past few decades, the concept of 'stress' outlined above has increasingly entered popular discourse, and is now commonly used in books, magazines, radio and television programmes. Lay concepts of stress are usually those of a diffuse and invisible 'force', somehow mediating between individuals (and their mental and physical state) and the social environment in which they live and work. In some ways it has become a secular version of more traditional concepts of witchcraft, sorcery and other forms of interpersonal malevolence, and of divine punishment, fate and possession by malign spirits (see Chapter 5). In a study[8] in Massachusetts, for example, 95% of a sample of 42 patients with psychosomatic disorders blamed their condition on 'stress', although they varied widely in what they meant by this term. In some cases it was described as an invisible force in the environment, pressing down on the individual (to be 'under acute stress'); or as an invisible and malevolent force, usually produced by other people, that enters your body and then causes disease ('stress can cause my bronchi to spasm', 'stress goes to the weakest organ. I let it get to me and eat me away'); or as something that 'builds up' inside you unless you can get it out ('a good relationship can make you stay healthy, because you can ventilate a lot of stress'). Although many other lay uses of the term stress exist in Western culture, these examples illustrate the extent to which Selye's original concept has entered popular culture, and how it has become blended there with older explanations for disease and other misfortune.

Recommended reading

Parkes C. M. (1971) Psycho-social transitions: a field for study. *Soc. Sci. Med.* **5**, 101–115

Selye H. (1976) Forty years of stress research: principal remaining problems and misconceptions. *Can. Med. Assoc. J.* **115**, 53–57

World Health Organisation (1971) Society, stress and disease. *WHO Chron.* **25**, 168–178

Young, A. (1980) The discourse on stress and the reproduction of conventional knowledge. *Soc. Sci. Med.* **14B**, 133–146. A critique of both medical and lay models of stress.

Helman, C. G. (1987) Heart disease and the cultural construction of time: the type A behaviour pattern as a Western culture-bound syndrome. *Soc. Sci. Med.* **25**, 969–979. The role of Western cultural values in coronary heart disease.

Eisenbruch, M. (1988) The mental health of refugee children and their cultural development. *Int. Migration Rev.* **22**, 282–300

Chapter 12

Cultural factors in epidemiology

Epidemiology is the study of the distribution and determinants of the various forms of disease in human populations. Its focus is not on the individual case of ill-health, but rather on groups of people, both healthy and diseased. When investigating a particular disease (such as lung cancer), epidemiologists try to relate its occurrence and distribution to a variety of factors associated with most victims of that condition (such as smoking behaviour) to discover its probable aetiology. The factors most commonly examined are the age, sex, marital status, occupation, socioeconomic position, diet, environment (both natural and man-made) and behaviour of the victims. Their aim is to uncover a causal link between one or more of these factors and the development of the disease.

Most epidemiological surveys utilize one of two approaches, or sometimes a combination of the two. The *case–control* method examines a sample of the population suffering from a particular disease, and compares them with a similar sample of those without the disease. If one can demonstrate a statistically significant correlation between certain factors and the occurrence of the disease – such as a long history of cigarette smoking in those suffering from lung cancer – a 'causal' link can be postulated. In the *cohort study* approach one begins with a healthy population – some of whom are associated with hypothetical risk factors, such as smoking – and follows them up over time, waiting for a particular disease to occur. If those associated with a particular risk factor are found to be more likely to develop the disease subsequently, one can postulate a causal link between the risk factor and the disease. In many of these epidemiological studies, however, the precise nature of this link cannot be explained, and must remain presumptive until further evidence is accumulated. In other cases, such as lung cancer and smoking, or congenital birth defects and thalidomide use during pregnancy, the aetiological link is much clearer, and can also be explained in physiological terms.

On an individual level, however, the notion of 'risk factors' has only a limited predictive value. For example, not all heavy smokers will develop lung cancer, not all immigrants will suffer a suicidal depression, nor will all type A personalities develop coronary heart disease. In understanding why a particular individual gets a particular disease at a particular time, a much wider range of factors – genetic, physical, sociocultural and psychological – must all be taken into account, as well as the interrelationships between them. This multi-factorial explanation of ill-health is often more useful than postulating a simple cause–effect relationship between one risk factor and one type of disease. As Kendell[1] has pointed out: 'In medicine, as in physics, specific causes have given way to complex chains of event sequences in constant interplay with one another. The very idea of "cause" has become meaningless, other than as a convenient designation for the point in these chain of event sequences at which intervention is most practicable.'

Both sociologists and anthropologists have made important contributions to the understanding of how these complex factors are related to disease. They have pointed out how such variables as social class, economic position, gender, life events and cultural beliefs and practices can be correlated with the incidence and distribution of certain diseases. Sociologists Murphy and Brown,[2] for example, in their study of 111 women in London, have demonstrated how both psychological and physical ill-health was preceded by one or more severe life events in the previous six months (see Chapter 11). On a more 'macro' level, the Black Report[3] in 1982 showed how in the UK there is a relationship between social class and health, and how members of the lower socioeconomic classses have poorer health, and a higher mortality, than their fellow citizens in the more affluent classes. In the developing world, too, there is a clear relationship between health and income. In many of these countries, much of the population, already weakened by poor nutrition, will suffer from infectious and other communicable diseases. These diseases are often transmitted with the help of polluted water supplies, poor sanitation and inadequate housing – all of which can only be improved by an adequate income.[4] Therefore, at a macro level, these types of economic and social factors – as well as the political organization of the society – must always be taken into account, before considering the exact role of cultural factors in health and illness.

In the developing world, anthropological insights have been especially useful in unravelling the causes of more exotic diseases, such as *kuru* (a progressive, degenerative disease of the brain), which epidemiological studies in the 1950s had found to be confined to women and children in a small area of the Eastern Highlands of New Guinea. The disease was virtually unknown among men. Various theories were advanced to explain this, but it was eventually found to be caused by a slow virus infection in the brain, which was transmitted by the ritual cannibalism on dead relatives practised only by some women and children in that area.[5] Other anthropological research has shed light on *why* people smoke, drink, take narcotic drugs, mutilate their bodies, avoid nutritious diets, have dangerous pastimes and follow stressful occupations or lifestyles. Marmot[6] has pointed out how cultural factors (as well as social and psychological ones) may influence much of this 'risk-related behaviour'. He notes how, in most medical epidemiological studies, the risks associated with such factors as smoking, intake of certain foods or obesity are examined, but often scant attention is paid to the *cultural* influences shaping dietary patterns, obesity or smoking. Studies that have looked at these cultural dimensions point out that cultural beliefs and practices are only part of the multi-factorial aetiology of disease. In the case of *kuru*, for example, the virus, the social division between the sexes, and the practice of cannibalism all share in its aetiology and explain its distribution.

In the industrialized world, anthropological insights are of particular relevance in Community Oriented Primary Care (COPC),[7] which focuses on the primary health care of individuals and families, but also on the health needs and health problems of their local community. Part of the continuing surveillance of the community's health involves an awareness of the role of cultural beliefs and behaviours, in either improving health or causing disease.

These cultural factors, where they can be identified, are often difficult to quantify and are therefore less attractive to medical epidemiologists and statisticians. Nor is there a neat, measurable dose–response relationship between a particular cultural factor and a particular disease – as there might be between a pathogenic organism (or chemical) and the disease that it causes. Nevertheless, despite this difficulty in quantifying cultural factors, there is sufficient evidence available to confirm their role in the development of disease – even if this role is contributory, rather than directly causative. It should also be noted that, in some cases, cultural factors may *protect* against ill-health. In the studies by Marmot and his colleagues,[8,9] quoted below, the rates of coronary heart disease were compared between samples of Japanese men living in Japan,

Hawaii and California. The degree of their adherence to traditional Japanese culture and world-view was correlated with their incidence of CHD; it was found that the rate of CHD among the Japanese Americans was the highest of the three groups, and this matched their increasing distance from their traditional culture. This type of study also has the value of pointing out the relative importance of genetic and environmental factors – of nature and nurture – in the causation of disease. If three groups of Japanese with similar genetic backgrounds have different rates of CHD, environmental influences must somehow be implicated.

Culture and the identification of disease

The cultural and social background of the epidemiologist, and of the populations studied, may affect the validity of the epidemiological data gathered. In the first instance, there are still differences in the diagnostic criteria used to define particular diseases, between epidemiologists in different countries. These differences in labelling policy may give an inaccurate picture of the incidence of certain diseases in different countries. For example, Fletcher et al.[10] examined the apparent predominance of 'chronic bronchitis' in the UK, and of 'emphysema' in North America. It was found that this was largely due to the fact that the *same* constellation of symptoms and signs was diagnosed as chronic bronchitis in the UK, but as 'emphysema' in the USA. Other studies, among British and American psychiatrists (see Chapter 10) have shown differences in diagnostic criteria between the two groups, with American psychiatrists diagnosing schizophrenia more readily than their British counterparts. A recent study[11] also showed marked differences in the rates of diagnosis of various diseases by doctors in five European countries. These differences, it was suggested, may either be the result of actual variations in disease morbidity in the five countries, or due to differences in the ways doctors in those countries actually *interpret* and diagnose certain symptoms and signs.

Zola[12] points out how the perceived incidence of a disease in a particular community depends on its actual incidence and the degree of its recognition (by patients or doctors) as being something abnormal. In the latter case, this depends on the social context in which the disease occurs, and whether there is a fit between the symptoms and signs and the society's definition of what constitutes abnormality. He quotes studies illustrating how Arapesh women report no pain during menstruation, though quite the contrary is reported in the USA. Other studies, quoted by Fox,[13] have shown how congenital dislocation of the hip is considered normal (though not necessarily good) among the Navaho Indians of the south-western USA, and how in 'Regionville' backache was consi-dered abnormal by the higher socioeconomic groups, but not by the lower socioeconomic class. Lay definitions of abnormality or disease determine, to some extent, whether these conditions find their way to doctors, and thus into the morbidity statistics. In Zola's words, 'a selective process might well be operating in what symptoms are brought to the doctor . . . it might be this selective process and not an etiological one which accounts for the many unexplained or overexplained epidemiological differ-ences observed between and within societies'.

Epidemiology is directed more towards the study of 'disease' rather than that of 'illness'. Its scientific approach leads to an emphasis on 'hard' or objectively verifiable data, such as abnormal blood pressure readings, blood tests or other measurable changes in the body's structure or function. However, this excludes the many forms of illness, particularly the culture-bound folk illnesses mentioned in Chapters 5 and 10, where physiological data are often absent. Anthropologists like Rubel have suggested that epidemiological techniques used to study such diseases as tuberculosis or syphilis can also be applied to folk illnesses such as *susto* in Latin America. These folk illnesses are perceived as real by members of these societies, just as medical epidemiologists see tuberculosis as real. They can also have marked effects on people's behaviour, and on their mental and physical health. In Rubel's view,[14] the unique constellation of cultural beliefs, symptoms, and behavioural changes that characterize *susto* recur with remarkable constancy among many Hispanic American groups, Indian and non-Indian alike. By studying ethnographic case histories of those suffering from the condition, Rubel is able to isolate certain variables usually associated with each occurrence of the illness. He has suggested that *susto*, and other folk illnesses, can be thought of as having a multi-factorial aetiology; that is, they result from the complex interplay of the victim's previous state of health, personality (including his self-perception of success or failure in the performance of social expectations), and social system in which he or she lives (particularly its role expecta-tions). *Susto* occurs in social situations which the individual finds stressful, such as an inability to meet the expectations of family, friends or employers, and is 'the vehicle by means of which people of Hispanic American peasant and urban societies manifest their reactions to some forms of self-perceived stressful situations'. While its identification rests mainly on folk perceptions, and the observations of anthropologists, the techniques of epidemiology should be valuable in relating its occurrence to social, cultural or psychological variables.

Cultural factors in the epidemiology of disease

As mentioned above, cultural factors can be either causal, contributory or protective in their relation to ill-health. In this section a number of these cultural factors are listed, many of which have already been described in more detail in previous chapters. The list is not meant to be exhaustive, but rather a selection of those factors most commonly examined by anthropologists and epidemiologists. Their relevance is illustrated later in the chapter by a number of case histories.

Economic situation

This includes whether wealth is evenly distributed throughout the society; whether the sample group are poor, or wealthy, relative to other members of the society; whether income is sufficient for adequate housing, nutrition and clothing; the cultural values associated with wealth, poverty, employment and unemployment; and whether the basic economic unit (of earning, accumulating and sharing wealth) is the individual, the family or a larger collectivity.

Family structure

This includes whether nuclear or extended families are the rule; the degree of interaction, cohesion and mutual support among family members; whether the emphasis is on familial rather than on individual achievements; and whether responsibility for child-rearing, the provision of food, and care of the elderly, sick or dying is shared among family members.

Gender roles

This includes the division of labour between the sexes, especially who works, who remains at home, who prepares the food, and who cares for the children; the social rights, obligations and expectations associated with the two gender roles; cultural beliefs about the behaviour appropriate to each gender (such as alcohol consumption, smoking and competitive behaviour being regarded as 'natural' for men, but not for women); and degree of 'medicalization' of the female life-cycle.

Marriage patterns

This includes whether polygamy or monogamy is encouraged; and whether marriage is *endogamous* (where the individual must marry within his family, clan or tribe) or *exogamous* (where he must choose a partner from outside these groups). In the case of endogamy, there is a greater likelihood of the 'pooling' of recessive genes, with a higher incidence of such inherited diseases as haemophilia, thalassaemia major, and Tay–Sachs disease.

Sexual behaviour

This includes whether promiscuity, premarital or extramarital sexual relations are encouraged or forbidden; whether these sexual norms apply to men or to women; whether special sexual norms (such as celibacy or promiscuity) are applied to restricted groups within the society (such as nuns or prostitutes); whether homosexuality, both male and female, is tolerated or forbidden; and whether there are taboos on sexual intercourse during pregnancy, menstruation or lactation.

Contraceptive patterns

This includes cultural attitudes towards contraception and abortion. A taboo on both of these enlarges family size, and in some cases may have a negative effect on maternal health. Certain forms of contraception, or abortion, may also be dangerous to maternal health, and attitudes to the use of condoms may influence the spread of sexually transmitted diseases, as well as hepatitis B and AIDS.

Population policy

This includes cultural beliefs about the optimal size of the family (such as the 'one-child' policy in China), and the gender of its children. For example, the incidence of infanticide and self-induced abortion may be related to these beliefs. Wagley[15] describes a Brazilian Indian tribe, the Tenetehara, who believe a woman should have no more than three children, and that these should not be all of the same sex. If a woman with two daughters gives birth to a third, the child is killed. Over time, such beliefs can affect the size and composition of local communities.

Pregnancy and childbirth practices

This includes changes in diet, dress or behaviour during pregnancy; the techniques used in childbirth, and the nature of the birth attendants; care of the umbilical cord (in some cultures, dung is applied as a dressing to the newly cut umbilical cord, thus increasing the risk of neonatal tetanus[16]); customs relating to the puerperium, such as social isolation or the observance of special taboos; and whether breast or artificial infant foods (such as powdered milk) are preferred.

Child-rearing practices

This includes the emotional climate of child-rearing, whether permissive or authoritarian; the degree of competitiveness encouraged among children (which may be related to mental illness, suicide attempts, development of the type A behaviour pattern in later life); the degree of physical or emotional abuse tolerated as normal; and initiation rituals carried out at puberty (such as circumcision and scarification).

Body image alterations

This includes culturally sanctioned bodily mutilations or alterations, such as male or female circumcision, scarification, tattooing, ear and lip piercing, foot-binding and forms of cosmetic surgery (like augmentation mammoplasty operations). Also, cultural values supporting, or discouraging, certain body shapes, such as slimness, tallness or obesity, especially among women.

Diet

This includes how food is prepared, stored and preserved; the utensils used in cooking and storing food; whether food is symbolically classified into food and non-food, sacred or profane food, or 'hot' and 'cold', irrespective of nutritional value; whether vegetarianism or meat-eating is the rule; whether special diets are followed during pregnancy, lactation, menstruation and ill-health; dietary fads and fashions; and the use of Western foodstuffs – with high salt, fat and refined carbohydrate levels – in non-Western communities, as a sign of 'modernization'.

Dress

This includes cultural prescriptions about forms of dress appropriate for men and women, and for special occasions; fashions of dress, such as tight dresses or corsets, high-heeled or 'platform'-heeled shoes – which may be related to the incidence of certain diseases or injuries; and body adornments, such as cosmetics, jewellery, perfume and hair dyes which may sometimes cause skin diseases. Long dresses which cover much of the body may predispose to certain conditions: for example, Underwood and Underwood[17] relate the long dress and veil worn by women in Yemen, as well as their confinement to 'harems', to their increased rate of osteomalacia, tuberculosis and anaemia. In the UK, the lack of sunlight combined with a vegetarian diet, confinement to home, and long dresses are all believed to contribute towards the high rate of osteomalacia in female Asian immigrants.[18]

Personal hygiene

This includes whether personal hygiene is neglected or encouraged; whether rituals of washing and purification are carried out on a regular basis; and whether bathing arrangements are private or communal.

Housing arrangements

This includes the construction, siting and internal division of living space; whether this space is occupied by members of the same family, clan or tribe; and the number of occupants per room, house or hut (which may influence the spread of infectious diseases).

Sanitation arrangements

This especially concerns the modes of disposal of human wastes; and whether they are disposed of near residences, food supplies or water sources.

Occupations

This includes whether men and women follow similar or different occupations; whether certain occupations are reserved for particular individuals, families or groups within the society – as in the traditional caste system in India, or the *apartheid* system in South Africa; whether certain occupations have a higher prestige and receive higher rewards in some societies (such as the type A executive in Western society); the use of certain techniques, such as traditional methods of hunting, fishing, agriculture or mining – which are associated with a high incidence of accidental death, trauma or infectious diseases; and some modern occupations, common in the industrialized world, which are also associated with certain diseases (such as pneumoconiosis in coal miners, bladder cancer in dye workers, or silicosis in metal grinders).

Religion

This includes whether a religion is characterized by a coherent, reassuring world-view; whether such religious practices as fasts, food taboos, ritual immersions, communal feasts, self-mutilations and flagellation, fire-walking and mass pilgrimages are required, all of which may be associated with the incidence of certain diseases.

Funerary customs

This concerns especially how, and by whom, the dead are disposed of; whether the corpse is buried or cremated immediately, or displayed in public for some time (which may aid the spread of infectious diseases); and the sites of burial, cremation or display of the corpse, and whether these are near to residences, food or water supplies.

Culturogenic stress

This includes whether culturogenic stress – and the *nocebo* effect – is induced or aggravated by the culture's values, goals, hierarchies of prestige, norms, taboos or expectations.

Migrant status

This includes whether migrants have adapted to their new culture in terms of behaviour, diet, language and dress; whether they are subject to discrimination, racism or persecution by the host community; and whether their familial structure and religious world-view remain intact after migration; and the culture of the 'host' community and its attitude to immigration.

Use of chemical comforters

This especially includes cultural values associated with smoking, alcohol, tea, coffee, prescribed and non-prescribed drugs, and the use of hallucinogens as sacramental drugs; the use of intravenous 'hard' drugs by an addict subculture, and the prevalence of needle sharing among those groups (relevant to the spread of both hepatitis B and AIDS).

Leisure pursuits

This includes the various forms of sport and recreation; whether these involve physical exercise or not; whether they are competitive or not; and whether they are associated with the risks of injury or disease.

Domestic animals and birds

This includes the nature and number of pets and domestic livestock; whether they are kept within the home or outside it; and the degree of direct physical contact between individuals and these animals. Various viral illnesses have been linked to domestic pets, such as benign lymphoreticulosis ('cat-scratch fever') and psittacosis ('parrot fever'), and also protozoal diseases such as toxoplasmosis, transmitted by cat faeces.

Self-treatment strategies and lay therapies

This includes all the treatments used within the popular and folk sectors, such as the use of herbal remedies, patent medicines, special diets, bodily manipulations, injections and cupping. Lay healing that takes place in a public ritual, rather than a private consultation, may predispose to the spread of infectious diseases. Certain alternative therapies, such as acupuncture, may be implicated in the spread of hepatitis B infection.

The above sections summarize some of the cultural factors that may be of relevance to epidemiologists. The importance of some of these factors to the study of the origin and distribution of disease is illustrated in the following case histories.

Case history: Cervical cancer in Latin America

Cervical cancer is a well documented example of the role of cultural factors – in this case, sexual norms and practices – in the distribution of a disease. Various studies have shown it to be rare in nuns, and common in prostitutes. It is extremely uncommon among Jewish, Mormon and Seventh Day Adventist women. Women with cervical cancer are more likely to have experienced early marriage, early commencement of coitus, multiple sexual partners and multiple marriages. It was originally thought that a woman's sexual behaviour could determine her risk of cervical cancer. However Skegg et al.[19] have also pointed out that its incidence is very high in Latin America, where women are expected to have only one sexual partner in their lives, and strong cultural sanctions exist against their having premarital or extramarital sexual relationships. They suggest that – if the hypothesis of the infective origin of cervical cancer is correct – then, in some communities, a woman's risk of getting the disease will depend less on her sexual behaviour than on that of her husband or male partner. One should therefore look at the patterns of sexual behaviour in a society as a whole, especially the sexual habits of the men. On this basis, they postulate three types of society: type A, where both men and women are strongly discouraged from premarital or extramarital relations (for example, Mormons or Seventh Day Adventists); type B, where only women are strongly discouraged from extramarital sexual relations, but men are expected to have many, especially with prostitutes, as in many Latin American societies, and in Europe last century; and type C, where both men and women have several sexual partners during their lives (as in the modern, Western 'permissive society'). The incidence of cervical cancer is lowest in type A, and highest in type B societies. In type A groups, such as Jews, Seventh Day Adventists and Mormons, the low incidence could be due to endogamous marriage and monogamous patterns of sexual behaviour, as well as to low recourse to prostitutes. In Latin America, in contrast, recourse to prostitutes is common. In one study quoted by Skegg, 91% of male Colombian students reported premarital intercourse, and 92% of these men had experienced intercourse with prostitutes. The authors suggest that this may account for the high incidence of cervical cancer in Latin America, as the prostitutes may act as a reservoir of infection. Similarly, the decline in mortality from the disease in the UK and USA (type C societies) may be due to changing patterns of sexual behaviour among men, with less recourse to prostitutes in a more 'permissive' society.

Case history: Hepatitis B

Brabin and Brabin[20] have reviewed the role of cultural factors in the transmission of the hepatitis B virus. The level of infection by the virus varies widely between countries, ethnic groups, tribes, and even neighbouring villages. Part of the reason for this is a number of cultural factors, including sexual behaviour patterns, family and marriage patterns, and cultural changes affecting women and their childbearing age. For example, the risk of infection with the virus varies with the level of promiscuity, and the spouses of promiscuous partners are therefore at greater risk from infection – which is particularly important in the case of pregnant women. They point out that marriage patterns which permit extramarital relations, poly-gamy, frequent divorces, or the exchange of partners may all contribute to spread of the virus – as may widespread recourse to prostitution, especially in tropical countries. Family patterns involving frequent adoption of children, their movement between households, and the movement of women in marriage between villages may also provide channels for the spread of infection. In contrast, marital patterns that forbid marriage between different communities, or segments of a community, may confine the infection to certain geographical or ethnic pockets; for example, Chinese immigrants in the UK and the USA, and Fijian Indians, all have low levels of HBsAG, characteristic of their homelands. Finally, social changes such as war, migrations, and social upheaval may break down barriers which contained the virus in a local environment, and spread it further afield. Because the prevalence of hepatitis B e antigen, which correlates with the rate of vertical transmission of the virus, declines with age, most vertical transmission occurs when women bear children at a younger age. Cultural changes which produce a later age of marriage and of childbearing will therefore reduce this transmission, and the spread of infection. The authors conclude that, especially in the case of hepatitis B, 'interpretation of epidemiologic data in non-Western societies demands a cultural perspective if modes of transmission are to be correctly defined and intervention planned'.

Case history: Coronary heart disease among Japanese in Japan, Hawaii and California

In a number of studies, Marmot and his colleagues[8,9] have examined the epidemiology of coronary heart disease, hypertension and stroke among 11 900 men of Japanese ancestry living in California, Hawaii and in Japan itself. The aim was to identify the influence of *non*-genetic factors on these three groups, by comparing disease rates of the two migrant groups and those of Japanese who had not emigrated. They found that there is a gradient in the occurrence of coronary heart disease between the three groups, with the lowest rate in Japan, intermediate in Hawaii, and highest in California. The influence of other risk factors commonly associated with high CHD rates, such as hypertension, diet, smoking, weight, blood sugar and serum cholesterol levels, were examined. It was found that the gradient in the incidence of CHD could *not* be explained only by the presence of these risk factors (for example, those who smoked similar amounts in the three groups still showed a gradient in the incidence of CHD). However, the incidence of CHD *was* found to be related to the degree of their adherence to the traditional Japanese culture they were all brought up in. The closer their adherence to these traditional values, the lower was their incidence of CHD. Within California, those Japanese Americans who had become most 'westernized' in outlook had higher rates than those immigrants who followed their more traditional lifestyle. Marmot and Syme[9] point out that 'these results support the hypothesis that the culture in which an individual is raised affects his likelihood of manifesting coronary heart disease in adult life', and that this relationship of culture of upbringing to CHD 'appears to be independent of the established coronary risk factors'. In the case of the Japanese, the cultural emphasis is on group cohesion, group achievement and social stability. In this cultural group, as in other traditional societies, it is suggested that 'a stable society whose members enjoy the support of their fellows in closely knit groups may protect against the forms of social stress that may lead to CHD'.

Case history: Parasitic diseases

Alland[21] has examined the relationships between certain cultural practices and the incidence, distribution and spread of parasitic diseases. Many of his findings apply also to infectious diseases. He notes how the arrangement of living space, the type and arrangement of houses, and the numbers of people per room or house, may all influence the spread or containment of disease. The social isolation of certain subgroups – such as a rigid caste system – may affect the spread of epidemics into certain communities. Population movements, such as a nomadic lifestyle, also help to spread parasitic and other infections, sometimes through the wider distribution of their human wastes. Certain cultural practices which separate man from the extra-human environment of some parasitic organisms also help to reduce infections. For example, the practice of digging deep latrines (as opposed to discharging waste products into rivers or streams) offers protection against those parasitic infections that are spread by urine or faeces. Contamination of water supplies is also prevented by its location far from domestic animals or human habitations, and by the separation of drinking sources from water used for bathing or laundering. Other cultural practices, such as frequent spitting, may increase the spread of viral and other infections through the community. Patterns of visiting the sick, or attending large public rites or festivals, may also be related to the spread of epidemics. Certain agricultural techniques, such as the cultivation of rice paddies, may increase the danger of schistosomiasis and other parasitic infestations. Certain forms of dress, such as tailored clothing, apparently provide a better environment for lice or fleas to live in than do loose togas, while the sharing of clothing within a family may also spread these infections. These and other cultural practices may influence the distribution of a wide range of parasitic, bacterial, viral and fungal infections.

In addition to these conditions, there is a considerable body of research that links migration to an increased incidence of certain illnesses, both mental and physical. These studies, some of which are quoted in the previous chapter, indicate a higher incidence of mental illness, attempted suicide and hypertension among some immigrants, compared with the incidence of these conditions in their countries of origin. As with coronary heart disease among Japanese Americans, it appears that the cultural lifestyles of both immigrant and host communities, as well as the fit (or lack of fit) between the two, coupled with the economic situation of the country and its attitudes towards newcomers, may all contribute towards the increased incidence of these stress-related conditions.

Variations in medical treatment and diagnosis

Epidemiological techniques can also be used in the study of differences in the diagnostic and treatment behaviour of doctors from various countries. Some of the differences between British and American psychiatrists – in the frequency with which they diagnose schizophrenia and affective disorders – have already been described in Chapter 10. In the case of medical treatments, one can compare the rate of a particular treatment (such as tonsillectomy) in two countries, with the actual prevalence (in both countries) of the condition (in this case recurrent tonsillitis) for which the treatment is usually prescribed. If the rate of tonsillectomies is much higher in one country, in the absence of a proportionately higher rate of tonsillitis, one can infer that cultural influences on both doctor and patient are responsible for this. Obviously both economic and technological factors, as well as the supply of both medical manpower and hospital facilities, play a part in this phenomenon, and such a study is more valid if carried out between countries with similar levels of social and industrial development.

Case history: Comparison of surgical rates in the USA, Canada, and England and Wales

Vayda et al.[22] compared overall surgical rates in Canada, England and Wales, and the USA, between 1966 and 1976. In particular, they examined the *relationship* between:

1. Operative rates per 100 000 population in the three countries.
2. Selected resources (surgical manpower and hospital beds).
3. National priorities, as measured by percentage of gross national product (GNP) spent on health care.
4. Disease prevalence, as measured by mortalities for selected diseases for which surgery is one form of treatment.

The rates of ten common operations were computed in the three countries, and compared. These were: lens extraction, tonsil surgery, prostatectomy, excision of knee cartilage, inguinal herniorraphy, cholecystectomy, colectomy, gastrectomy, hysterectomy, and Caesarian section. During the ten years studied, overall surgical rates in England and Wales were found to have remained constant, while Canadian rates were also relatively constant, but US rates increased by about 25%. Canadian rates, though, continued to be 60% higher than the British rates, and the US rates, which were 80% greater than those in England and Wales in 1966, were 125% greater than in England and Wales in 1976. Caesarian sections increased in all three countries from 53% to 126%. In 1976, about 12% of all Canadian and American births were delivered in this way, but only 7% were in England and Wales. Hysterectomy rates were twice as high in Canada and the USA than in the British sample. In comparing the availability of hospital beds, the British sample had the lowest number (and the lowest number of operations) of the three in 1976, and while Canada had 30% more hospital beds than the USA, overall US operative rates were 40% higher than Canada's rate. In the decade under study, England and Wales spent about 5% of their GNP on health care, while Canada spent about 7% and the USA about 9% The study could find no clear correlation between operative rates in the three countries and the availability of either hospital beds or medical manpower; nor were they related to differing mortality rates (as a measure of prevalence) of the selected diseases, between the countries. Instead, the differences were due to 'differing treatment styles and philosophies of patient management', the different value systems of these countries, the priority they assign to health care (as reflected in the percentage of GNP allocated to health care), and changes in technology (especially the increases in cardiac, vascular and thoracic surgery in the USA and Canada). The authors note that 'differing operative rates are more a reflection of consumer and provider prefer- ences; consequently, outcomes must be measured in terms of quality of life and postoperative morbidity rather than by mortality'. This is because most operations done are 'elective' or 'discretionary', and not done for any potentially fatal condition; this explains why the differences in operative rates were *not* related to differing mortalities from the selected conditions. The study demonstrated, therefore, that 'at least three industrialized Western countries have tolerated substantial differences in their frequencies of surgery without consistent unfavourable outcom- es'. To some extent, therefore, the cultural values of the surgeon, the patient, and the society in which they live play a part in determining the frequency with which surgery is used as a treatment for certain conditions.

Culture and ecology

Future research in both epidemiology and medical anthropology is likely to focus on the role of certain cultural factors which damage not only individual health, but also the health of the human species as a whole. This will involve adopting a more global perspective, including the cultures, economic systems, political organization and ecology of the planet as a whole. For example, the widespread use of chlorofluorocarbons (CFCs) in both refrigerators and aerosols has been found to be one of the causes of both the thinning of the ozone layer and global warming – the so-called 'greenhouse effect' – both of which can seriously damage human health. Although economic factors (such as the profits involved in producing, promoting and selling these products) play a major role, so do *culturally* influenced beliefs and behaviours. In the case of those aerosols containing CFCs which are used as deodorants, air cleaners, hair lacquers and furniture polish, for example, use of these preparations is also influenced by certain *cultural* values, especially in the Western industrialized world. These values stress the importance of living in an odour-free world – with an absence of both natural body odour and extraneous smells within the home. They promote certain hair styles and colours (particularly those hairstyles that suggest a youthful appearance) and emphasize shiny, reflecting surfaces on furniture within the home as a sign of both order and affluence.

As this small example indicates, therefore, there is often a connection – direct or indirect – between human cultural beliefs and behaviours, the ecology of the planet, and the health of its inhabitants. Other human practices which involve polluting the environment, deforestation, the use of nuclear power and weaponry, the extinction of many species of wildlife, and the emphasis on short-term profits and political power over the long-term interests of humanity all need to be considered by the medical anthropologist of the future – because human culture influences how those problems are produced, whether they are recognized, and whether or not they are dealt with.

Recommended reading

Brabin, L. and Brabin, B.J. (1985) Cultural factors and transmission of hepatitis B virus. *Am. J. Epidemiol.* **122,** 725–730

Marmot, M. (1981) Culture and illness: epidemiological evidence. In: Christie, M. J. and Mellett, P. G. (eds) *Foundations of Psychosomatics.* Chichester: Wiley, pp. 323–340

Marmot, M. G. and Syme, S. L. (1976) Acculturation and coronary heart disease in Japanese Americans. *Am. J. Epidemiol.* **104,** 225–247

Skegg, D. C. G., Corwin, P. A., Paul, C. and Doll, R. (1982) Importance of the male factor in cancer of the cervix. *Lancet* **ii,** 581–583

Appendix

Clinical questionnaires

In this section short questionnaires are included on the topic of each chapter of the book. These questionnaires can be used in two ways. Faced with a clinical situation where sociocultural factors might be relevant, the health professional can ask himself or herself these questions, as a way of increasing awareness of these factors, and acting accordingly. Each set of questions can provide the basis for a small research project on a particular topic, within the wider field of applied medical anthropology. In this latter case, it is suggested that the books and journals recommended at the end of each chapter be consulted for further theoretical background before the project is attempted.

Chapter 2: Cultural definitions of anatomy and physiology

1. What alterations in the shape, size, clothing and surface of the patient's body can be ascribed to their sociocultural background?
2. How does the patient conceptualize the inner structure (including the location of organs) of his/her body?
3. How does the patient conceptualize the inner workings of his/her body?
4. To what extent do 1, 2 and 3 affect:
   (a) the clinical presentation of the patient's condition,
   (b) the patient's attitude towards the origin, treatment and prognosis of his/her condition?
5. To what extent do 1, 2 and 3 affect the health of the patient?
6. To what extent do 1, 2 and 3 affect compliance with medical treatment or advice?
7. Is medical diagnosis, treatment or advice congruent with 1, 2 and 3?
8. In pregnancy/menstruation/lactation, to what extent do 1, 2 and 3 affect:

(a) the behaviour and diet of the woman,
(b) the health of the woman,
(c) the health of the fetus or infant?

Chapter 3: Diet and nutrition

1. Is the patient's diet nutritionally adequate (and is there evidence of malnutrition)?
2. If the diet is inadequate (or if malnutrition is present), are foodstuffs being excluded from the diet because they are not available?
3. Are foodstuffs being excluded from the diet because the patient cannot afford to buy them, even though they are available?
4. Are foodstuffs being excluded from the diet because they are classified as:

   (a) non-food,
   (b) profane food,
   (c) 'hot' (or 'cold') food,
   (d) medicine,
   (e) low social value food (not signalling correct status, caste, ethnicity, region, etc.)?

5. Are foodstuffs included in the diet because they are classified as:

   (a) food,
   (b) sacred food,
   (c) 'hot' (or 'cold') food,
   (d) medicine,
   (e) high social value food?

6. What forms of eating are defined as 'meals' and 'snacks'?
7. In 'meals', what social function does the content, order, preparation and timing of the meal perform for those who take part in it? What does it signal to them, and to others, about the types of relationships between those who take part in it?
8. In pregnancy/menstruation/lactation, is the woman's diet nutritionally adequate?
9. If not, is this because of 2, 3, 4 or 5, or combinations of these?
10. In infant feeding, how do sociocultural factors affect:

    (a) the choice of breast or artificial feeding,

(b) the length of breast or artificial feeding,
(c) the techniques of weaning, and types of weaning foods used,
(d) maternal beliefs about the optimal size, shape and weight of their infants?

11. In infant feeding, how do economic factors affect:

(a) the choice of breast or artificial feeding,
(b) the length of breast or artificial feeding,
(c) the techniques of weaning and types of weaning food used?

Chapter 4: Caring and curing: the sectors of health care

1. What sectors of health care can be identified in your society?
2. Within these sectors, who are the patients and who are the healers? How does one become a patient or a healer? How can the health care provided by each sector be compared as far as:

(a) availability of healers,
(b) cost of consultations,
(c) formality or informality of consultations,
(d) length of consultations
(e) types of data considered relevant to the consultation,
(f) whether the consultation is private or public,
(g) how diagnosis and treatment are carried out,
(h) who attends the consultation,
(i) effectiveness (or dangers) in treating 'disease',
(j) effectiveness (or dangers) in treating 'illness'?

3. What sources of advice has the patient sought before consulting a health professional?
4. If non-professional advice was sought:

(a) Why were they consulted?
(b) What do they provide that professional advice cannot (the perceived benefits of the advice)?
(c) Was the advice effective or dangerous to health?

5. If advice from health professionals was sought:

(a) Why were they consulted?
(b) What do they provide that non-professionals cannot (the perceived benefits of the advice)?
(c) Was the advice effective or dangerous to health?

Chapter 5: Doctor–patient interactions

1. In what ways are the health professional's perception, diagnosis and treatment of ill-health influenced by his/her:

   (a) Individual attributes (age, gender, personality, experience, prejudices),
   (b) education or subculture (ethnic, religious or professional),
   (c) cultural background,
   (d) socioeconomic status?

2. Can the aetiology (or presentation) of the patient's ill-health be related to his/her:

   (a) individual attributes (age, gender, personality, experience, prejudices),
   (b) education or subculture (ethnic, religious or professional),
   (c) cultural background,
   (d) socioeconomic status?

3. How does the patient view the meaning and significance of his/her ill-health?

4. What explanatory model does he/she use? What are his or her answers to the following questions:

   (a) What has happened (labelling the condition)?
   (b) Why has it happened (aetiology)?
   (c) Why to me (relation to diet, behaviour, personality, heredity)?
   (d) Why now (timing, mode of onset)?
   (e) What would happen to me if nothing was done about it (its likely course, outcome, prognosis and dangers)?
   (f) What are its likely effects on other people (family, friends, neighbours, employers, etc.)?
   (g) What should I do about it – or to whom should I turn for further help (self-treatment, consultations with lay advisers, folk healers or health professionals)?

5. Does the patient believe that he/she is suffering from a folk illness?

6. How do the patient's family and friends view his/her ill-health? What explanatory models do they use?

In the consultation:

7. Does the patient have 'illness' as well as 'disease'?

8. Does the patient have 'illness', but no 'disease'?
9. Does the patient have 'disease', but no 'illness'?
10. Is the patient's 'illness' being treated, as well as his/her 'disease'?
11. Is the diagnosis/treatment/prognosis given to the patient congruent with his/her explanatory model? Is consensus between health professional and patient achieved regarding the diagnosis/treatment/prognosis of the patient's ill-health?

After the consultation:

12. Is there compliance with the health professional's advice or treatment? If not, why not?
13. Is there satisfaction with the health professional's advice or treatment? If not, why not?
14. What is the *impact* of the medical diagnoses/medical tests/medical treatments on the individual patient's:

   (a) physical state,
   (b) psychological state,
   (c) behaviour,
   (d) social relationships,
   (e) employment,
   (f) economic status?

Chapter 6: Gender and reproduction

1. What elements define the patient's gender as either 'male' or 'female'? Their:

   (a) genetic gender,
   (b) somatic gender,
   (c) psychological gender,
   (d) social gender?

2. How does the patient's own gender culture define his/her appropriate:

   (a) behaviour,
   (b) emotions,
   (c) dress,
   (d) occupation,
   (e) leisure activities,
   (f) use of alcohol, tobacco and drugs?

3. What aspects of the patient's gender culture can be considered either pathogenic or protective of health?

4. Can the origin, presentation or prognosis of the patient's ill-health be related to their gender culture?
5. What is the relation of the patient's gender to his/her sexual behaviour?
6. To what extent is the patient's sexual behaviour tolerated, or tabooed, by his/her own cultural group?
7. In the patient's own cultural group, is gender defined more by biological criteria (genetic and somatic gender) or by sexual behaviour?
8. What aspects of the patient's life can be considered to be medicalized?

   (a) menstruation,
   (b) childbirth,
   (c) menopause,
   (d) social problems,
   (e) economic problems?

9. How does the patient's birth culture define the nature, and requirements of:

   (a) conception,
   (b) pregnancy,
   (c) childbirth,
   (d) puerperium?

10. What rituals, and ritual symbols are a feature of the birth cultures of:

   (a) the patient,
   (b) the health professional?

11. What are the advantages and disadvantages for the patient of delivery by:

   (a) an obstetrician?
   (b) a traditional birth attendant?

12. Are there physical or psychological symptoms suggestive of the couvade syndrome?
13. Are certain beliefs and behaviour prescribed as part of the ritual couvade?

Chapter 7: Pain and culture

1. What is the recognized pattern of pain behaviour (language of distress) in the sociocultural milieu of:

(a) the health professional,
(b) the patient?

2. Is the patient suffering private pain, but not translating it into public pain? If not, why not?
3. Is the patient displaying public pain? If so:

(a) Does he/she also have private pain?
(b) What does he/she intend to signal or achieve by the use of pain behaviour?

4. In the patient's sociocultural background, is pain behaviour accepted/encouraged/responded to or not?
5. In the clinical setting, is pain behaviour accepted/encouraged/responded to or not?
6. How does the patient view the origin, significance and prognosis of the pain?
7. How do the patient's family and friends view the origin, significance and prognosis of the pain?
8. Is treatment with analgesics sufficient or should the illness associated with the pain be treated as well?

Chapter 8: Culture and pharmacology

1. What factors are contributing towards the total drug effect? The attributes of:

(a) the drug itself,
(b) the patient,
(c) the prescriber,
(d) the setting?

2. To what extent is there a placebo element in:

(a) drug treatment,
(b) surgical or other treatment,
(c) hospital tests,
(d) the relationship with the health professional?

Psychological dependence:

3. What symbolic role does the drug or other treatment play in the patient's:

(a) daily activities,
(b) self-image,
(c) social relationships,
(d) relationships with health professionals?

4. Does the patient feel he/she has control over the drug treatment (its dosage, time of ingestion, effects on self or others) or not?
5. Is the drug taken for its effect on:

   (a) the patient himself/herself,
   (b) relationships with other people?

Physical addiction:

6. Does the patient belong to an addict subculture?
7. If so, what are its values and standards of behaviour?
8. How does he/she view:

   (a) other addicts,
   (b) non-addicts?

9. If there is evidence of stereotyping in 8, how does this affect treatment of his/her addiction?
10. In intravenous drug abuse, do the addicts practise needle sharing among themselves?

Alcoholism:

11. In the patient's sociocultural milieu, what values govern:

   (a) normal drinking,
   (b) abnormal drinking?

12. In normal drinking, what are the rules about:

   (a) who is allowed to drink (age, sex, ethnicity, class),
   (b) in whose company drinking is allowed to take place,
   (c) what can be drunk,
   (d) at what times drinking can take place,
   (e) in what settings drinking can take place,
   (f) the relation of drinking to religious and social festivals?

13. What does the alcohol symbolize to the drinker? What symbolic role does it play in his/her:

   (a) daily activities,
   (b) self-image,
   (c) social relationships,
   (d) relationships with health professionals?

14. What symbolic role does cigarette smoking play in the patient's:

   (a) daily activities,

(b) self-image,
(c) social relationships?

Chapter 9: Ritual and the management of misfortune

1. What rituals (social, religious, personal) exist in the patient's daily life? Do rituals play a central, pervasive role in his/her life, and do they deal adequately with misfortune, illness and death?

In the consultation:

2. What aspects of the health professional's behaviour, speech, dress and techniques have a ritual aspect?
3. What ritual symbols are used?
4. What associations do these ritual symbols have for:

   (a) the patient,
   (b) his/her family or friends,
   (c) the health professional?

5. Does the ritual, or its absence, positively affect the patient's mental or physical health, or his/her social relationships?
6. Does the ritual serve to integrate the patient back into his/her community, or to alienate him/her from it?
7. Does the ritual signal a biological and/or social transition in the patient's life?
8. What is the effect of the ritual, or its absence, on the psychological state of the health professional?

In hospital:

9. What aspects of the patient's admission procedure, dress, behaviour, diet, medication and control over time and space have a ritual significance for the patient and for the professional staff?
10. To what extent do these rituals accelerate, or impede, the patient's return to health?

In major life changes (pregnancy, birth, bereavement):

11. What rituals are used to symbolize the patient's biological and social transition in:

    (a) his/her sociocultural background,
    (b) the clinical setting?

12. Is this ritual – or its absence – advantageous (or dangerous)

to the patient's mental or physical health, or social relationships?

13. Should more ritual be used to place the transition in a wider social, moral or religious context?

Chapter 10: Cross-cultural psychiatry

1. In psychiatric diagnosis, what influences on the *diagnostician* may affect the validity of psychiatric diagnoses:
   (a) cultural factors,
   (b) social factors,
   (c) moral attitudes,
   (d) political pressures?

In cross-cultural diagnosis:

2. In the patient's sociocultural background, what are the definitions of normal and abnormal social behaviour?
3. Are the patient's beliefs and/or behaviour abnormal by the standards of his own community? If they are, is it controlled or uncontrolled abnormality?
4. Do the patient's family and/or friends regard this abnormality as beneficial or dangerous to them (or to the wider community)?
5. Are the specific clusters of symptoms and signs interpreted by the patient (or by family or friends) as evidence of a culture-bound psychological disorder?
6. Is the clinical presentation of the disorder shaped by cultural factors into a culture-bound disorder (such as *susto* or somatization)?
7. What role do cultural factors play in the aetiology of the disorder?

In cross-cultural treatment:

8. Is the illness of the disorder being treated, as well as the disease?
9. Should the patient's family and/or friends be asked to take part in the treatment process?
10. Should a folk healer, priest or exorcist be used by the patient (and/or his family) as a complementary form of treatment?
11. What could such healers provide that Western psychiatrists could not?

In family therapy:

12. Are the family dynamics evidence of:

    (a) cultural costume,
    (b) cultural camouflage?

13. In what ways are the structure and dynamics of the family the result of:

    (a) psychopathology,
    (b) cultural background,
    (c) economic status,
    (d) external social pressures?

Chapter 11: Cultural aspects of stress

1. Has the patient experienced any major life changes in the past year?
2. Is there any evidence of the giving-up-given-up complex?
3. What cultural factors could have contributed to the patient's stress response?
4. What cultural factors would protect the patient against developing the stress response?

In migrant communities:

5. What sources of stress for the migrant can be identified in:

    (a) the host community,
    (b) the migrant community,
    (c) the changes in life space involved in migration?

6. Is there evidence of cultural bereavement in the migrant, or his/her community?
7. What is meant by the term 'stress', when used by:

    (a) the patient,
    (b) their family and friends,
    (c) the health professional?

Chapter 12: Cultural factors in epidemiology

1. To what extent does the perceived incidence of the disease depend on:

    (a) its actual incidence,

(b) its recognition by the population as abnormal,
(c) its recognition by the researcher as abnormal?

2. What role do cultural factors play in 1(a), (b) and (c)?
3. What cultural factors can be linked to the occurrence and/or distribution of the disease in a causal way?
4. What cultural factors can be linked to the spread of the disease within the population?
5. What cultural factors may protect some members of the population from the disease?
6. What damage to the environment can be related to cultural beliefs and behaviour of:

(a) the patient,
(b) the health professional?

References

Chapter 1

1. Editorial (1980) More anthropology and less sleep for medical students. *Br. Med. J.* **281**, 1662
2. Keesing, R. M. (1981) *Cultural Anthropology: A Contemporary Perspective*. New York: Holt, Rinehart and Winston, p. 518
3. Tylor, E. B. (1871) *Primitive Culture: Research into the Development of Mythology, Philosophy, Religion, Art and Customs*. London: John Murray
4. Keesing, R. M. (1981) *op. cit.* p. 68
5. Kaufman, S. R. (1986) *The Ageless Self*. New York: Meridian
6. Leach, E. (1982) *Social Anthropology*. Glasgow: Fontana, pp. 41–43
7. Townsend, P. and Davidson, N. (eds) (1982) *Inequalities in Health: The Black Report*. Harmondsworth: Penguin
8. Zaidi, S. A. (1988) Poverty and disease: need for structural change. *Soc. Sci. Med.* **27**, 119–127
9. Lopez, S. and Hernandez, P. (1986) How culture is considered in evaluations of psychopathology. *J. Nerv. Ment. Dis.* **176**, 598–606
10. Foster, G. M. and Anderson, B. G. (1978) *Medical Anthropology*. New York: Wiley, pp. 2–3
11. Agency for International Development (1983) *Proceedings of the International Conference on Oral Rehydration Therapy (ICORT)*, 7–10 June 1983. Washington: Agency for International Development
12. Weiss, M. G. (1988) Cultural models of diarrhoeal illness: conceptual framework and review. *Soc. Sci. Med.* **27**, 5–16
13. Mull, J. D. and Mull, D. S. (1988) Mothers' concept of childhood diarrhoea in rural Pakistan: what ORT program planners should know. *Soc. Sci. Med.* **27**, 53–67

Chapter 2

1. Fisher, S. (1968) Body image. In: Sills, D. (ed.) *International Encyclopaedia of the Social Sciences*. New York: Free Press/Macmillan, pp. 113–116
2. Polhemus, T. (1978) Body alteration and adornment: a pictorial essay. In: Polhemus, T. (ed.) *Social Aspects of the Human Body*. Harmondsworth: Penguin, pp. 154–173
3. Jeffcoate, T. N. A. (1962) *Principles of Gynaecology*, 2nd ed. London: Butterworths, pp. 279–280
4. Jeffcoate, T. N. A. (1962) *op. cit.*, pp. 447–448
5. Garner, D. M. and Garfinkel, P. E. (1980) Socio-cultural factors in the development of anorexia nervosa. *Psychol. Med.* **10**, 647–656
6. Swartz, L. (1985) Anorexia nervosa as a culture-bound syndrome. *Soc. Sci. Med.* **20**, 725–730

7. Orbach, S. (1986) *Hunger Strike: The Anorectic's Struggle as a Metaphor for our Age.* New York: W.W. Norton
8. Polhemus, T. (1978) Introduction. In: Polhemus, T. (ed.) *Social Aspects of the Human Body.* Harmondsworth: Penguin, pp. 23–25
9. Ritenbaugh, C. (1982) Obesity as a culture-bound syndrome. *Cult. Med. Psychiatry* **6**, 347–361
10. Helman, C. G. (1978) 'Feed a cold, starve a fever': folk models of infection in an English suburban community, and their relation to medical treatment. *Cult. Med. Psychiatry* **2**, 107–137
11. Douglas, M. (1973) *Natural Symbols.* Harmondsworth: Penguin, pp. 93–112
12. Scheper-Hughes, N. and Lock, M. M. (1987) The mindful body: a prolegomenon to future work in medical anthropology. *Med. Anthropol. Q.* (New Series) **1**, 6–41
13. Boyle, C. M. (1970) Difference between patients' and doctors' interpretation of some common medical terms. *Br. Med. J.* **ii**, 286–289
14. Pearson, J. and Dudley, H. A. F. (1982) Bodily perceptions in surgical patients. *Br. Med. J.* **284**, 1545–1546
15. Tait, C. D. and Ascher, R. C. (1955) Inside-of-the-body test. *Psychosom. Med.* **17**, 139–148
16. Cassell, E. J. (1976) Disease as an 'It': concepts of disease revealed by patients' presentation of symptoms. *Soc. Sci. Med.* **10**, 143–146
17. Helman, C. G. (1985) Psyche, soma, and society: the social construction of psychosomatic disorders. *Cult. Med. Psychiatry* **9**, 1–26
18. Waddell, G., McCulloch, J. A., Kummel, E. and Venner, R. M. (1980) Nonorganic physical signs in low-back pain. *Spine* **5**, 117–125
19. Walters, A. (1961) Psychogenic regional pain alias hysterical pain. *Brain* **84**, 1–18
20. Kleinman, A., Eisenberg, L. and Good, B. (1978) Clinical lessons from anthropologic and cross-cultural research. *Ann. Int. Med.* **88**, 251–258
21. Colson, A. B. and de Armellado, C. (1983) An Amerindian derivation for Latin American Creole illnesses and their treatment. *Soc. Sci. Med.* **17**, 1229–1248
22. Foster, G. M. (1987) On the origin of humoral medicine in Latin America. *Med. Anthropol. Q.* (New Series) **1**, 355–393
23. Logan, M. H. (1975) Selected references on the hot–cold theory of disease. *Med. Anthropol. Newsletter* **6**, 8–14
24. Snow, L. F. and Johnson, S. M. (1978) Folklore, food, female reproductive cycle. *Ecol. Food Nutr.* **7**, 41–49
25. Greenwood, B. (1981) Cold or spirits? Choice and ambiguity in Morocco's pluralistic medical system. *Soc. Sci. Med.* **15B**, 219–235
26. Obeyesekere, G. (1977) The theory and practice of Ayurvedic medicine. *Cult. Med. Psychiatry* **1**, 155–181
27. Macdonald, A. (1984) *Acupuncture.* London: Allen and Unwin
28. Jeffreys, M., Brotherston, J. H. F. and Cartwright, A. (1960) Consumption of medicines on a working-class housing estate. *Br. J. Prev. Soc. Med.* **14**, 64–76
29. Helman, C. G. (1988) Dr Frankenstein and the industrial body: reflections on 'spare-part' surgery. *Anthropology Today* **4**, 14–16
30. Turkle, S. (1984) *The Second Self: Computers and the Human Spirit.* London: Granada, pp. 281–318
31. Homans, H. (1982) Pregnancy and birth as rites of passage for two groups of women in Britain. In: MacCormack, C.P. (ed.) *Ethnography of Fertility and Birth.* London: Academic Press, pp. 231–268
32. Snow L. F., Johnson, S. M. and Mayhew, H. E. (1978) The behavioral implications of some Old Wives Tales. *Obstet. Gynecol.* **51**, 727–732

33. Snow, L. F. and Johnson, S. M. (1977) Modern day menstrual folklore. *JAMA* **237**, 2736–2739
34. Turner, V. W. (1974) *The Ritual Process*. Harmondsworth: Penguin, pp. 48–49
35. Skultans, V. (1970) The symbolic significance of menstruation and the menopause. *MAN* **5**, 639–651
36. Ngubane, H. (1977) *Body and Mind in Zulu Medicine*. London: Academic Press, pp. 79, 164
37. Delaney, J., Lupton, M. J. and Toth, E. (1976) *The Curse: A Cultural History of Menstruation*. New York: Dutton
38. Snow, L. F. (1976) 'High blood' is not high blood pressure. *Urban Health* **5**, 5–55
39. Like, R. and Ellison, J. (1981) Sleeping blood, tremor and paralysis: a transcultural approach to an unusual conversion reaction. *Cult. Med. Psychiatry* **5**, 49–63
40. Foster, G. M. and Anderson, B. G. (1978) *Medical Anthropology*. New York: Wiley, p. 227

Chapter 3

1. Lévi-Strauss, C. (1970) *The Raw and the Cooked*. London: Jonathan Cape, pp. 142, 164
2. Ember, C. R. and Ember, M. (1985) *Cultural Anthropology*. Englewood Cliffs, NJ: Prentice-Hall, pp. 138–147
3. Jelliffe, D. B. (1967) Parallel food classifications in developing and industrialized countries. *Am. J. Clin. Nutr.* **20**, 279–281
4. Foster, G. M. and Anderson, B. G. (1978) *Medical Anthropology*. New York: Wiley, pp. 263–279
5. Hunt, S. (1976) The food habits of Asian immigrants. In: *Getting the Most out of Food*. Burgess Hill: Van den Berghs & Jurgens, pp. 15–51
6. Littlewood, R. and Lipsedge, M. (1982) *Aliens and Alienists*. Harmondsworth: Penguin, pp. 28–30
7. Twigg, J. (1979) Food for thought: purity and vegetarianism. *Religion* **9**, 13–35
8. Greenwood, B. (1981) Cold or spirits? Choice and ambiguity in Morocco's pluralistic medical system. *Soc. Sci. Med.* **15B**, 219–235
9. Harwood, A. (1971) The hot–cold theory of disease: implications for treatment of Puerto Rican patients. *JAMA* **216**, 1153–1158
10. Tann, S. P. and Wheeler, E. F. (1980) Food intakes and growth of young Chinese children in London. *Community Med.* **2**, 20–24
11. Snow, L. F. and Johnson, S. M. (1978) Folklore, food, female reproductive cycle. *Ecol. Food Nutr.* **7**, 41–49
12. Etkin, N. L. and Ross, P. J. (1982) Food as medicine and medicine as food: an adaptive framework for the interpretation of plant utilization among the Hausa of Northern Nigeria. *Soc. Sci. Med.* **16**, 1559–1573
13. Farb, P. and Armelagos, G. (1980) *Consuming Passions: The Anthropology of Eating*. Boston: Houghton Mifflin, p. 103
14. Belshaw, C. S. (1965) *Traditional Exchange and Modern Markets*. Englewood Cliffs, NJ: Prentice-Hall, pp. 12–20
15. Trowell, H. C. and Burkitt, D. P. (eds) (1981) *Western Diseases: Their Emergence and Prevention*. London: Edward Arnold

16. Jerome, N. W. (1969) Northern urbanization and food consumption patterns of southern-born Negroes. *Am. J. Clin. Nutr.* **22**, 1667–1669
17. Douglas, M. and Nicod, M. (1974) Taking the biscuit: the structure of British meals. *New Society* **30**, 744–747
18. Farb, P. and Armelagos, G. (1980) *op. cit.* p. 98
19. Charsley, S. (1987) Interpretation and custom: the case of the wedding cake. *MAN* **22**, 93–110
20. Keesing, R. M. (1981) *Cultural Anthropology*. New York: Holt, Rinehart and Winston, pp. 459–462
21. Artley, A. (1987) Out of sight, out of mind. *Spectator* **258**, 8–10
22. Stroud, C. E. (1971) Nutrition and the immigrant. *Br. J. Hosp. Med.* **5**, 629–634
23. Ward, P. S., Drakeford, J. P., Milton, J. and James, J. A. (1982) Nutritional rickets in Rastafarian children. *Br. Med. J.* **285**, 1242–1243
24. Editorial (1981) Asian rickets in Britain. *Lancet* **ii**, 402
25. Lennon, D. and Fieldhouse, P. (1979) *Community Dietetics*. London: Forbes, pp. 78–91
26. Mares, P., Henley, A. and Baxter, C. (1985) *Health Care in Multiracial Britain*. Cambridge: Health Education Council/National Extension College, p. 49
27. Farb, P. and Armelagos, G. (1980) *op. cit.* p. 78
28. Foster, G.M. and Anderson, B.G. (1978) *Medical Anthropology*. New York: Wiley, pp. 277–278
29. Goel, K. M., House, F. and Shanks, R. A. (1978) Infant-feeding practices among immigrants in Glasgow. *Br. Med. J.* **ii**, 1181–1183
30. Jones, R. A. K. and Belsey, E. M. (1977) Breast feeding in an Inner London borough: a study of cultural factors. *Soc. Sci. Med.* **11**, 175–179
31. Taitz, L. S. (1971) Infantile overnutrition among artificially fed infants in the Sheffield region. *Br. Med. J.* **i**, 315–316
32. Burkitt, D. P. (1973) Some diseases characteristic of modern Western civilization. *Br. Med. J.* **i**, 274–278
33. Lowenfels, A. B. and Anderson, M. E. (1977) Diet and cancer. *Cancer* **39**, 1809–1814
34. Newberne, P. M. (1978) Diet and nutrition. *Bull. N. Y. Acad. Med.* **54**, 385–396
35. Kolonel, L. N., Nomura, A. M. Y., Hirohata, T., Hankin, J. H. and Hinds, M. W. (1981) Association of diet and place of birth with stomach cancer incidence in Hawaii Japanese and Caucasians. *Am. J. Clin. Nutr.* **34**, 2478–2485

Chapter 4

1. Landy, D. (1977) Medical systems in transcultural perspective. In: Landy, D. (ed.) *Culture, Disease, and Healing: Studies in Medical Anthropology*. New York: Macmillan, pp. 129–132
2. Kleinman, A. (1980) *Patients and Healers in the Context of Culture*. Berkeley: University of California Press, pp. 49–70
3. Chrisman, N. J. (1977) The health seeking process: an approach to the natural history of illness. *Cult. Med. Psychiatry* **1**, 351–377
4. Kleinman, A., Eisenberg, L. and Good, B. (1978) Culture, illness, and care: clinical lessons from anthropologic and cross-cultural research. *Ann. Intern. Med.* **88**, 251–258
5. McGuire, M. B. (1988) *Ritual Healing in Suburban America*. New Brunswick: Rutgers University Press

6. Turner, V. W. (1974) *The Ritual Process*. Harmondsworth: Penguin, p. 14
7. Lewis, I. M. (1971) *Ecstatic Religion*. Harmondsworth: Penguin
8. Kleinman, A. (1980) *op. cit.* p. 200
9. Snow, L. F. (1978) Sorcerers, saints and charlatans: black healers in urban America. *Cult. Med. Psychiatry* **2**, 69–106
10. Ngubane, H. (1981) Aspects of clinical practice and traditional organization of indigenous healers in South Africa. *Soc. Sci. Med.* **15B**, 361–365
11. Underwood, P. and Underwood, Z. (1981) New spells for old: expectations and realities of Western medicine in a remote tribal society in Yemen, Arabia. In: Stanley, N. F. and Joshe, R. A. (eds), *Changing Disease Patterns and Human Behaviour*. London: Academic Press, pp. 271–297
12. Kimani, V. N. (1981) The unsystematic alternative: towards plural health care among the Kikuyu of central Kenya. *Soc. Sci. Med.* **15B**, 333–340
13. Lewis, I. M. (1971) *op. cit.*, pp. 49–57
14. Martin, M. (1981) Native American healers: thoughts for posttraditional healers. *JAMA* **245**, 141–143
15. Fabrega, H. and Silver, D. B. (1973) *Illness and Shamanistic Curing in Zinacantan*. Stanford: Stanford University Press, pp. 218–223
16. World Health Organisation (1978) *The Promotion and Development of Traditional Medicine*. WHO Tech. Rep. Ser. 622
17. World Health Organisation (1980) Health personnel and hospital establishments. *World Health Stat. Ann.*
18. Stacey, M. (1988) *The Sociology of Health and Healing*. London: Unwin Hyman, p. 258
19. Stacey, M. (1988) *op. cit.*, pp. 177–193
20. Littlewood, R. and Lipsedge, M. (1982) *Aliens and Alienists*. Harmondsworth: Penguin
21. Wing, J. K. (1978) *Reasoning about Madness*. Oxford: Oxford University Press
22. Illich, I. (1976) *Limits to Medicine*. London: Marion Boyars
23. Stacey, M. (1988) *op. cit.* pp. 229–260
24. Crawford, R. (1977) You are dangerous to your health: the ideology and politics of victim blaming. *Int. J. Health Serv.* **7**, 663–680
25. O'Brien, B. (1984) *Patterns of European Diagnoses and Prescribing*. London: Office of Health Economics
26. Maretzki, T. W. (1989) Cultural variations in biomedicine: the *kur* in West Germany. *Med. Anthropol. Q.* (New Series) **3**, 22–35
27. Payer, L. (1988) *Medicine and Culture*. New York: Henry Holt
28. Foster, G. M. and Anderson, B. G. (1978) *Medical Anthropology*. New York: Wiley, pp. 175–186
29. Pfifferling, J. H. (1980) A cultural prescription for medicocentrism. In: Eisenberg, L. and Kleinman, A. (eds) *Relevance of Social Science for Medicine*. Dordrecht: Reidel, pp. 197–222
30. Goffman, E. (1961) *Asylums*. Harmondsworth: Penguin
31. Scott, C. S. (1974) Health and healing practices among five ethnic groups in Miami, Florida. *Public Health Rep.* **89**, 524–532
32. Stimson, G. V. (1974) Obeying doctor's orders: a view from the other side. *Soc. Sci. Med.* **8**, 97–104
33. Stacey, M. (ed.) (1976) *The Sociology of the National Health Service*. London: Croom Helm
34. Levitt, R. (1976) *The Reorganised National Health Service*. London: Croom Helm
35. Elliott-Binns, C. P. (1973) An analysis of lay medicine. *J. R. Coll. Gen. Pract.* **23**, 255–264

36. Elliott-Binns, C. P. (1986) An analysis of lay medicine: fifteen years later. *J. R. Coll. Gen. Pract.* **36**, 542–544
37. Dunnell, K. and Cartwright, A. (1972) *Medicine Takers, Prescribers and Hoarders.* London: Routledge and Kegan Paul
38. Sharpe, D. (1979) The pattern of over-the-counter 'prescribing'. *MIMS Magazine,* 15 September, 39–45
39. Jefferys, M., Brotherston, J. H. F. and Cartwright, A. (1960) Consumption of medicines on a working-class housing estate. *Br. J. Prev. Soc. Med.* **14**, 64–76
40. Hindmarch, I. (1981) Too many pills in the cupboard. *New Society* **55**, 142–143
41. Warburton, D. M. (1978) Poisoned people: internal pollution. *J. Biosoc. Sci.* **10**, 309–319
42. Blaxter, M. and Paterson, E. (1980) *Attitudes to Health and Use of Health Services in Two Generations of Women in Social Classes 4 and 5.* Report to DHSS/SSRC Joint Working Party on Transmitted Deprivation. Unpublished
43. Pattison, C. J., Drinkwater, C. K. and Downham, M. A. P. S. (1982) Mothers' appreciation of their children's symptoms. *J. R. Coll. Gen. Pract.* **32**, 149–162
44. *Pulse* (1982) Self-help groups for your patients. *Pulse* 29 May, 51–52
45. Levy, L. (1982) Mutual support groups in Great Britain. *Soc. Sci. Med.* **16**, 1265–1275
46. *Self-help.* Undated booklet. Hayes: Leo Laboratories, p. 25
47. Robinson, D. and Henry, S. (1977) *Self-help and Health: Mutual Aid for Modern Problems.* London: Martin Robertson
48. Fulder, S. (1988) *Handbook of Complementary Medicine.* London: Oxford University Press
49. National Institute of Medical Herbalists. Undated *Information Leaflet.* Newcastle-upon-Tyne: NIMH
50. Community Health Foundation. Undated pamphlet. *Your Guide to Healthy Living.* London: Community Health Foundation
51. Hyde, F. F. (1978) The origin and practice of herbal medicine. *MIMS Magazine,* 1 February, 127–136
52. National Federation of Spiritual Healers. Undated pamphlet. *About the National Federation of Spiritual Healers.* Sunbury-on-Thames: NFSH
53. Tod, J. (ed.) (1982) *Someone to Talk to: A Directory of Self-help and Support Services in the Community.* London: Mental Health Foundation, p. 57
54. de Jonge, P. (1981) Magical world of Wicca in a Sheffield semi. *Doctor,* 2 July, 30
55. Royal London Homeopathic Hospital (1978) *One Hundred and Nineteenth Annual Report.*
56. Advertisement (1981) *Horoscope* **29**, p. 36
57. CCAM Undated Pamphlet. *CCAM: Council for Complementary and Alternative Medicine.* London: CCAM
58. Research Council for Complementary Medicine (1988) *The First Five Years: 1983–1988.* London: RCCM
59. Davies, P. (1984) *Report on Trends in Complementary Medicine.* London: Institute for Complementary Medicine
60. What is the British Holistic Medical Association? (1989) *Holistic Health* No. 22, 36
61. Fulder, S. and Monro, R. (1981) *The Status of Complementary Medicine in the UK.* London: Threshold Foundation
62. Wadsworth, M. E. J., Butterfield, W. J. H. and Blaney, R. (1971) *Health and Sickness: the Choice of Treatment.* London: Tavistock
63. Office of Health Economics (1981) *OHE Compendium of Health Statistics, 1981,* 4th ed. London: OHE

64. Levitt, R. (1976) *op. cit.*, p. 179
65. Fry, J., Brooks, D. and McColl, I. (1984) *NHS Data Book*. Lancaster: MTP Press
66. Levitt, R. (1976) *op. cit.*, p. 99
67. Chaplin, N. W. (ed.) (1976) *The Hospital and Health Services Year Book*. London: The Institute of Health Service Administrators, pp. 374–377
68. White, A. E. (1978) The vital role of the cottage-community hospital. *J. R. Coll. Gen. Pract.* **28**, 485–491
69. Harris, C. M. (1980) *Lecture Notes on Medicine in General Practice*. Oxford: Blackwell, p. 27
70. Hunt, J. H. (1964) The renaissance of general practice. In: Farndale, J. (ed.) *Trends in the National Health Service*. London: Pergamon Press, pp. 161–181
71. Levitt, R. (1976) *op. cit.* p. 95
72. Morrell, D. C. (1971) Expressions of morbidity in general practice. *Br. Med. J.* **ii**, 454

Chapter 5

1. Gordon, D. R. (1988) Tenacious assumptions in Western medicine. In: Lock, M. and Gordon, D. R. (eds) *Biomedicine Examined*. Dordrecht: Kluwer, pp. 19–56
2. Eisenberg, L. (1977) Disease and illness: distinctions between professional and popular ideas of sickness. *Cult. Med. Psychiatry* **1**, 9–23
3. Kleinman, A., Eisenberg, L. and Good, B. (1978) Culture, illness and care: clinical lessons from anthropologic and cross-cultural research. *Ann. Int. Med.* **88**, 251–258
4. Good, B. J. and Good, M. D. (1981) The meaning of symptoms: a cultural hermeneutic model for clinical practice. In: Eisenberg, L. and Kleinman, A. (eds) *The Relevance of Social Science for Medicine*. Dordrecht: Reidel, pp. 165–196
5. Feinstein, A. R. (1975) Science, clinical medicine, and the spectrum of disease. In: Beeson, P. B. and McDermott, W. (eds) *Textbook of Medicine*. Philadelphia: Saunders, pp. 4–6
6. Fabrega, H. and Silver, D. B. (1973) *Illness and Shamanistic Curing in Zinacantan: An Ethnomedical Analysis*. Stanford: Stanford University Press, pp. 218–223
7. Engel, G. L. (1980) The clinical applications of the biopsychosocial model. *Am. J. Psychiatry* **137**, 535–544
8. Cassell, E. J. (1976) *The Healer's Art: A New Approach to the Doctor–Patient Relationship*. New York: Lippincott, pp. 47–83
9. Fox, R. C. (1968) Illness. In: Sills, D. (ed.) *International Enyclopaedia of the Social Sciences*. New York: Free Press/Macmillan, pp. 90–96
10. World Health Organisation (1946) *Constitution of the World Health Organisation*. Geneva: WHO
11. Blaxter, M. and Paterson, E. (1980) *Attitudes to Health and Use of Health Services in Two Generations of Women in Social Classes 4 and 5*. Report to DHSS/SSRC Joint Working Party on Transmitted Deprivation. Unpublished
12. Dunnell, K. and Cartwright, A. (1972) *Medicine Takers, Prescribers and Hoarders*. London: Routledge & Kegan Paul, p. 13
13. Apple, D. (1960) How laymen define illness. *J. Health Soc. Behav.* **1**, 219–225
14. Guttmacher, S. and Elinson, J. (1971) Ethno-religious variations in perceptions of illness. *Soc. Sci. Med.* **5**, 117–125
15. Lewis, G. (1981) Cultural influences on illness behaviour. In: Eisenberg, L.

and Kleinman, A. (eds) *The Relevance of Social Science for Medicine*. Dordrecht, Reidel, pp. 151–162

16. Kleinman, A. (1980) *Patients and Healers in the Context of Culture*. Berkeley: University of California Press, pp. 104–118
17. Helman, C. G. (1984) The role of context in primary care. *J. R. Coll. Gen. Pract.* **34**, 547–550
18. Helman, C. G. (1981) Disease *versus* illness in general practice. *J. R. Coll. Gen. Pract.* **31**, 548–552
19. Rubel, A. J. (1977) The epidemiology of a folk illness: Susto in Hispanic America. In: Landy, D. (ed.) *Culture, Disease, and Healing: Studies in Medical Anthropology*. New York: Macmillan, pp. 119–128
20. Good, B. (1977) The heart of what's the matter: the semantics of illness in Iran. *Cult. Med. Psychiatry* **1**, 25–58
21. Kleinman, A. (1980) *op. cit.*, pp. 149–158
22. Frankenberg, R. (1980) Medical anthropology and development: a theoretical perspective. *Soc. Sci. Med.* **14B**, 197–207
23. Sontag, S. (1978) *Illness as Metaphor*. New York: Vintage
24. Peters-Golden, H. (1982) Breast cancer: varied perceptions of social support in the illness experience. *Soc. Sci. Med.* **16**, 483–491
25. Henahan, J. F. (1988) AIDS' economic, political aspects become as global as medical problem. *JAMA* **259**, 3377
26. Daniels, V. S. (1987) *AIDS*. London: MTP Press
27. Cassens, B. J. (1985) Social consequences of the acquired immunodeficiency syndrome. *Ann. Int. Med.* **103**, 768–771
28. Warwick, I., Aggleton, P. and Homans, H. (1988) Young people's health beliefs and AIDS. In: Aggleton, P. and Homans, H. (eds) *Social Aspects of AIDS*. London: Falmer Press, pp. 106–125
29. Wellings, K. (1988) Perceptions of risk – media treatment of AIDS. In: Aggleton, P. and Homans, H. *op. cit.*, pp. 65–82
30. Watney, S. (1988) AIDS, 'moral panic' theory and homophobia. In: Aggleton, P. and Homans, H. *op. cit.*, pp. 52–64
31. Cominos, E. D., Gottschang, S. K. and Scrimshaw, S. C. M. (1989) Kuru, AIDS and unfamiliar social behaviour – biocultural consideration in the current epidemic: discussion paper. *J. R. Soc. Med.* **82**, 95–98
32. Chrisman, N. J. (1981) *Analytical Scheme for Health Relief Research*. Unpublished
33. Snow L. F. (1976) 'High blood' is not high blood pressure. *Urban Health* **5**, 54–55
34. Snow, L. F. and Johnson, S. M. (1978) Folklore, food, female reproductive cycle. *Ecol. Food Nutr.* **7**, 41–49
35. Pill, R. and Stott, N. C. H. (1982) Concepts of illness causation and responsibility: some preliminary data from a sample of working class mothers. *Soc. Sci. Med.* **16**, 43–52
36. Greenwood, B. (1981) Cold or spirits? Choice and ambiguity in Morocco's pluralistic medical system. *Soc. Sci. Med.* **15B**, 219–235
37. Landy, D. (1977) Malign and benign methods of causing and curing illness. In: Landy D. (ed.) *Culture, Disease, and Healing: Studies in Medical Anthropology*. New York: Macmillan, pp. 195–197
38. Snow, L. F. (1978) Sorcerers, saints and charlatans: black folk healers in urban America. *Cult. Med. Psychiatry* **2**, 69–106
39. Spooner, B. (1970) The evil eye in the Middle East. In: Douglas, M. (ed.) *Witchcraft Confessions and Accusations*. London: Tavistock, pp. 311–319
40. Underwood, P. and Underwood, Z. (1981) New spells for old: expectations

and realities of Western medicine in a remote tribal society in Yemen, Arabia. In: Stanley, N. F. and Joshe, R. A. (eds) *Changing Disease Patterns and Human Behaviour.* London: Academic Press, pp. 271–297

41. Lewis, I. M. (1971) *Ecstatic Religion.* Harmondsworth: Penguin
42. Blaxter, M. (1979) Concepts of causality: lay and medical models. In: Osborne, D. J. (ed.) *Research in Psychology and Medicine,* Vol. 2. London: Academic Press, pp. 154–161
43. Foster, G. M. and Anderson, B. G. (1978) *Medical Anthropology.* New York: Wiley, pp. 53–70
44. Young, A. (1983) The relevance of traditional medical cultures to modern primary health care. *Soc. Sci. Med.* **17**, 1205–1211
45. Brody, H. (1987) *Stories of Sickness.* New Haven: Yale University Press
46. Blumhagen, D. (1980) Hyper-tension: a folk illness with a medical name. *Cult. Med. Psychiatry* **4**, 197–227
47. Helman, C. G. (1978) 'Feed a cold, starve a fever': folk models of infection in an English suburban community, and their relation to medical treatment. *Cult. Med. Psychiatry* **2**, 107–137
48. Zola, I. K. (1973) Pathways to the doctor: from person to patient. *Soc. Sci. Med.* **7**, 677–689
49. Zola, I. K. (1966) Culture and symptoms: an analysis of patients' presenting complaints. *Am. Sociol. Rev.* **31**, 615–630
50. Hackett, T. P., Gassem, N. H. and Raker, J. W. (1973) Patient delay in cancer. *N. Engl. J. Med.* **289**, 14–20
51. Olin, H. S. and Hackett, T. P. (1964) The denial of chest pain in 32 patients with acute myocardial infarction. *JAMA* **190**, 977–981
52. Scott, C. S. (1964) Health and healing practices among five ethnic groups in Miami, Florida. *Public Health Rep.* **89**, 524–532
53. Zborowski, M. (1952) Cultural components in responses to pain. *J. Soc. Issues* **8**, 16–30
54. Helman, C. G. (1985) Disease and pseudo-disease: a case history of pseudo angina. In: Hahn, R. A. and Gaines, A. D. (eds) *Physicians of Western Medicine: Anthropological Approaches to Theory and Practice.* Dordrecht: Reidel, pp. 293–331
55. Mechanic, D. (1972) Social psychologic factors affecting the presentation of bodily complaints. *N. Engl. J. Med.* **286**, 1132–1139
56. Stimson, G. V. and Webb, B. (1975) *Going to see the Doctor: The Consultation Process in General Practice.* London: Routledge & Kegan Paul
57. Balint, M. (1964) *The Doctor, his Patient and the Illness.* Tunbridge Wells: Pitman, pp. 21–25
58. Bell, C. (1984) A hundred years of *Lancet* language. *Lancet* **ii**, 1453
59. Boyle, C. M. (1970) Differences between patients' and doctors' interpretation of some common medical terms. *Br. Med. J.* **ii**, 286–289
60. Pearson, D. and Dudley, H. A. F. (1982) Bodily perceptions in surgical patients. *Br. Med. J.* **284**, 1545–1546
61. Leff, J. P. (1978) Psychiatrists' *versus* patients' concepts of unpleasant emotions. *Br. J. Psychiatry* **133**, 306–313
62. Stimson, G. V. (1974) Obeying doctor's orders: a view from the other side. *Soc. Sci. Med.* **8**, 97–104
63. Waters, W. H. R., Gould, N. V. and Lunn, J. E. (1976) Undispensed prescriptions in a mining general practice. *Br. Med. J.* **i**, 1062–1063
64. Harwood, A. (1971) The hot–cold theory of disease: implications for treatment of Puerto Rican patients. *JAMA* **216**, 1153–1158
65. Cay, E. L., Philip, A. E., Small, W. P., Neilson, J. and Henderson, M. A.

(1975) Patient's assessment of the result of surgery for peptic ulcer. *Lancet* **i**, 29–31

66. Hall, E. T. (1977) *Beyond Culture*. New York: Anchor Books, pp. 85–103

Chapter 6

1. Keesing, R. M. (1981) *Cultural Anthropology*. New York: Holt, Rinehart and Winston, pp. 27–29
2. MacCormack, C. P. and Strathern, M. (eds) (1981) *Nature, Culture and Gender*. Cambridge: Cambridge University Press
3. Ganong, W. F. (1983) *Review of Medical Physiology*. Los Altos: Lange Medical Publications, pp.342–343
4. Keesing, R. M. (1981) *op. cit.*, pp. 301–310
5. Keesing, R. (1981) *op. cit.*, p 150
6. Goddard, V. (1987) Honour and shame: the control of women's sexuality and group identity in Naples. In: Caplan, P. (ed.) (1987). *The Cultural Construction of Sexuality*. London: Tavistock, pp. 166–192
7. Dunk, P. (1989) Greek women and broken nerves in Montreal. *Med Anthropol.* **11**, 29–45
8. Shepherd, G. (1987) Rank, gender, and homosexuality: Mombasa as a key to understanding sexual options. In: Caplan, P. (ed.) *op. cit.*, pp. 240–270
9. Ember, C. R. and Ember, M. (1985) *Cultural Anthropology*. Englewood Cliffs, NJ: Prentice-Hall, pp. 137–156
10. Rosaldo, M. Z. and Lamphere, L. (1974) *Women, Culture, and Society*. Stanford: Stanford University Press
11. Caplan, P. (1987) Introduction. In: Caplan, P. (ed.) *op. cit.*, pp. 1–30
12. Devisch, R. and Gailly, A. (1985) A therapeutic self-help group among Turkish women: Dertleşmek: 'The sharing of sorrow'. *Psichiatrica e Psicoterapia analitica*, **4**, 133–152
13. Lewis, I. M. (1971) *Ecstatic Religion*. Harmondsworth: Penguin
14. McGuire, M. B. (1988) *Ritual Healing in Suburban America*. New Brunswick: Rutgers University Press
15. Stacey, M. (1988) *The Sociology of Health and Healing*. London: Unwin Hyman, pp. 78–97
16. Stacey, M. (1988) *op. cit.*, pp. 177–193
17. Fry, J., Brooks, D. and McColl, I. (1984) *NHS Data Book*. Lancaster: MTP Press
18. Gamarnikow, E. (1978) Sexual division of labour: the case of nursing. In: Kuhn, A. and Wolpe, A. M. (eds) *Feminism and Materialism*. London: Routledge and Kegan Paul, pp. 96–123
19. Krantzler, N. (1986) Media images of physicians and nurses in the United States. *Soc. Sci. Med.* **22**, 933–952
20. Littlewood, J. (1989) A model for nursing using anthropological literature. *Int. J. Nurs. Stud.* **26**, 221–229
21. Illich, I. (1976) *Limits to Medicine*. London: Marion Boyars
22. Gabe, J. and Calnan, M. (1989) The limits of medicine: women's perception of medical technology. *Soc. Sci. Med.* **28**, 223–231
23. Stacey, M. (1989) *op. cit.*, pp. 253–254
24. Cooperstock, R. (1976) Psychotropic drug use among women. *Can. Med. Assoc. J.* **115**, 760–763
25. Stimson, G. (1975) The message of psychotropic drug ads. *J. Commun.* **25**, 153–160

26. Titmuss, R. M. (1984) The position of women: some vital statistics. In: Black, N., Boswell, D., Gray. A., Murphy, S. and Popay, J. (eds) *Health and Disease.* Milton Keynes: Open University Press, pp. 71–75
27. Dalton, K. (1964) *The Premenstrual Syndrome.* London: Heinemann
28. Gottlieb, A. (1988) American premenstrual syndrome. *Anthropol. Today* **4,** 10–13
29. Lock, M. M. (1982) Models and practice in medicine: menopause as syndrome or life transition? *Cult. Med. Psychiatry* **6,** 261–280
30. Kaufert, P. A. and Gilbert, P. (1986) Women, menopause and medicalisation. *Cult. Med. Psychiatry* **10,** 7–21
31. Waldron, I. (1978) Type A behavior pattern and coronary heart disease in men and women. *Soc. Sci. Med.* **12B,** 167–170
32. Low, S. M. (1989) Health, culture and the nature of nerves. *Med. Anthropol.* **11,** 91–95
33. U205 Course Team (1985) *Medical Knowledge: Doubt and Certainty.* Milton Keynes: Open University Press, pp. 73–81
34. Hahn, R. A. and Muecke, M. A. (1987) The anthropology of birth in five US ethnic populations: implications for obstetrical practice. *Curr. Probl. Obstet. Gynecol. Fertil.* **10,** 133–171
35. Stacey, M. (1988) *op. cit.,* p. 52
36. Leavitt, J. W. (1987) The growth of medical authority: technology and morals in turn-of-the-century obstetrics. *Med. Anthropol. Q.* (New Series) **1,** 230–255
37. Davis-Floyd, R. E. (1987) The technological model of birth. *J. Am. Folklore* **100,** 479–495
38. Graham, H. and Oakley, A. (1981) Competing ideologies of reproduction: medical and maternal perspectives on pregnancy. In: Roberts, H. (ed.) *Women, Health and Reproduction.* London: Routledge and Kegan Paul, pp. 99–118
39. Kitzinger, S. (1982) The social context of birth: some comparisons between childbirth in Jamaica and Britain. In: MacCormack, C.P. (ed.) *Ethnography of Fertility and Birth.* London: Academic Press, pp. 181–203
40. MacCormack, C. P. (1982) Biological, cultural and social adaptation in human fertility and birth: a synthesis. In: MacCormack, C. P. (ed.) *op. cit.,* pp. 1–23
41. McGilvray, D. B. (1982) Sexual power and fertility in Sri Lanka: Batticaloa Tamils and Moors. In: MacCormack, C. P. (ed.) *op. cit.,* pp. 25–73
42. Pillsbury, B. L. K. (1984) 'Doing the month': confinement and convalescence of Chinese women after childbirth. In: Black, N., Boswell, D., Gray, A., Murphy, S. and Popay, J. (eds) *Health and Disease.* Milton Keynes: Open University Press, pp. 17–24
43. World Health Organisation (1978) *The Promotion and Development of Traditional Medicine.* Technical Report Series 622. Geneva: World Health Organisation
44. World Health Organisation (1979) *Traditional Birth Attendants: An Annotated Bibliography on their Training, Utilization and Evaluation.* Geneva: World Health Organisation
45. Cosminsky, S. (1982) Childbirth and change: a Guatemalan study. In: MacCormack, C. P. (ed.) *op. cit.,* pp. 205–239
46. Keesing, R, M. (1981) *op. cit.,* p. 161
47. Heggenhougen, H. K. (1980) Fathers and childbirth: an anthropological perspective. *J. Nurse Midwifery* **25,** 21–26
48. Lipkin, M. and Lamb, G. S. (1982) The couvade syndrome: an epidemiological study. *Ann. Intern. Med.* **96,** 509–511

Chapter 7

1. Morrell, D. C. (1977) Symptom interpretation in general practice. *J. R. Coll. Gen. Pract.* **22,** 297–309
2. Weinman, J. (1981) *An Outline of Psychology as Applied to Medicine.* Bristol: Wright, p. 5
3. Engel, G. L. (1950) 'Psychogenic' pain and the pain-prone patient. *Am. J. Med.* **26,** 899–909
4. Fabrega, H. and Tyma, S. (1976) Language and cultural influences in the description of pain. *Br. J. Med. Psychol.* **49,** 349–371
5. Hoebel, E. A. (1960) *The Cheyenne. Indians of the Great Plains.* New York: Holt, Rinehart and Winston, pp. 11–16
6. Zola, I. K. (1966) Culture and symptoms: an analysis of patients' presenting complaints. *Am. Sociol. Rev.* **31,** 615–630
7. Boyle, C. M. (1970) Difference between patients' and doctors' interpretation of some common medical terms. *Br. Med. J.* **ii,** 286–289
8. Helman, C. G. (1985) Disease and pseudo-disease: a case history of pseudo-angina. In: Hahn, R. and Gaines, A. (eds) *Physicians of Western Medicine: Anthropological Perspectives on Theory and Practice.* Dordrecht: Reidel, pp. 293–331
9. Zborowski, M. (1952) Cultural components in responses to pain. *J. Soc. Issues* **8,** 16–30
10. Wolff, B. B. and Langley, S. (1977) Cultural factors and the response to pain. In: Landy, D. (ed.) *Culture, Disease, and Healing: Studies in Medical Anthropology.* New York: Macmillan, pp. 313–319
11. Lewis, G. (1981) Cultural influences on illness behaviour: a medical anthropological approach. In: Eisenberg, L. and Kleinman, A. (eds) *The Relevance of Social Science for Medicine.* Dordrecht: Reidel, pp. 151–162
12. Levine, J. D., Gordon, N. C. and Fields, H. L. (1978) The mechanism of placebo analgesia. *Lancet* **ii,** 654–657
13. Landy, D. (1977) In: Landy, D. (ed.) *Culture, Disease, and Healing: Studies in Medical Anthropology.* New York: Macmillan, p. 313
14. le Barre, W. (1947) The cultural basis of emotions and gestures. *J. Pers.* **16,** 49–68
15. Hawkins, C. F. (1975) The alimentary system. In: Mann, W. N. (ed.) *Conybeare's Textbook of Medicine.* London: Churchill Livingstone, p. 326
16. Kleinman, A. (1980) *Patients and Healers in the Context of Culture.* Berkeley: University of California Press, pp. 138–145
17. Skultans, V. (1976) Empathy and healing: aspects of spiritualist ritual. In: Loudon, J. B. (ed.) *Social Anthropology and Medicine.* London: Academic Press, pp. 190–221

Chapter 8

1. Claridge, G. (1970) *Drugs and Human Behaviour.* London: Allen Lane
2. Wolf, S. (1959) The pharmacology of placebos. *Pharmacol. Rev.* **11,** 689–705
3. Shapiro, A. K. (1959) The placebo effect in the history of medical treatment: implications for psychiatry. *Am. J. Psychiatry* **116,** 298–304
4. Benson, H. and Epstein, M. D. (1975) The placebo effect: a neglected asset in the care of patients. *JAMA* **232,** 1225–1227
5. Editorial (1972) *Lancet* **ii,** 122–123

6. Editorial (1972) *op. cit.*, p. 123
7. Levine, J. D., Gordon, N. C. and Fields, H. L. (1978) The mechanism of placebo analgesia. *Lancet* ii, 654–657
8. Adler, H. M. and Hammett, V. O. (1973) The doctor–patient relationship revisited: an analysis of the placebo effect. *Ann. Intern. Med.* 78, 595–598
9. Joyce, C. R. B. (1969) Quantitative estimates of dependence on the symbolic function of drugs. In: Steinberg, H. (ed.) *Scientific Basis of Drug Dependence*. London: Churchill, pp. 271–280
10. Schapira, K., McClelland, H. A., Griffiths, N. R. and Newell, D. J. (1970) Study on the effects of tablet colour in the treatment of anxiety states. *Br. Med. J.* ii, 446–449
11. Branthwaite, A. and Cooper, P. (1981) Analgesic effects of branding in treatment of headaches. *Br. Med. J.* 282, 1576–1578
12. Jefferys, M., Brotherston, J. H. F. and Cartwright, A. (1960) Consumption of medicines on a working-class housing estate. *Br. J. Prev. Soc. Med.* 14, 64–76
13. Helman, C. G. (1981) 'Tonic', 'fuel' and 'food': social and symbolic aspects of the long-term use of psychotropic drugs. *Soc. Sci. Med.* 15B, 521–533
14. Claridge, G. (1970) *op. cit.*, p. 25
15. Claridge, G. (1970) *op. cit.*, p. 126
16. Benson, H. and McCallie, D. P. (1979) Angina pectoris and the placebo effect. *N. Engl. J. Med.* 300, 1424–1429
17. Lader, M. (1979) Spectres of tolerance and dependence. *MIMS Magazine*, 15 August, 31–35
18. Parish, P. A. (1971) The prescribing of psychotropic drugs in general practice. *J. R. Coll. Gen. Pract.* 21, Suppl. 4
19. Trethowan, W. H. (1975) Pills for personal problems. *Br. Med. J.* iii, 749–751
20. Hall, R. C. W. and Kirkpatrick, B. (1980) The benzodiazepines. *Am. Fam. Physician* 17, 131–134
21. Editorial (1973) Benzodiazepines: use, overuse, misuse, abuse? *Lancet* i, 1101–1102
22. Parish, P. A. (1971) *op. cit.*, pp. 29–30
23. Williams, P. (1981) Areas of concern in the prescription of psychotropic drugs. *MIMS Magazine* 1 January, 37–43
24. Smith, M. C. (1980) The relationship between pharmacy and medicine. In: Mapes, R. (ed.) *Prescribing Practice and Drug Usage*. London: Croom Helm, pp. 157–200
25. Cooperstock, R. and Lennard, H. L. (1979) Some social meanings of tranquillizer use. *Soc. Health Illness* 1, 331–345
26. Pellegrino, E. D. (1976) Prescribing and drug ingestion: symbols and substances. *Drug Intell. Clin. Pharmacol.* 10, 624–630
27. Warburton, D. M. (1978) Poisoned people: internal pollution. *J. Biosoc. Sci.* 10, 309–319
28. Jones, D. R. (1979) Drugs and prescribing: what the patient thinks. *J. R. Coll. Gen. Pract.* 29, 417–419
29. Tyrer, P. (1978) Drug treatment of psychiatric patients in general practice. *Br. Med. J.* ii, 1008–1010
30. Claridge, G. (1970) *op. cit.*, p. 231
31. Burr, A. (1984) The ideologies of despair: a symbolic interpretation of punks and skinheads' usage of barbiturates. *Soc. Sci. Med.* 19, 929–938
32. Plummer, K. (1988) Organizing AIDS. In: Aggleton, P. and Homans, H. (eds) *Social Aspects of AIDS*. Lewes: Falmer Press, pp. 20–51
33. Robins, L. N., Davis, D. H. and Goodwin, D. W. (1974) Drug use by US Army enlisted men in Vietnam: a follow-up on their return home. *Am. J. Epidemiol.* 99, 235–249

34. Jackson, B. (1978) Deviance as success: the double inversion of stigmatised roles. In: Babcock, B. A. (ed.) *The Reversible World: Symbolic Inversion in Art and Society*. Ithaca: Cornell University Press, pp. 258–271
35. Freeland, J. B. and Rosenstiel, C. R. (1974) A socio-cultural barrier to establishing therapeutic rapport: a problem in the treatment of narcotic addicts. *Psychiatry* **37**, 215–220
36. Knupfer, G. and Room, R. (1967) Drinking patterns and attitudes of Irish, Jewish and White Protestant American men. *Q. J. Studies Alcohol* **28**, 676–699
37. Kunitz, S. J. and Levy, J. E. (1981) Navajos. In: Harwood, A. (ed.) *Ethnicity and Medical Care*. Cambridge, Mass: Harvard University Press, 337–396
38. O'Connor, J. (1975) Social and cultural factors influencing drinking behaviour. *Irish J. Med. Sci.* Suppl. (June), 65–71
39. Greeley, A. M. and McCready, W. C. (1978) A preliminary reconnaissance into the persistence and explanation of ethnic subcultural drinking patterns. *Med. Anthropol.* **2**, 31–51
40. Thomas, A. E. (1978) Class and sociability among urban workers. *Med. Anthropol.* **2**, 9–30
41. Hunt, G. and Satterlee, S. (1986) Cohesion and division: drinking in an English village. *MAN* **21**, 521–537
42. United States Department of Health and Human Services (1984) *A Report of the Surgeon General: Chronic Obstructive Lung Disease*. Publication 84–56205. Washington: Office of the Assistant Secretary for Health
43. United States Department of Health, Education, and Welfare (1979) *A Report of The Surgeon General: Smoking and Health*. Publication 79–50066. Washington: Office of the Assistant Secretary for Health
44. Reeder, L. G. (1977) Socio-cultural factors in the etiology of smoking behaviour: an assessment. *Natl. Inst. Drug Abuse Res. Monogr. Ser.* **17**, 186–201
45. Marsh, A. and Matheson, J. (1983) *Smoking Attitudes and Behaviour: an Enquiry Carried Out on behalf of the Department of Health and Social Security*. London: HMSO
46. Doherty, W. J. and Whitehead, D. (1986) The social dynamics of cigarette smoking: a family systems perspective. *Family Process* **25**, 453–459
47. Tobacco use and world health: a situation analysis. (1986) *Bull. Pan Am. Health Organ.* **20**, 409–417
48. Dobkin de Rios, M. (1973) Curing with *ayahuasca* in an urban slum. In: Harner, M. J. (ed.) *Hallucinogens and Shamanism*. London: Oxford University Press, pp. 67–85
49. Littlewood, R. and Lipsedge, M. (1982) *Aliens and Alienists*. Harmondsworth: Penguin, p. 34
50. La Barre, W. (1969) *The Peyote Cult*. New York: Schocken Books
51. Harner, M. J. (1973) Common themes in South American Indian *yage* experiences. In: Harner, M. J. *op. cit.*, pp. 155–175
52. Schultes, R. E. (1976) *Hallucinogenic Plants*. New York: Golden Press, pp. 142–147

Chapter 9

1. Loudon, J. B. (1966) Private stress and public ritual. *J. Psychosom. Res.* **10**, 101–108

2. Turner, V. W. (1968) *The Drums of Affliction*. Oxford: Clarendon Press and IAI, pp. 1–8
3. Leach, E. (1968) Ritual. In: Sills, D. L. (ed.) *International Encyclopaedia of the Social Sciences*. New York: Free Press/Macmillan, pp. 520–526
4. Turner, V. W. (1969) The Ritual Process. Harmondsworth: Penguin, pp. 48–49
5. Ngubane, H. (1977) *Body and Mind in Zulu Medicine*. London: Academic Press, pp. 111–139
6. Standing, H. (1980) Beliefs about menstruation and pregnancy. *MIMS Magazine* 1 June, 21–27
7. Leach, E. (1976) *Culture and Communication*. Cambridge: Cambridge University Press, pp. 33–36, 77–79
8. Van Gennep, A. (1960) *The Rites of Passage*. (Transl. by Vizedom, M. D. and Caffee, G. L.) London: Routledge & Kegan Paul
9. Ngubane H. (1977) *op. cit.*, pp. 78–79
10. Davis-Floyd, R. E. (1987) The technological model of birth. *J. Am. Folklore* **100**, 479–495
11. Kitzinger, S. (1982) The social context of birth: some comparisons between childbirth in Jamaica and Britain. In: MacCormack, C. P. (ed.) *Ethnography of Fertility and Birth*. London: Academic Press, pp. 181–203
12. Hertz, R. (1960) *Death and the Right Hand*. London: Cohen and West, pp. 27–86
13. Eisenbruch, M. (1984) Cross-cultural aspects of bereavement. II. Ethnic and cultural variations in the development of bereavement practices. *Cult. Med. Psychiatry* **8**, 315–347
14 Skultans, V. (1980) A dying ritual. *MIMS Magazine* 15 June, 43–47
15. Eisenbruch, M. (1984) Cross-cultural aspects of bereavement. I. A conceptual framework for comparative analysis. *Cult. Med. Psychiatry* **8**, 283–309
16. Foster, G. M. and Anderson, B. G. (1978) *Medical Anthropology*. New York: Wiley, pp. 115–117
17. Beattie, J. (1967) Divination in Bunyoro, Uganda. In: Middleton, J. (ed.) *Magic, Witchcraft and Curing*. Austin: University of Texas Press, pp. 211–231
18. Balint, M. (1974) *The Doctor, his Patient and the Illness*. London: Pitman, p. 5
19. Balint, M. (1974) *op. cit.*, pp. 24–25
20. Rose, L. (1971) *Faith Healing*. Harmondsworth: Penguin, p. 62
21. Parkes, C. M. (1975) *Bereavement*. Harmondsworth: Penguin
22. Turner, V. W. (1964) An Ndembu doctor in practice. In: Kiev, A. (ed.) *Magic, Faith and Healing*. New York: Free Press, pp. 230–263
23. Bosk, C. L. (1980) Occupational rituals in patient management. *New Engl. J. Med.* **303**, 71–76
24. Katz, P. (1981) Ritual in the operating room. *Ethnology* **20**, 335–350
25. Douglas, M. (1973) *Natural Symbols*. Harmondsworth: Penguin, pp. 19–39
26. Byrne, P. (1976) Teaching and learning verbal behaviours. In: Tanner, B. (ed.) *Language and Communication in General Practice*. London: Hodder and Stoughton, pp. 52–70
27. Foster, G. M. and Anderson, B. G. (1978) *op. cit.*, p. 119

Chapter 10

1. Babcock, B. A. (1978) Introduction. In: Babcock, B. A. (ed.) *The Reversible World: Symbolic Inversion in Art and Society*. Ithaca: Cornell University Press, pp. 13–36

2. Abrahams, R. D. and Bauman, R. (1978) Ranges of festival behaviour. In: *The Reversible World: Symbolic Inversion in Art and Society*. Ithaca: Cornell University Press, pp. 193–208

3. Lewis, I. M. (1971) *Ecstatic Religion*. Harmondsworth: Penguin, pp. 178–205

4. Littlewood, R. and Lipsedge, M. (1982) *Aliens and Alienists*. Harmondsworth: Penguin, pp. 171–177

5. Foster, G. M. and Anderson, B. G. (1978) *Medical Anthropology*. New York: Wiley, pp. 81–100

6. Kiev, A. (1964) Implications for the future. In: Kiev, A. (ed.) *Magic, Faith and Healing*. New York: Free Press, pp. 454–64

7. Edgerton, R. B. (1977) Conceptions of psychosis in four East African societies. In: Landy, D. (ed.) *Culture, Disease and Healing: Studies in Medical Anthropology*. New York: Macmillan, pp. 358–367

8. Landy, D.(1977) Emotional states and cultural constraints. In: Landy, D. (ed.) *Culture, Disease and Healing: Studies in Medical Anthropology*. New York: Macmillan, pp. 333–335

9. Littlewood, R. and Lipsedge, M. (1982) *op. cit.*, pp. 184–209

10. Kiev, A. (1972) *Transcultural Psychiatry*. Harmondsworth: Penguin, pp. 11–25

11. Kiev, A. (1972) *op. cit.*, pp. 78–108

12. Kleinman, A. (1980) *Patients and Healers in the Context of Culture*. Berkeley: University of California Press, pp. 176–177

13. Kleinman, A. (1987) Anthropology and psychiatry. *Br. J. Psychiatry* **151**, 447–454

14. Littlewood, R. (1989) From categories to contexts: a decade of the new cross-cultural psychiatry. *Br. J. Psychiatry*. In Press

15. Waxler, N. (1977) Is mental illness cured in traditional societies? A theoretical analysis. *Cult. Med. Psychiatry* **1**, 233–253

16. Rubel, A. (1977) The epidemiology of folk illness: *susto* in hispanic America. In: Landy, D. (ed.) *Culture, Disease and Healing: Studies in Medical Anthropology*. New York: Macmillan, pp. 119–128

17. Pichot, P. (1982) The diagnosis and classification of mental disorders in French-speaking countries: background, current views and comparison with other nomenclatures. *Psychol. Med.* **12**, 475–492

18. Merskey, H. and Shafran, B. (1986) Political hazards in the diagnosis of 'sluggish schizophrenia'. *Br. J. Psychiatry* **148**, 247–256

19. Kendell, R. E. (1975) *The Role of Diagnosis in Psychiatry*. Oxford: Blackwell, pp. 70–71

20. Kendell, R. E. (1975) *op. cit.*, pp. 49–59

21. Temerlin, M. K. (1968) Suggestion effects in psychiatric diagnosis. *J. Nerv. Ment. Dis.* **147**, 349–353

22. Kendell, R. E. (1975) *op. cit.*, pp. 9–26

23. Eisenberg, L. (1977) Disease and illness: distinctions between professional and popular ideas of sickness. *Cult. Med. Psychiatry* **1**, 9–23

24. Szasz, T. (1989) Psychiatric justice. *Br. J. Psychiatry* **154**, 864–869

25. Wing, J. K. (1978) *Reasoning about Madness*. Oxford: Oxford University Press, pp. 167–193

26. Littlewood, R. and Lipsedge, M. (1982) *op. cit.*, pp. 238–242

27. Blackburn, R. (1988) On moral judgements and personality disorders: the myth of the psychopathic personality revisited. *Br. J. Psychiatry* **153**, 505–512

28. Cooper, J. E., Kendell, R. E., Gurland, B. J., Sartorius, N. and Farkas, T. (1969) Cross-national study of diagnosis of the mental disorders: some results from the first comparative investigation. *Am. J. Psychiatry* **125**, Suppl., 21–29

29. Katz, M. M., Cole, J. O. and Lowery, H. A. (1969) Studies of the diagnostic

process: the influence of symptom perception, past experience, and ethnic background on diagnostic decisions. *Am. J. Psychiatry* **125,** 109–119

30. Copeland, J. R. M., Cooper, J. E., Kendell, R. E. and Gourlay, A. J. (1971) Differences in usage of diagnostic labels among psychiatrists in the British Isles. *Br. J. Psychiatry* **118,** 629–640

31. Littlewood, R. and Lipsedge, M. (1982) *op. cit.,* p. 119

32. Scheper-Hughes, N. (1978) Saints, scholars, and schizophrenics: madness and badness in Western Ireland. *Med. Anthropol.* **2,** 59–93

33. Littlewood, R. and Lipsedge, M. (1982) *op. cit.* pp. 210–231

34. Littlewood, R. (1980) Anthropology and psychiatry: an alternative approach. *Br. J. Med. Psychol.* **53,** 213–225

35. Kleinman, A. and Kleinman, J. (1985) In: Kleinman, A. and Good, B. (eds) *Culture and Depression.* Berkeley: University of California Press, pp. 429–490

36. Kleinman, A. (1980) *op. cit.* pp. 146–178

37. Helman, C. G. (1985) Psyche, soma and society: the social construction of psychosomatic disorders. *Cult. Med. Psychiatry* **9,** 1–26

38. Lau, B. W. K., Kung, N. Y. T. and Chung, J. T. C. (1983) How depressive illness presents in Hong Kong. *Practitioner* **227,** 112–114

39. Hussain, M. F. and Gomersall, J. D. (1978) Affective disorder in Asian immigrants. *Psychiatria Clin.* **11,** 87–89

40. Simons, R. C. and Hughes, C. C. (eds) (1985) *The Culture-Bound Syndromes.* Dordrecht: D. Reidel

41. Littlewood, L. and Lipsedge, M. (1987) The butterfly and the serpent: culture, psychopathology and biomedicine. *Cult. Med. Psychiatry* **11,** 289–335

42. De La Cancela, V., Guarnaccia, P. J. and Carillo, E. (1986) Psychosocial distress among Latinos: a critical analysis of *ataques de nervios. Humanity Soc.* **10,** 431–447

43. Dow, J. (1986) Universal aspects of symbolic healing: a theoretical synthesis. *Am. Anthropol.* **88,** 56–69

44. Kleinman, A. (1980) *op. cit.,* pp. 82, 360

45. Lewis, I. M. (1971) *op. cit.,* pp. 37–65

46. Murphy, J. M. (1964) Psychotherapeutic aspects of Shamanism on St. Lawrence Island, Alaska. In: Kiev, A. (ed.) *Magic, Faith and Healing.* New York: Free Press, pp. 53–83

47. Finkler, K. (1981) Non-medical treatments and their outcomes. Part Two. Focus on the adherents of spiritualism. *Cult. Med. Psychiatry* **5,** 65–103

48. Kleinman, A. (1980) *op. cit.,* pp. 319–352

49. Christie-Seely, J. (1981) Teaching the family system concept in family medicine. *J. Fam. Pract.* **13,** 391–401

50. Minuchin, S., Rosman, B. L. and Baker, L. (1978) *Psychosomatic Families.* Cambridge: Harvard University Press

51. Byng-Hall, J. (1988) Scripts and legends in families and family therapy. *Fam. Proc.* **27,** 167–179

52. Prince-Embury, S. (1984) The family health tree: a form of identifying physical symptom patterns within the family. *J. Fam. Pract.* **18,** 75–81

53. McGoldrick, M., Pearce, J. K. and Giordano, J. (eds) (1982) *Ethnicity and Family Therapy.* New York: Guildford Press

54. Maranhao, T. (1984) Family therapy and anthropology. *Cult. Med. Psychiatry* **8,** 255–279

55. DiNicola, V. F. (1986) Beyond Babel: family therapy as cultural transition. *Int. J. Fam. Therapy* **7,** 179–191

56. Lau, A. (1984) Transcultural issues in family therapy. *J. Fam. Therapy* **6,** 91–112

57. Barot, R. (1988) Social anthropology, ethnicity and family therapy. *J. Fam. Therapy* **10**, 271–282
58. Krupinski, J. (1967) Sociological aspects of mental health in migrants. *Soc. Sci. Med.* **1**, 267–281
59. Cox, J. L. (1977) Aspects of transcultural psychiatry. *Br. J. Psychiatry* **130**, 211–221
60. Schaechter, F. (1965) Previous history of mental illness in female migrant patients admitted to the psychiatric hospital, Royal Park. *Med. J. Aust.* **2**, 277–279
61. Littlewood, R. and Lipsedge, M. (1982) *op. cit.*, pp. 87–106
62. Wright, C. M. (1981) Pakistani family life in Newcastle. *J. Maternal Child Health* **6**, 427–430
63. Gelder, M., Gath, D. and Mayou, R. (eds) (1983) *Oxford Textbook of Psychiatry*. London: Oxford University Press, p. 289
64. Burke, A. W. (1984) Racism and psychological disturbance among West Indians in Britain. *Int. J. Soc. Psychiatry* **30**, 50–68
65. Lopez, S. and Hernandez, P. (1976) How culture is considered in evaluations of psychotherapy. *J. Nerv. Ment. Dis.* **176**, 598–606

Chapter 11

1. Selye, H. (1936) A syndrome produced by diverse nocuous agents. *Nature* **138**, 32
2. Selye, H. (1976) Forty years of stress research: principal remaining problems and misconceptions. *Can. Med. Assoc. J.* **115**, 53–57
3. Bridges, P. K. (1982) The physiology and biochemistry of stress: some practical aspects. *Practitioner* **226**, 1575–1579
4. Weinman, J. (1981) *An Outline of Psychology as Applied to Medicine*. Bristol: Wright, pp. 60–84
5. Young, A. (1980) The discourse on stress and the reproduction of conventional knowledge. *Soc. Sci. Med.* **14B**, 133–146
6. Parkes, C. M. (1971) Psycho-social transitions: a field for study. *Soc. Sci. Med.* **5**, 101–115
7. World Health Organisation (1971) Society, stress, and disease. *WHO Chron.* **25**, 168–178
8. Helman, C. G. (1985) Psyche, soma and society: the social construction of psychosomatic disorders. *Cult. Med. Psychiatry* **9**, 1–26
9. Tyrrell, D. A. J. (1981) Respiratory infection: new agents and new concepts. *J. R. Coll. Physicians Lond.* **15**, 113–115
10. Baker, G. H. B. and Brewerton, D. A. (1981) Rheumatoid arthritis: a psychiatric assessment. *Br. Med. J.* **282**, 2014
11. Trimble, M. R. and Wilson-Barnet, J. (1982) Neuropsychiatric aspects of stress. *Practitioner* **226**, 1580–1586
12. Parkes, C. M., Benjamin, B. and Fitzgerald, R. G. (1969) Broken heart: a statistical study of increased mortality among widowers. *Br. Med. J.* **i**, 740–743
13. Murphy, F. and Brown, G. W. (1980) Life events, psychiatric disturbance and physical illness. *Br. J. Psychiatry* **136**, 326–338
14. Engel, G. (1968) A life setting conducive to illness: the giving up–given up complex. *Ann. Intern. Med.* **69**, 293–300
15. Karasek, R. A., Russell, R. S. and Theorell, T. (1982) Physiology of stress and regeneration in job-related cardiovascular illness. *J. Hum. Stress* **8**, 29–42

16. Brown, G. W. and Harris, T. (1979) *Social Origins of Depression*. London: Tavistock
17. Kiritz, S. and Moos, R. H. (1974) Physiological effects of social environments. *Psychosom. Med.* **36,** 96–113
18. Guthrie, G. M., Verstraete, A., Deines, M. M. and Stern, R. M. (1975) Symptoms of stress in four societies. *J. Soc. Psychol.* **95,** 165–172
19. Foster, G. M. and Anderson, B. G. (1978) *Medical Anthropology*. New York: Wiley, pp. 93–94
20. Hahn, R. A. and Kleinman, A. (1983) Belief as pathogen, belief as medicine: 'voodoo death' and the 'placebo phenomenon' in anthropological perspective. *Med. Anthropol. Q.* **14,** 3
21. Landy, D. (ed.) (1977) *Culture, Disease and Healing: Studies in Medical Anthropology*. New York: Macmillan, p. 327
22. Lévi-Strauss, C. (1967) *Structural Anthropology*. New York: Anchor Books, pp. 161–162
23. Engel, G. L. (1971) Sudden and rapid death during psychological stress: folklore or folk wisdom? *Ann. Intern. Med.* **74,** 771–782
24. Cannon, W. (1942) Voodoo death. *Am. Anthropol.* **44,** 169–181
25. Engel, G. L. (1978) Psychologic stress, vasopressor (vasovagal) syncope, and sudden death. *Ann. Intern. Med.* **89,** 403–412
26. Lex, B. W. (1977) Voodoo death: new thoughts on an old explanation. In: Landy, D. (ed.) *Culture, Disease and Healing: Studies in Medical Anthropology*. New York: Macmillan, pp. 327–331
27. Hertz, R. (1960) *Death and the Right Hand*. London: Cohen and West, pp. 27–86
28. Goffman, E. (1961) *Asylums*. Harmondsworth: Penguin
29. Cassens, B. J. (1985) Social consequences of the acquired immunodeficiency syndrome. *Ann. Intern. Med.* **103,** 768–771
30. Waxler, N. E. (1981) The social labelling perspective on illness and medical practice. In: Eisenberg, L. and Kleinman, A. (eds) *The Relevance of Social Science for Medicine*. Dordrecht: Reidel, pp. 283–306
31. Haynes, R. B., Sackett, D. L., Taylor, D. W., Gibson, E. S. and Johnson, A. L. (1978) Increased absenteeism from work after detection and labeling of hypertensive patients. *N. Engl. J. Med.* **299,** 741–744
32. Friedman, M. and Rosenman, R. H. (1959) Association of specific overt behaviour pattern with blood and cardiovascular findings. *JAMA* **169,** 1286–1296
33. Rosenman, R. H. (1978) Role of type A behavior pattern in the pathogenesis of ischaemic heart disease, and modification for prevention. *Adv. Cardiol.* **25,** 35–46
34. Appels, A. (1972) Coronary heart disease as a cultural disease. *Psychother. Psychosom.* **22,** 320–324
35. Waldron, I. (1978) Type A behavior pattern and coronary heart disease in men and women. *Soc. Sci. Med.* **12B,** 167–170
36. Weber, M. (1948) *The Protestant Ethic and the Spirit of Capitalism*. London: Allen and Unwin
37. Helman, C. G. (1987) Heart disease and the cultural construction of time: the type A behaviour pattern as a Western culture-bound syndrome. *Soc. Sci. Med.* **25,** 969–979
38. Eitinger, L. (1960) The symptomatology of mental illness among refugees in Norway. *J. Ment. Sci.* **106,** 947–966
39. Eisenbruch, M. (1988) The mental health of refugee children and their cultural development. *Int. Migration Rev.* **22,** 282–300
40. Cassell, J. (1975) Studies of hypertension in migrants. In: Paul, O. (ed.) *Epidemiology and Control of Hypertension*. New York: Stratton, pp. 41–61

41. Carpenter, L. and Brockington, I. F. (1980) A study of mental illness in Asians, West Indians and Africans living in Manchester. *Br. J. Psychiatry* **137**, 201–205
42. Hitch, P. J. and Rack, P. H. (1980) Mental illness among Polish and Russian refugees in Bradford. *Br. J. Psychiatry* **137**, 206–211
43. Burke, A. W. (1976) Attempted suicide among the Irish-born population in Birmingham. *Br. J. Psychiatry* **128**, 534–537
44. Burke, A. W. (1976) Attempted suicide among Asian immigrants in Birmingham. *Br. J. Psychiatry* **128**, 528–533
45. Burke, A. W. (1976) Socio-cultural determinants of attempted suicide among West Indians in Birmingham: ethnic origin and immigrant status. *Br. J. Psychiatry* **129**, 261–266

Chapter 12

1. Kendell, R. E. (1975) *The Role of Diagnosis in Psychiatry.* Oxford: Blackwell, p. 64
2. Murphy, E. and Brown, G. W. (1980) Life events, psychiatric disturbance and physical illness. *Br. J. Psychiatry* **136**, 326–338
3. Townsend, P. and Davidson, N. (eds) (1982) *Inequalities of Health: The Black Report.* Harmondsworth: Penguin
4. Zaidi, S. A. (1988) Poverty and disease: need for a structural change. *Soc. Sci. Med.* **27**, 119–127
5. Gadjusek, D. C. (1963) Kuru. *Trans. R. Soc. of Tropical Med. Hyg.* **57**, 151–169
6. Marmot, M. (1981) Culture and illness: epidemiological evidence. In: Christie, M. J. and Mellett, P. G. (eds) *Foundations of Psychosomatics.* Chichester: Wiley, pp. 323–340
7. Kark, S. (1981) *The practice of community-oriented primary care.* New York: Appleton-Century-Crofts
8. Marmot, M. G., Syme, S. L., Kagan, A., Kato, H., Cohen, J. B. and Belsky, J. (1975) Epidemiological studies of coronary heart disease and stroke in Japanese men living in Japan, Hawaii and California: prevalence of coronary and hypertensive heart disease and associated risk factors. *Am. J. Epidemiol.* **102**, 514–525
9. Marmot, M. G. and Syme, S. L. (1976) Acculturation and coronary heart disease in Japanese Americans. *Am. J. Epidemiol.* **104**, 225–247
10. Fletcher, C. M., Jones, N. L., Burrows, B. and Niden, A. H. (1964) American emphysema and British bronchitis: a standardized comparative study. *Am. Rev. Resp. Dis.* **90**, 1–13
11. O'Brien, B. (1984) *Patterns of European Diagnoses and Prescribing.* London: Office of Health Economics
12. Zola, I. K. (1966) Culture and symptoms: an analysis of patients' presenting complaints. *Am. Soc. Rev.* **31**, 615–630
13. Fox, R. (1968) Illness. In: Sills, D. (ed.) *International Encyclopaedia of the Social Sciences.* New York: Free Press/Macmillan, pp. 90–96
14. Rubel, A. J. (1977) The epidemiology of a folk illness: *susto* in Hispanic America. In: Landy, D. (ed.) *Culture, Disease and Healing: Studies in Medical Anthropology.* New York: Macmillan, pp. 119–128
15. Wagley, C. (1969) Cultural influences on population: a comparison of two Tupi tribes. In: *Environment and Cultural Behavior.* New York: Natural History Press, pp. 268–279

16. MacCormack, C. P. (1982) Biological, cultural and social adaptation in human fertility and birth: a synthesis. In: MacCormack, C.P. (ed.) *Ethnography of Fertility and Birth*. London: Academic Press, pp. 1–23
17. Underwood, P. and Underwood, Z. (1981) New spells for old: expectations and realities of Western medicine in a remote tribal society in Yemen, Arabia. In: Stanley, N. F. and Joshe, R. A. (eds) *Changing Disease Patterns and Human Behaviour*. London: Academic Press, pp. 271–297
18. Qureshi, S. M. (1980) Health problems of Asian immigrants. *Medicos* 5, 19–21
19. Skegg, D. C. G., Corwin, P. A., Paul, C. and Doll, R. (1982) Importance of the male factor in cancer of the cervix. *Lancet* ii, 581–583
20. Brabin, L. and Brabin, B. J. (1985) Cultural factors and transmission of hepatitis B virus. *Am. J. Epidemiol.* 122, 725–730
21. Alland, A. (1969) Ecology and adaptation to parasitic diseases. In: Vayda, A. P. (ed.) *Environment and Cultural Behavior*. New York: Natural History Press, pp. 80–89
22. Vayda, E., Mindell, W. R. and Rutkow, I. M. (1982) A decade of surgery in Canada, England and Wales, and the United States. *Arch. Surg.* 117, 846–853

Index

319

Baptism, 200
Barot, R., family culture, 244
Bauman, R., festival behaviour, 216
Baxter, C., health care, 46
Beattie, J., rituals, 205, 208
Behaviour
  abnormal
    controlled, 216–218
      glossolalia, 217–218
      spirit possession, 217
    culture-bound, 219
    language of distress, 216
    overlap with religious practises,
      219
    spectrum, 218–219
  competitive, and disease, 273, 274
  medicalization and control of, 66
  nature/nurture controversy, 127–
    128
  normal, 215
    rites of reversal, 215–216
    social definition, 215
  pain and changes in, 161, 164
Belgium, Turkish women self-help
    groups, 135
Belladona (Atropa belladona), 190
Belsey, E. M., 49
Belshaw, C. S., food, 40
Belsky, J., CHD in Japanese, 269–270,
    280
Belsnickling, 216
Benson, H., placebo effect, 170
Benzodiazepines, 177–179
Bereavement
  cultural, 262
  death rate in widowers, 252
  life space, 252
  stress, 250, 251, 252
  see also Death, Mourning rituals
Birth cultures
  and epidemiology of disease, 274
  father's role, 155
  labour pain, Poland/USA, 161
  non-Western, 150–151
  position during, 150
  post-partum period, 150, 151
  rituals, 198, 200–201, 209
  traditional attendants, 135, 146, 150,
    151–153
    see Traditional birth attendants
  Western, 145–146, 145–150
    criticisms, 147
    episiotomies, 148

Birth cultures (cont.)
  Western (cont.)
    father's role, 155
    hospital obstetrics
      growth of, 146–147
      rituals, 149, 200–201
    medicalization, 66, 142–143, 148–
      150
    obstetrician/mother's assessment,
      149
    obstetrics, social transition
      rituals, 149
    origins of, 147–148
    puerperium, 151
    technological model, 148
Black Report, The, 5, 268
Blackburn, R., psychiatric diagnosis,
  227
Blaxter, M.
  ill-health, 92
  lay causes of illness, 110
  popular health care, 73
Blood
  beliefs, case-histories, 26–29
  high/low, 26, 28, 38, 56, 97, 120
  impurities, 26
  index of emotional states, 26
  living (sangue vivo), 29
  menstrual beliefs, 26–28
  as non-regenerative liquid, 29
  polluting power, 26
  as potent symbol, 26
  sleeping (sangue dormido), 29
  symbols, 26
  thin, 26
Blumhagen, D., lay/medical
    understanding, 111, 121
Body
  beliefs about blood, 25–26
  case histories, 26–29
  clinical questionnaire, 285–286
  during pregnancy, 23–25
  functioning
    balance and imbalance, 17–21
    lay beliefs, 17–23
    as machine, 22–23
    plumbing model, 21–22
  image, 4, 11
    alterations, 12–14
    case history, 16–17
    clothing, 14
    dieting, 13
    epidemiology of disease, 274

Obeyesekere, G., Ayurvedic
   medicine, 20
Occupation
   body language, 12
   epidemiology of disease, 276
   gender and, 132
   redundancy, stress of, 252, 255
Occupational therapists, 68, 79
O'Connor, J., alcohol use, 183–184,
   186
Olin, H. S., seeking medical aid, 116
Oral rehydration therapy (ORT), 9–10
Orbach, S., anorexia nervosa, 13
Organic brain disorders, 220, 223
Osteomalacia, 45–46
   in female Asian UK immigrants, 275
   in Yemen women, 275
Osteopathy, 76, 78
Overnutrition, 47, 50

Pain
   behaviour
      Anglo-Saxon 'stiff upper lip', 159
      Cheyenne Indians, 159–160
      child-rearing and effect on, 166–
         167
      guilt and, 166
      healers available and display of,
         162
      involuntary, 159
      mimicking, 164
      non-verbal, 164
      private, 159–160
      public, 159, 160–165
         presentation, 163–165
         social aspects, 165–167
      somatization, 164
      tolerance to, 162–163
      voluntary, 159
   clinical questionnaire, 290–291
   description of, 165
   expectation, 161
   misfortune linked with, 161–162
   physiological perspective, 158
   placebo analgesia, 63, 171
   significance
      body structure beliefs and, 160
      dysmenorrhoea, 160
      normal/abnormal, 160
Pakistan
   hot–cold foods, 36
   oral rehydration therapy, 9–10
Papua, New Guinea, see New Guinea

Paraguay, Chiriguano Indians,
   childbirth, 155
Paramedical professions, 63, 68
   see also specific professions
Parasitic diseases
   cultural factors, 280–281
   lay aetiologies, 106
Parasuicide, 235
Parish, P. A.
   drug prescriptions, 179
   psychotropic prescriptions, 177
Parkes, C. M.
   grieving, 207
   life changes, 252
   stress, 250
Parteras, 151
Paterson, E.
   ill-health, 92
   popular health care, 73
Pattison, C. J., popular health care,
   73
Paul, C., cervical cancer, 278–289
Payer, L., medical system, 67–68
Pearce, J. K., family culture, 243
Pearson, J.
   lay concepts of body, 15
   medical terms, 121
Pellegrino, E. D., chemical coping,
   178
Penicillin, as a 'hot' drug, 123
Peptic ulcer, placebo effect, 171
Peru
   body alteration, 12
   hallucinogenics, 190, 191
Peters-Golden, H., breast cancer, 100
Pets, epidemiology of disease, 277
Peyote cactus (Lophophora williamsii),
   190
Pfifferling, J. H., medical profession,
   69
Pharmacists, 72, 79
Philippines
   cash crops, 44
   father and childbirth, 155
Physiotherapists, 68, 79
Pill, R., lay theories of illness, 104–105
Placebo effect
   analgesia, 163, 171
   angina pectoris, 175–176
   brand-name, 173
   characteristics of drug, 173
   culture-bound, 171–172
      world-view, 172
   drug attributes and, 173